Biostatistics for Clinical and Public Health Research

Biostatistics for Clinical and Public Health Research

Melody S. Goodman

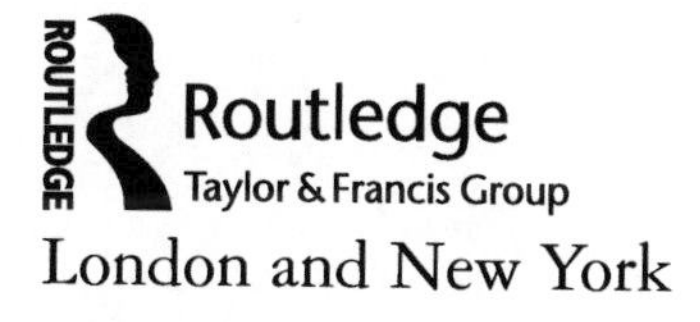

London and New York

First published 2018
by Routledge
711 Third Avenue, New York, NY 10017

and by Routledge
2 Park Square, Milton Park, Abingdon, Oxon, OX14 4RN

Routledge is an imprint of the Taylor & Francis Group, an informa business

Library of Congress Cataloging-in-Publication Data

Names: Goodman, Melody S., author.
Title: Biostatistics for clinical and public health research / Melody S. Goodman.
Description: Milton Park, Abingdon, Oxon ; New York, NY : Routledge, 2018. |
Includes bibliographical references and index.
Identifiers: LCCN 2017025994| ISBN 9781498784801 (hbk) | ISBN 9781138196353 (pbk) |
ISBN 9781315155661 (ebk)
Subjects: LCSH: Public health--Research--Statistical methods. | Biometry.
Classification: LCC RA440.85 .G66 2018 | DDC 362.1072/7--dc23
LC record available at https://lccn.loc.gov/2017025994

ISBN: 978-1-4987-8480-1 (hbk)
ISBN: 978-1-138-19635-3 (pbk)
ISBN: 978-1-315-15566-1 (ebk)

Please visit the eResources at: www.routledge.com/9781138196353

This book is dedicated to all of my students, past, present, and future. To all of the introduction to biostatistics instructors who believe in the "I hear, I forget, I do, I understand" approach to teaching this material. I hope this "old-school" workbook helps with learning and teaching.

It is also dedicated in loving memory of my mother, Linder White-Goodman. You were my first teacher, best friend, loudest cheerleader, and greatest critic. Thanks for always telling me I can do, be, and achieve anything I want. For believing in me when I didn't believe in myself and reassuring me that I was great but could always do better. For showing me that education was a viable path to success and could be used as a tool to change my life circumstances. You touched many lives but none more profoundly than mine, your only daughter. As hard as I tried not to follow in your footsteps, I too am an educator—just in a different context. This book is one of my greatest teaching accomplishments.

Contents

Acknowledgments

It takes a village to write a book even if there is only one name on the cover. I want to thank the Goodman Lab team at the Washington University School of Medicine (Nicole Ackermann, Goldie Komaie, Sarah Lyons, and Laurel Milam). Although I often get the credit and accolades, you make it possible for me to look good. You are an amazing group of women and have been an enormous support to me, for which I am forever grateful. I know that working for me can be challenging. This was especially the case when I decided to write two books in addition to everything else that we already had going on as a team, but you smiled through it all.

A special thanks to the talented young female statisticians who worked in the Goodman Lab and served as teaching assistants for my course. Each of you made significant contributions that helped turn my course notes into an actual book: Nicole Ackermann (Chapters 1 through 5, 15, and Lab A), Sarah Lyons (Chapters 11 through 13), and Laurel Milam (Chapters 6 through 10, 14, and Labs B through E). Thank you for creating examples, datasets, code books, figures, tables, and callout boxes; thank you for truly making this a team effort.

Thanks to Sharese T. Wills for being brave enough to take on the challenge of editing a biostatistics book. You took what I thought were solid drafts and completely reworked them, making them much better.

To my family, friends, mentors, and colleagues who have supported me through this journey—there are too many of you to name (not really; I am just too private to do so), but I hope that you know who you are. It is rare for someone to have such strong personal and professional support systems, and I am lucky to have both. It is great to feel wanted in your department and supported by your institution, but I think it is rare to feel supported by your profession. Thank you to all the academics who have helped me to get to the point of publishing this workbook on biostatistics. It was not an easy journey, and there is still more on the road ahead. However, I never would have made it this far without you.

Author

Dr. Melody S. Goodman, is an associate professor in the Department of Biostatistics at New York University College of Global Public Health. She is a biostatistician with experience in study design, developing survey instruments, data collection, data management, and data analysis for public health and clinical research projects. She has taught introductory biostatistics for masters of public health and medical students for over 10 years at multiple institutions (Stony Brook University School of Medicine, Washington University in St. Louis School of Medicine, New York University College of Global Public Health).

List of abbreviations

ACS American Community Survey
BMI Body mass index
BRFSS Behavioral Risk Factor Surveillance System
CBT Cognitive behavioral therapy
CDC Centers for Disease Control and Prevention
CDF Cumulative distribution function
CL Confidence limit
CLM Confidence limit for mean
CLT Central limit theorem
CRP C-reactive protein
df Degrees of freedom
DRE Digital rectal examination
ED Emergency department
GED General education diploma
GIS Graphical information system
HIV Human immunodeficiency virus
LCLM Lower confidence limit
MRCI Medication Regimen Complexity Index
mRFEI Modified retail food environment index
MSA Metropolitan Statistical Area
NATA National Air Toxics Assessment
NHANES National Health and Nutrition Examination Survey
NIH National Institutes of Health
PDF Probability density function
PK Pyruvate kinase
PSA Prostate-specific antigen
ROC Receiver operating characteristic
RR Relative risk
RT-PCR Reverse transcription polymerase chain reaction
SEM Standard error of the mean
SES Socioeconomic status
SSA Social Security Administration
TRUS Transrectal ultrasound
UCLM Upper confidence limit
VPA Vigorous physical activity
YRBSS Youth Risk Behavior Surveillance System

Introduction

This workbook started as a set of course notes and handouts that I used while teaching Introduction to Biostatistics. Although I love technology, I just think that "old school" is better for some things. I remember learning math in elementary school with workbooks. I am almost sure that none of my current students have even seen a workbook. Nonetheless, there is something about working through problems that helps people to grasp the concepts. We try to use examples in this workbook that are easy to understand, and we walk through problems step by step.

This introductory workbook is designed like a good set of notes from the best student in the class—the professor. Its outline format at the beginning of each chapter points to key concepts in a concise way, and chapters include highlights, bold text, and italics to point out other areas of focus. In addition, tables provide important information. Labs that include real-world clinical and public health examples walk readers through exercises, ensuring that students learn essential concepts and know how to apply them to data. The workbook provides the reader with the statistical foundation needed to pass medical boards and certification exams in public health. Also, those enrolled in online courses may find this workbook to be a great resource to supplement course textbooks. Researchers in the field, particularly those new to quantitative methods and statistical software (e.g., SAS or Stata), will find that this book starts at an appropriate level and covers a breadth of needed material with proper depth for a beginner. The workbook will also serve as a great reference to consult after the initial reading.

The workbook provides a solid foundation of statistical methods, allowing math-phobic readers to do basic statistical analyses, know when to consult a biostatistician, understand how to communicate with a biostatistician, and interpret quantitative study findings in the contexts of the hypotheses addressed. Many introductory biostatistics books spend considerable time explaining statistical theory, but what students and researchers really need to know is how to apply these theories in practice. This workbook walks readers through just that, becoming a lifelong reference.

This workbook covers the basics—from descriptive statistics to regression analysis—providing a survey of topics, including probability, diagnostic testing, probability distributions, estimation, hypothesis testing (one-sample, two-sample, means proportions, nonparametric, and categorical), correlation, regression (linear and logistic), and survival analysis. Examples are used to teach readers how to conduct analyses and interpret the results. There is no fluff or extra verbiage. The workbook provides readers with exactly what they need to know and shows them how to apply their knowledge to a problem.

The workbook not only provides the reader with an introduction to statistical methods but also a step-by-step how-to guide for using SAS and Stata statistical software packages to apply these methods to data, using lots of practical hands-on examples.

Statistical package: A collection of statistical programs that describe data and perform various statistical tests on the data.

Some of the most widely used statistical packages include the following:

- SAS—used in this book
- R
- Stata—used in this book
- SPSS
- MATLAB®
- Mathematica
- Minitab
- Excel

In addition, this workbook provides a solid foundation with concisely written text and minimal reading required. Although it is designed for an academic course, the workbook can be used as a self-help book that allows the user to learn by doing. The real-world practical examples show the user how to place results in context and that outcomes of analysis do not always go the way that the researcher predicts.

The workbook walks the readers through problems, both by hand and with statistical software. Readers can learn how the software performs the calculations, and they can gain the ability to read and interpret SAS and Stata output. The SAS and Stata code provided in the workbook provide readers with a solid foundation from which to start other analyses and apply to their own datasets.

General overview

What is statistics?

Statistics

1 "The science whereby inferences are made about specific, random phenomena on the basis of relatively limited sample material."[1]
2 "The art of learning from data. It is concerned with the collection of data, their subsequent description, and their analysis, which often lead to the drawing of conclusions."[2]

The two main branches of statistics

1 ***Mathematical statistics:*** The branch of statistics concerned with the development of new methods of statistical inference and requires detailed knowledge of abstract mathematics for its implementation.
2 ***Applied statistics:*** The branch of statistics involved with applying the methods of mathematical statistics to specific subject areas such as medicine, economics, and public health.

A **Biostatistics:** The branch of applied statistics that applies statistical methods to medical, biological, and public health problems. The study of biostatistics explores the collection, organization, analysis, and interpretation of numerical data.

Basic problem of statistics

Consider a sample of data $x_1, x_2, \ldots, x_n$ where x_1 corresponds to the first sample point and x_n corresponds to the nth sample point. Presuming that the sample is drawn from some population P, what inferences or conclusions can be made about P from the sample? (See figure below.)

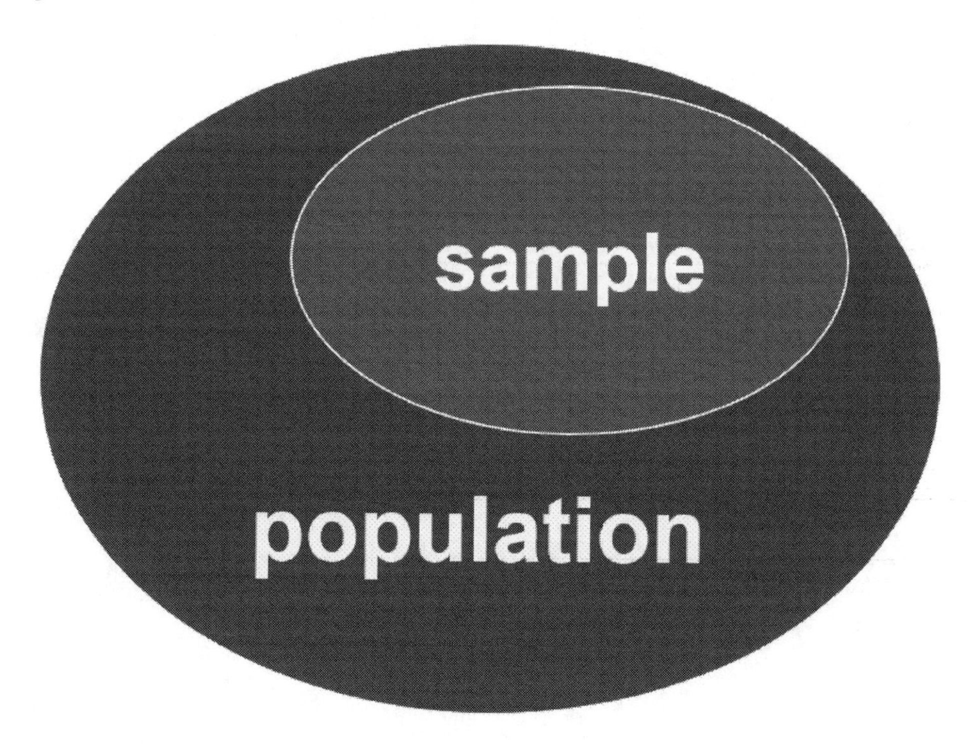

Data

Data are often used to make key decisions. Such decisions are said to be *data driven*. With the use of technology, we are able to collect, merge, and store large amounts of data from multiple sources. Data are often the core of any public health or clinical research study, which often starts with a research question and the collection and analysis of data to answer that question. It is important for researchers and practitioners to understand how to collect (or extract from other sources), describe, and analyze data. Furthermore, the ability to understand and critique data and methods used by others is increasing in importance as the volume of research studies increases while the quality remains inconsistent.

Units and variables

In most instances, a dataset is structured as a data matrix with the unit of analysis (e.g., research participants, schools, research papers) in the rows and the variables in the columns.

- ***Units (cases):*** The research participants or objects for which information is collected.
- ***Variables:*** Systematically collected information on each unit or research participant.

Types of variables

- ***Nominal:*** Unordered categories (e.g., male, female).
- ***Ordinal:*** Ordered categories (e.g., mild, moderate, severe).
- ***Ranked:*** Data transformation where numerical or ordinal values are replaced by the rank when the data are sorted (e.g., top five causes of death, top three favorite movies).
- ***Discrete:*** Has a finite number of values where both ordering and magnitude are important (e.g., number of accidents, number of new AIDS cases in a one-year period).
- ***Continuous:*** Has an infinite number of possible values between its minimum and maximum values (e.g., volume of tumor, cholesterol level, time).

In this book, we will discuss ways to describe and analyze a single variable and the relationship between two or more variables. We demonstrate and walk through key principles by hand and supplement this with the use of a statistical package. A statistical package does what the user tells it to do. It is important to understand key concepts so that you can arrive at accurate outcomes from a software package, read statistical output, and properly interpret the results. In Chapter 1, we discuss methods for describing sample data, and, in the rest of the chapters, we discuss ways of analyzing data to test hypotheses.

References

1. Rosner B. *Fundamentals of Biostatistics.* 8th ed. Boston, MA: Cengage Learning. 2016.
2. Ross SM. *Introductory Statistics.* 2nd ed. Burlington, MA: Elsevier Academic Press. 2005.

1 Descriptive statistics

This chapter will focus on descriptive statistics and will include the following:

- Measures of central tendency (measures of location)
- Measures of spread (measures of dispersion)
- Measures of variability
- Graphic methods
- Outliers and standard distribution rules

Terms

- arithmetic mean (average)
- bar graph
- box plot
- Chebyshev Inequality
- decile
- descriptive statistics
- empirical rule
- geometric mean
- GIS map
- histogram
- interquartile range
- median
- mode
- outlier
- percentiles
- quartile
- quintile
- range
- scatterplot
- standard deviation
- stem-and-leaf plot
- tertile
- variance

Introduction

A complete statistical analysis of data has several components. A good first step in data analysis is to describe the data in some concise way, which allows the data analyst a chance to learn about the data being considered. ***Descriptive statistics*** is the part of statistics that is concerned with the description and summarization of data. Initial descriptive analysis quickly provides the researcher an idea of the principal trends and suggests where a more detailed look is necessary. The measures used in describing data include measures of central tendency, spread, and the variability of the sample. All of these measures can be represented in both tabular and graphic displays. We will go over different types of graphs and displays in this chapter.

Measures of central tendency (Measures of location)

One type of measure that is useful for summarizing data defines the center, or middle, of the sample. Thus, this type of measure is called a measure of central tendency (also "measure of location"). Several measures of central tendency exist, but four measures of central tendency will be discussed in this section:

1 Arithmetic mean (average)
2 Median
3 Mode
4 Geometric mean

Arithmetic Mean: The sum of all observations divided by the number of observations.

- The arithmetic mean is what is commonly referred to as an *average*.
- This is the most widely used measure of central tendency. However, the arithmetic mean, or average, is oversensitive to extreme values, meaning that the mean can be influenced by a value that is much higher or much lower as compared to other values in the dataset.
- We use the notation μ to denote the mean of a population and $\bar{x}$ to denote the mean of a sample.

Equation 1.1 shows the calculation of the arithmetic mean.

$$\bar{x} = \frac{1}{n}\sum_{i=1}^{n} x_i = \frac{x_1 + x_2 + \ldots + x_n}{n} \tag{1.1}$$

Because the mean is based on summation, knowing several properties of summation is often useful as you begin to analyze data, specifically as the data relate to the mean.

BOX 1.1 PROPERTIES OF THE SAMPLE MEAN

Equation 1.2 shows the multiplicative property of summations:

$$\sum_{i=1}^{n} cx_i = c\sum_{i=1}^{n} x_i \tag{1.2}$$

Three important properties of the arithmetic mean:

1. If $y_i = x_i + c$ where i = 1,…,n then $\bar{y} = \bar{x} + c$
2. If $y_i = cx_i$ where i = 1,…,n then $\bar{y} = c\bar{x}$
3. If $y_i = c_1x_i + c_2$ where i = 1,…,n then $\bar{y} = c_1\bar{x} + c_2$

Median: The median is the value in the middle of the sample variable such that 50% of the observations are greater than or equal to the median and 50% of the observations are less than or equal to the median.

- The median is an alternate measure of central tendency (measure of location) and is second to the arithmetic mean in familiarity.
- The median is useful in data that have outliers and extreme values; the median is insensitive to these values.
- Calculation of the median uses only the middle points in a sample and is less sensitive to the actual numeric values of the remaining data points.

Calculation: Suppose that there are n observations in a sample and that these observations are ordered from smallest (1) to largest (n). The sample median is defined as follows:

If n is odd,

$$\text{Median} = \text{the} \left(\frac{n+1}{2}\right)^{th} \text{observation}$$

If n is even,

$$\text{Median} = \text{the average of the} \left(\frac{n}{2}\right)^{th} \text{plus the} \left(\frac{n}{2}+1\right)^{th} \text{observations}$$

EXAMPLE PROBLEM 1.1

Calculate the arithmetic mean and median of Sample 1.
Sample 1: 2.15, 2.25, 2.30

To find the mean, we add all the values and divide the sum by n, which equals 3.

$$\text{Mean} = \frac{2.15+2.25+2.30}{3} = \frac{6.7}{3} = 2.23$$

To find the median, we put all values in numerical order and find the $\left(\frac{3+1}{2}\right)^{th}$ = 2nd value.

Median = 2nd value of Sample 1 (2.15, 2.25, 2.30) = 2.25.

PRACTICE PROBLEM 1.1

Calculate the arithmetic mean and median of Sample 2.
Sample 2: 2.15, 2.25, 2.30, 2.60

Mode: The mode is the observation that occurs most frequently.

- This measure of central tendency (measure of location) is not a useful measure if there are a large number of possible values, each of which occurs infrequently.
- Some distributions can have more than one mode. We can classify a distribution by the number of modes in the data.

- If there is one mode, the distribution is unimodal. For example, in the following sequence of numbers, there is one mode because 7 appears the most out of any data value:
  - 1 2 3 5 7 7 7 8 8 9
- If there are two modes, the distribution is bimodal. For example, the following sequence of numbers has two modes because 5 and 6 both appear the most out of any data value in the sequence:
  - 2 3 4 5 5 6 6 7 10
- If there are three modes, the distribution is trimodal. For example, the following sequence of numbers has three modes because 1, 2, and 6 appear the most out of any data value in the sequence:
  - 1 1 2 2 5 6 6 8 9

Arithmetic mean versus median

Because the mean is sensitive to outliers and extreme values, it is important to determine when to use the arithmetic mean versus the median. The distribution of the data is a key factor in making this decision.

Arithmetic mean

For a symmetric distribution, the arithmetic mean is approximately the same as the median.

For a positively skewed distribution, the arithmetic mean tends to be larger than the median.

For a negatively skewed distribution, the arithmetic mean tends to be smaller than the median.

Median

If the distribution is symmetric, the relative position of the points on each side of the sample median is the same. The mean or median can be used to describe this sample.

If the distribution is positively skewed (skewed to the right), the points above the median tend to be farther from the median in absolute value than points below the median. This is sometimes referred to as "having a heavy right tail."

If a distribution is negatively skewed (skewed to the left), points below the median tend to be farther from the median in absolute value than points above the median. This is sometimes referred to as "having a heavy left tail."

See Figure 1.1 for a demonstration of the relationship between the arithmetic mean and the median and the skewed versus nonskewed distributions. The mode is also represented in the symmetric distribution on the figure.

Geometric Mean: The geometric mean is the antilogarithm of $\overline{\log x}$ (see Equation 1.3).

This measure of central tendency is not often used in practice but can be useful when dealing with biological or environmental data that are based on concentrations (e.g., biomarkers, blood lead levels, C-reactive protein [CRP], cortisol).

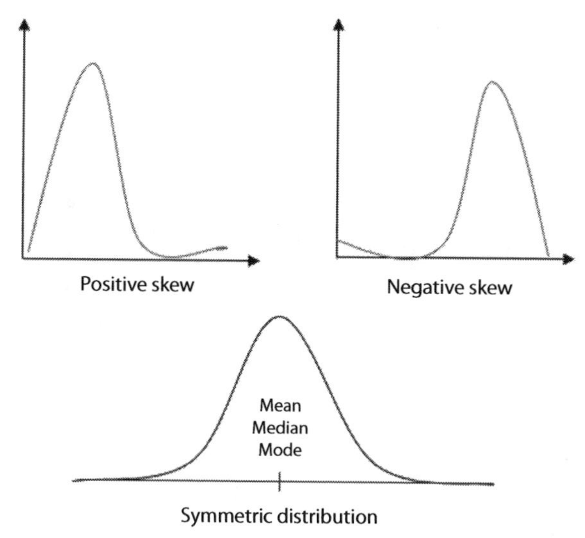

Figure 1.1 **Positively and negatively skewed distribution.** In the distribution with a positive skew (top left) and the distribution with a negative skew (top right), the median is a better measure of central tendency than the mean. The mean more accurately captures the central tendency of the data when the distribution is symmetric (center bottom) with thin tails versus when the data is skewed. The mean follows the tail of a skewed distribution. The relationship between the sample mean and the sample median can be used to assess the symmetry of a distribution.

Equation 1.3 shows the $\overline{\log x}$ calculation.

$$\overline{\log x} = \frac{1}{n}\sum_{i=1}^{n} \log x_i \tag{1.3}$$

Example of geometric mean using data from the 2014 National Health and Nutrition Examination Survey

The 2014 National Health and Nutrition Examination Survey (NHANES) measures participants' blood lead levels.[1] Using these data, we computed the geometric mean for the participants. The geometric mean for blood lead levels for the entire group of 2014 participants with nonmissing data was 0.83 ug/mL compared to the arithmetic mean of 1.1 ug/mL. We also categorized participants into age groups and computed the geometric mean of blood lead levels by age category (see Figure 1.2).

EXAMPLE PROBLEM 1.2

Calculate the geometric mean for the dataset in Sample 1 from Example Problem 1.1.

Log (2.15) = 0.33
Log (2.25) = 0.35
Log (2.30) = 0.36

$$\overline{\log x} = \frac{0.33+0.35+0.36}{3} = \frac{1.04}{3} = 0.3467$$

Geometric mean = antilog(0.3467) = $10^{0.3467}$ = 2.22

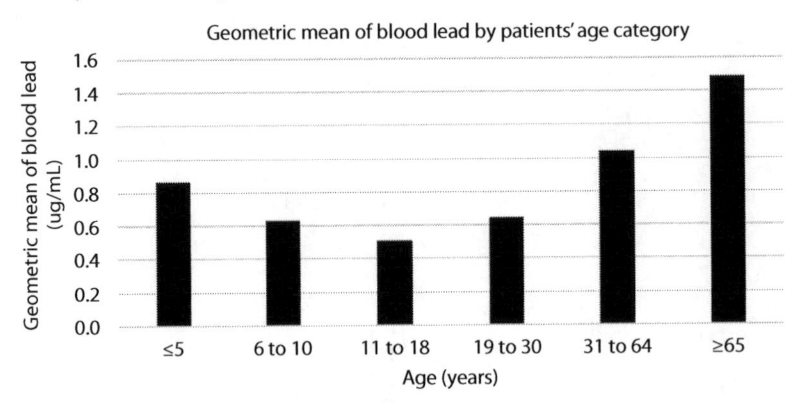

Figure 1.2 **Geometric mean of blood lead levels by patients' age category for participants of the 2014 National Health and Nutrition Examination Survey (NHANES).** (Data from the National Health and Nutrition Examination Survey, Centers for Disease Control and Prevention website, https://wwwn.cdc.gov/Nchs/Nhanes/Search/nhanes13_14.aspx, accessed February 23, 2016.)

PRACTICE PROBLEM 1.2

Calculate the geometric mean of Sample 2.

Measures of spread

Many variables can be well described by a combination of a measure of central tendency (measure of location) and a measure of spread. Measures of spread tell us how far or how close together the data points are in a sample. Six measures of spread will be discussed in this section:

1. Range
2. Quantiles
3. Percentiles
4. Interquartile range
5. Variance
6. Standard deviation

Range: The range is the difference between the largest and smallest observations of a variable.

The range measures the spread of a variable as the distance from the minimum to the maximum value. Although the range is very easy to compute, it is sensitive to extreme observations. The range depends on the sample size (n). The larger the n, the larger the range tends to be. This makes it hard to compare ranges from datasets of different sizes.

Quantiles and Percentiles: Quantiles and percentiles are measures of spread that are determined by the numerical ordering of the data. They are cut points that divide the frequency distribution into equal groups, each containing the same fraction of the total population.

Quantiles and percentiles can also be used to describe the spread of a variable. They are less sensitive to outliers and are not greatly affected by the sample size, which is an advantage over the range.

- The most useful percentiles are often determined by the sample size and subject matter.
- The pth percentile is the value V_p such that p percent of the sample points is less than or equal to V_p.
- The median, which we learned about previously in this chapter, is the 50th percentile.
- Other frequently used percentiles include the following:
    - ***Tertiles:*** Two points that divide and order a sample variable into three categories, each containing a third of the population (e.g., high, medium, low). The 33rd and 66th percentiles of a sample variable are used to categorize it into tertiles.
    - ***Quartiles:*** Three points that divide and order a sample variable into four categories, each containing a fourth of the population. The 25th, 50th, and 75th percentiles of a variable are used to categorize it into quartiles.
    - ***Quintiles:*** Four points that divide and order a sample variable into five categories, each containing a fifth of the population. The 20th, 40th, 60th, and 80th percentiles of a variable are used to categorize it into quintiles.
    - ***Deciles:*** Nine points that divide and order a sample variable into ten categories, each containing a tenth of the population. The 10th, 20th, 30th, 40th, 50th, 60th, 70th, 80th, and 90th percentiles of a variable are used to categorize it into deciles.

The pth percentile is defined by the following:

1. The $(k + 1)th$ largest sample point if $np/100$ is not an integer. (k is the largest integer less than $np/100$).
2. The average of the $\left(\frac{np}{100}\right)^{th}$ and the $\left(\frac{np}{100}+1\right)^{th}$ largest observations if $np/100$ is an integer.

Interquartile Range: The interquartile range is between the 75th and 25th percentiles. This measure of spread encompasses the middle 50% of observations and is not easily influenced by extreme values.

EXAMPLE PROBLEM 1.3

Calculate the range and interquartile range using the dataset in Sample 1 in Example Problem 1.1.

$$\text{Range} = 2.30 - 2.15 = 0.15$$

$$75^{th}\ p = \frac{np}{100} = \frac{3\times 75}{100} = 2.25 \rightarrow V_{75} = 2.30$$

$$25^{th}\ p = \frac{np}{100} = \frac{3\times 25}{100} = 0.75 \rightarrow V_{25} = 2.15$$

$$V_{75} - V_{25} = 2.30 - 2.15 = 0.15$$

The range is equal to 0.15, and the interquartile range is also equal to 0.15.

PRACTICE PROBLEM 1.3

Calculate the range and interquartile range for the dataset in Sample 2 from Practice Problem 1.1.

Measures of variability

- Measures of variability are measures of spread that tell us how varied our data points are from the average of the sample.
- Measures of variability include the variance and the standard deviation (S).

Variance: The variance is a measure that will inform us how values in our dataset differ from the mean.

- A high variance indicates a wide range of values; a low variance indicates that values are closer to the mean.
- Equation 1.4 shows us how to calculate the variance.

$$S^2 = \frac{\sum_{i=1}^{n} (x_i - \bar{x})^2}{n-1} \tag{1.4}$$

where x_i is the sample observation for variable X, $\bar{x}$ is the mean of X, and n is the number of units (observations) in the sample. Variance is also noted as σ^2 in some instances; S^2 refers to a sample variance, and σ^2 refers to a population variance.

Standard Deviation: The standard deviation is the square root of the variance.

- The standard deviation is similar to the variance in that it also tells us how much variation around the mean there is in the dataset. The standard deviation is more commonly used than the variance because, in many cases, the standard deviation has the same units as the mean, whereas the variance has units squared, which can complicate interpretation.
- Equation 1.5 shows us how to calculate the standard deviation. Similar to the notation of variance, in some instances, the standard deviation will be noted as σ, which refers to the population standard deviation. When the standard deviation for a sample is being referred to, S is typically used.

$$S = \sqrt{\frac{\sum_{i=1}^{n} (x_i - \bar{x})^2}{n=1}} = \sqrt{Variance} \tag{1.5}$$

BOX 1.2 PROPERTIES OF THE SAMPLE VARIANCE

1. Suppose there are two samples, $x_1,\ldots,x_n$ and $y_1,\ldots,y_n$, where $y_i = x_i + c$, $i = 1,\ldots,n$, and S_x^2 and S_y^2 are the respective variances, then $S_x^2 = S_y^2$.
2. Suppose there are two samples, $x_1,\ldots,x_n$ and $y_1,\ldots,y_n$, where $y_i = cx_i$, $i = 1,\ldots,n$, and S_x^2 and S_y^2 are the respective variances, then $S_y^2 = c^2S_x^2$ and $S_y = cS_x$ if $c > 0$ or $S_y = -cS_x$ if $c < 0$.

EXAMPLE PROBLEM 1.4

Calculate the variance and standard deviation of the dataset in Sample 1 in Example Problem 1.1.

$$S^2 = \frac{(2.15-2.23)^2+(2.25-2.23)^2+(2.30-2.23)^2}{3-1}$$

$$= \frac{0.0064+0.0004+0.0049}{2} = \frac{0.0117}{2} = 0.00585$$

$$S = \sqrt{0.00585} = 0.076$$

PRACTICE PROBLEM 1.4

Calculate the variance and standard deviation of Sample 2 from Practice Problem 1.1.

Grouped Data: Grouped data refers to data that are given as a count of observations within an interval of a continuous variable.

Suppose that data were given to us in a frequency table, such as the data in Table 1.1, but we wanted to know the mean and variance of those data. Table 1.1 contains a pair of frequency distributions of weight (lbs.) for a group of people who reported asthma and a group of people who reported no asthma. These data are from the 2014 Behavioral Risk Factor Surveillance System (BRFSS)[2] data and are limited to participants residing in the state of Missouri.

Note that the continuous measure of weight for each subject is not given; instead, the weight of each subject is within one of three ranges of weight. Suppose that you want to calculate the mean and standard deviation for these subjects. You can do this by using the formulas for the grouped mean and grouped variance.

Grouped mean

Equation 1.6 shows us how to calculate the grouped mean.

$$\bar{x} = \frac{\sum_{i=1}^{k} m_i f_i}{\sum_{i=1}^{k} f_i} \tag{1.6}$$

where k is the number of intervals, m_i is the midpoint of the ith interval, and f_i is the frequency associated with the ith interval.

Table 1.1 Asthma status by weight group

Weight group, lbs	*Weight group midpoint*	*Asthma* *(n = 890)*	*No asthma* *(n = 5834)*
70–150	110	206	1786
151–205	178	394	2699
206–730	468	290	1349

Source: Behavioral Risk Factor Surveillance System (BRFSS), Centers for Disease Control and Prevention, http://www.cdc.gov/brfss/annual_data/annual_2014.html, 2014. Accessed February 23, 2016.

Note: The 2014 Behavioral Risk Factor Surveillance System (BRFSS) survey asked participants if they were "(ever told) you had asthma?" The response values were *yes*, *no*, *don't know/not sure*, or *refused*. Those who answered the latter two responses were excluded from the data presented in Table 1.1. Survey participants were also asked, "About how much do you weigh without shoes?" Those who did not give weight were excluded from the data presented in Table 1.1. Also, weights given in kilograms were converted to pounds. The data presented in Table 1.1 are limited to residents of the state of Missouri.[2]

BOX 1.3 SIDE NOTE ON GROUPED MEAN

Side Note: $\sum_{i=1}^{k} f_i = n$, where n is the number of observations in the sample.

Side Note: Zero is an integer; it is not a positive integer.

Grouped variance

Equation 1.7 shows us how to calculate grouped variance.

$$s^2 = \frac{\sum_{i=1}^{k} (m_i - \bar{x})^2 f_i}{\left(\sum_{i=1}^{k} f_i\right) - 1} \tag{1.7}$$

To get the grouped standard deviation, we could simply take the square root of the grouped variance.

EXAMPLE PROBLEM 1.5

Calculate the grouped mean and grouped standard deviation for the group with asthma (Table 1.1).

$$\bar{x} = \frac{110(206) + 178(394) + 468(290)}{890} = \frac{22660 + 70132 + 135720}{890}$$

$$= \frac{228512}{890} = 256.8 \textit{ lbs}$$

$$s^2 = \frac{(110 - 256.8)^2 \times 206 + (178 - 256.8)^2 \times 394 + (468 - 256.8)^2 \times 290}{890 - 1}$$

$$= \frac{(-146.8)^2 \times 206 + (-78.8)^2 \times 394 + (211.2)^2 \times 290}{889}$$

$$= \frac{21550.24 \times 206 + 6209.44 \times 394 + 44605.44 \times 290}{889}$$

$$= \frac{4439349.44 + 2446519.36 + 1295577.6}{889}$$

$$= 22296.3\ lbs^2$$

$$S = \sqrt{22296.3}$$

$$= 149.3\ lbs$$

PRACTICE PROBLEM 1.5

Calculate the grouped mean and grouped standard deviation for the group without asthma (Table 1.1).

Types of graphs

- Graphic displays provide a quick overall impression of the data, which is sometimes difficult to obtain with numeric measures.
- Several types of graphs are shown in this section, including bar graphs, histograms, stem-and-leaf plots, scatterplots, box plots, and GIS maps.

What makes a good graphic or tabular display?

To make a good graphic or tabular display, the material should be as self-contained as possible and should be understandable without the need for additional text. These attributes require clear labeling, including the title, units, and axes on graphs or figures. The statistical terms used in tables and figures should be well defined. Keep in mind these important attributes of good displays.

Bar Graph: A widely used method for displaying grouped data, a bar graph is a pictorial representation of a frequency distribution for either nominal or ordinal data.

- Nominal data are represented by categories that have no order. An example of nominal data is type of food. We could have categories of spicy, bland, or flavorful.
- Ordinal data are also represented in categories; however, the categories are ordered. An example of ordinal data is price category of food. The dishes can be cheap, affordable, moderately expensive, or pricey.

With nominal or ordinal data, the bar graph is constructed by dividing the data into groups. For each group, a rectangle is constructed with a base of a constant width and a height proportional to the frequency within that group. The main problem with using a bar graph to present nominal or ordinal data is that the sense of the actual sample points in the respective groups is lost.

Figure 1.3 shows an example of a bar graph with nominal data. In this graph, we can see that family practitioners perform the majority of care for most of the respondents in the sample, and general practitioners/internists are in a close second.

Histogram: The most commonly used type of graph, the histograms depicts the symmetry and spread of a single variable. It shows the frequency distribution for discrete or continuous data. It allows for identification of intervals with high levels of frequency, gaps in the data, and values that are far from others.

- *Discrete* or *continuous* are ways to classify numerical data (see also Chapter 4).
- Whereas discrete variables can have only whole number values, continuous variables can have decimals.

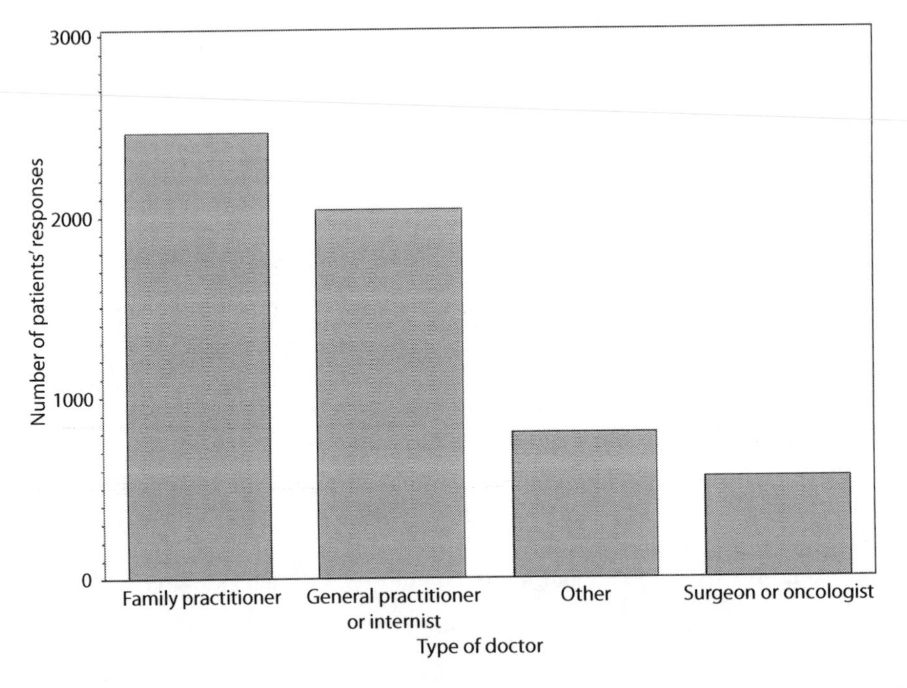

Figure 1.3 **Type of doctor providing the majority of care per patients' responses.** Data used to create the figure are from participants' responses to the question, "What type of doctor provides the majority of your healthcare?" The responses were *cancer surgeon, family practitioner, general surgeon, gynecologic oncologist, general practitioner/internist, plastic surgeon/reconstructive surgeon, medical oncologist, radiation oncologist, urologist, other,* or *don't know/not sure*. Some did not answer the question. Note that *urologist* and *other* were combined to make the *other* category in the figure. Don't know/not sure and abstentions were excluded from the figure. (Data from the Behavioral Risk Factor Surveillance System (BRFSS), Centers for Disease Control and Prevention website, http://www.cdc.gov/brfss/annual_data/annual_2014.html, 2014, accessed February 23, 2016.)

- Examples of discrete data include the following:
  - The number of Zika virus cases in a state. These would be discrete numerical data because we can have only a whole number of Zika cases (e.g., 12 Zika cases). It would not be possible to have 11.6 Zika cases in a state.
  - The number of live births at a hospital in a given year.
  - The temperature of the water in a river on a given day.
- Examples of continuous data include the following:
  - Concentration of lead in the blood of a patient.
  - Parts per million of water contamination.
  - Length of time a cancer patient survives after diagnosis.
- When there are a large number of discrete possibilities, the line between discrete and continuous data can be blurry. Rounding of measurement can also make continuous data appear discrete.

On the basis of the histogram in Figure 1.4, would you say the distribution of age in this sample is skewed or symmetric?[3–6]

This is a random sample that is based on a modest sample size (n = 93) from a real dataset; nevertheless, the distribution is fairly symmetric. However, the left tail is heavier than the right tail, suggesting a left skew.

Stem-and-Leaf Plot: In this type of plot, the actual sample values are preserved, and a grouped display of the data is presented. The collection of leaves takes on the general shape of the distribution of sample points. The stem-and-leaf plot can be used to overcome problems with bar graphs. From the stem-and-leaf plot, it is easy to compute the median and other quantiles.

To construct a stem-and-leaf plot, follow these steps:

1. Separate each data point into a stem component and a leaf component.
   a. The stem component consists of the number formed by all but the rightmost digit.
   b. The leaf component consists of the rightmost digit.
2. Write the smallest stem in the dataset in the upper left-hand corner of the plot.
3. Write the second stem, first stem + 1, below the first stem.
4. Continue with Step 3 until you reach the largest stem in the dataset.
5. Draw a vertical bar to the right of the column of stems.
6. For each number in the dataset, find the appropriate stem, and write the leaf to the right of the vertical bar.

The data[3–6] on age of the sample of patients from Figure 1.4 were used to create the stem-and-leaf plot in Figure 1.5.

EXAMPLE PROBLEM 1.6

Create a stem-and-leaf plot for Sample 3, which consists of the following observed data points: 234, 235, 243, 246, 247, 248, 250, 263, 274, 275.

To create the stem-and-leaf plot pictured in Figure 1.6, we first start by separating all of the data points into stem-and-leaf components. Here, we have stems of 23, 24, 25, 26, and 27. Next, we place the stems in numerical order—which they already happen to be in—starting with the top of the left column labeled *Stem*. Now, we draw our

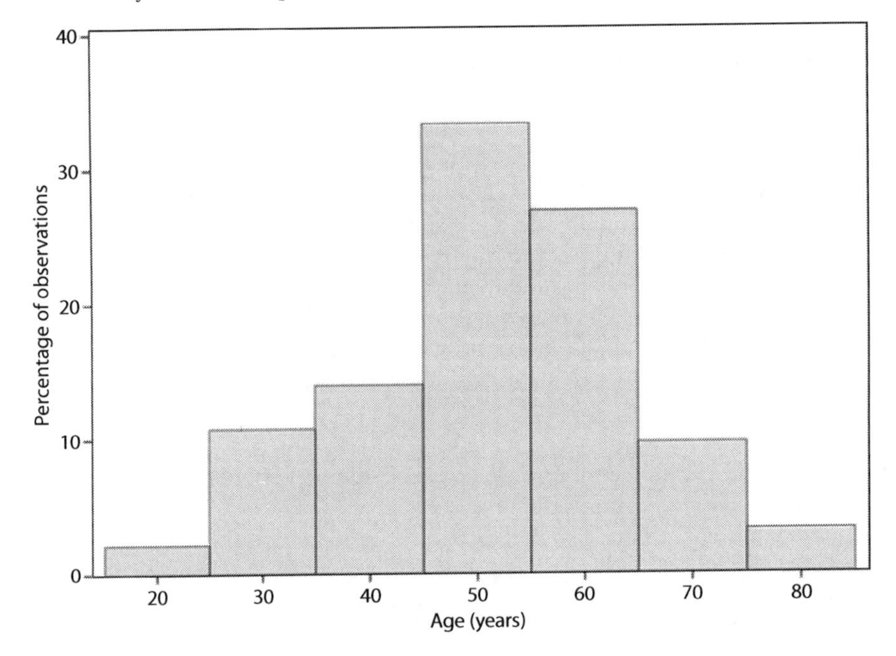

Figure 1.4 **Age of a random sample (n = 93) of primary care clinic patients seen between July 2013 and April 2014.** The data are from a random sample of 93 participants in a study conducted in a primary care clinic in St. Louis, MO. Participants were recruited from the waiting room of the clinic, and they completed the survey in English. A total of 1380 patients participated in the study. (From Goodman, M. S., Griffey, R. T., Carpenter, C. R., Blanchard, M., and Kaphingst, K. A., *J Am Board Fam Med.*, 28(5), 584–594, 2015, doi:10.3122/jabfm.2015.05.150037.)

Stem	Leaf
2	0376
3	011233445557789
4	01223456788999
5	00000011122222223334444455666666777889
6	0001222244456667
7	00127
8	23

Figure 1.5 **Stem-and-leaf plot of age of sample of primary care clinic patients.** The data are from the same random sample of 93 patients (from a total of 1380 patients) represented in Figure 1.4. (From Goodman, M. S., Griffey, R. T., Carpenter, C. R., Blanchard, M., and Kaphingst, K. A., *J Am Board Fam Med.*, 28(5), 584–594, 2015, doi:10.3122/jabfm.2015.05.150037.)

vertical bar to the right of the stem values and fill in the leaf for each data point in the column we label *Leaf*.

PRACTICE PROBLEM 1.6

Create a stem-and-leaf plot for Sample 4, which consists of the following observed data points: 348, 345, 342, 347, 374, 369, 350, 368, 364, 358, 359, 365, 373, 354, 352, 358, 372, 366, 364, 355.

Stem	Leaf
23	45
24	3678
25	0
26	3
27	45

Figure 1.6 **Stem-and-leaf plot of Sample 3.** The stem-and-leaf plot shows the distribution of the data in Sample 3 from Example Problem 1.6.

Box Plots: Box plots show the relationship among the median, upper quartile (75th percentile), and lower quartile (25th percentile) to demonstrate the skewness of a distribution. The box represents the middle 50% of observations (interquartile range) with the lower end of the box at the 25th percentile and the upper end of the box at the 75th percentile. The line in the middle of the box is the median (50th percentile). From the bottom of the box is a line with a horizontal bar at the 5th percentile, and from the top of the box is a line with a horizontal bar at the 95th percentile.

If the distribution is symmetric, the 75th and 25th percentiles should be approximately equally spaced from the median.

If the 75th percentile is farther from the median than the 25th percentile, the distribution is positively skewed.

If the 25th percentile is farther from the median than the 75th percentile, the distribution is negatively skewed.

Box plots will also show the presence of outliers. In the box plot in Figure 1.7, we can see that there is one outlier in the non-Hispanic white category. This is represented by the point above the upper horizontal bar representing the 95th percentile.

- Does the box plot in Figure 1.7 give you a sense of the mean of the BMI in the two groups?
  - Yes, the mean is represented by the small diamonds inside the box plots.
- Does the box plot in Figure 1.7 give you a sense of the median BMI in the two groups?
  - Yes, the median is represented by the bars through the middle of the boxes.
- Does the box plot in Figure 1.7 give you a sense of the mode(s) of BMI in the two groups?
  - No, we do not get a sense of the mode from a box plot.
- How would you compare the distribution of BMI among non-Hispanic white participants and non-Hispanic black participants based on Figure 1.7?
  - The distributions appear similar between the two groups. The BMI distribution for non-Hispanic blacks has a larger spread than the BMI distribution for non-Hispanic whites.

Scatterplots: Scatterplots represent data by depicting single points for each observation.

- There are two types of scatterplots: a one-way scatterplot and a two-way scatterplot.
  - A *one-way scatterplot* uses a single horizontal axis to display the relative position of each data point in a group. This plot is not often used in practice.
  - A *two-way scatterplot* is used to depict the relationship between two continuous measurements. Each point on the graph represents a pair of values.

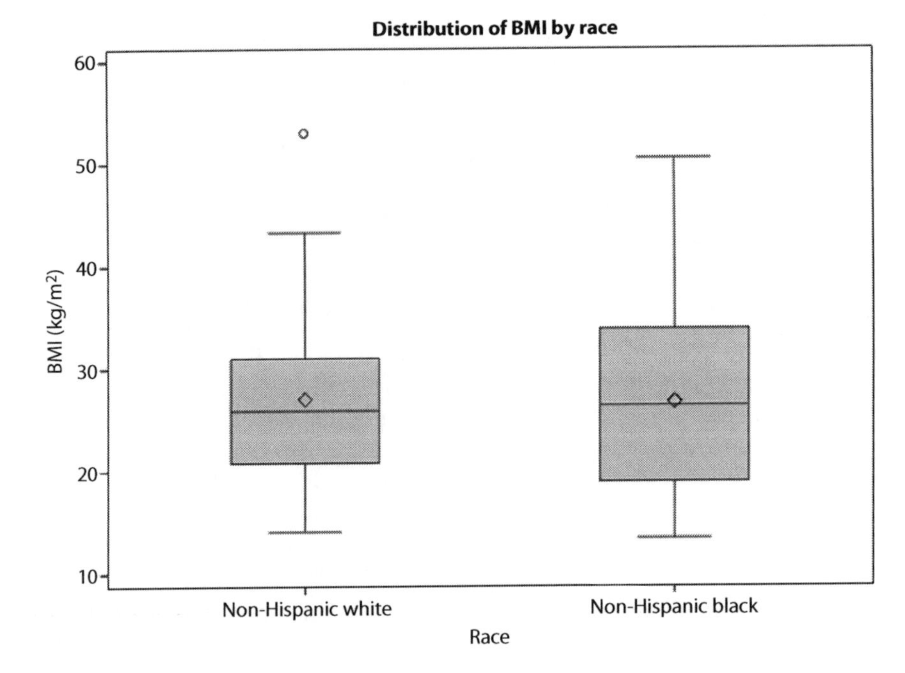

Figure 1.7 **Distribution of BMI by race.** BMI indicates body mass index. The box plot shows BMI by race for a random sample (n = 100) of non-Hispanic white and non-Hispanic black participants in the 2014 NHANES survey. (Data from the National Health and Nutrition Examination Survey, Centers for Disease Control and Prevention website, https://wwwn.cdc.gov/Nchs/Nhanes/Search/nhanes13_14.aspx, accessed February 23, 2016.)

Figure 1.8 shows an example of a two-way scatterplot. The two continuous variables being represented in the graph are waist circumference and body mass index.

Is there a relationship between the two variables?

We can see, on the basis of the scatterplot, that as body mass index goes up, waist circumference also goes up.

GIS Map: Graphical information system (GIS) maps show data that have some kind of geospatial attribute.

- There are two main types of geospatial data: Vector data and raster data.
  - Types of vector data:
    - Points, such as longitude and latitude
    - Polygons, such as city boundaries
    - Lines, such as streets
  - Types of raster data:
    - Elevations
    - Temperature
- Figure 1.9 shows an example of a GIS map from a study on playground safety in the neighborhoods of St. Louis, Missouri.[7]

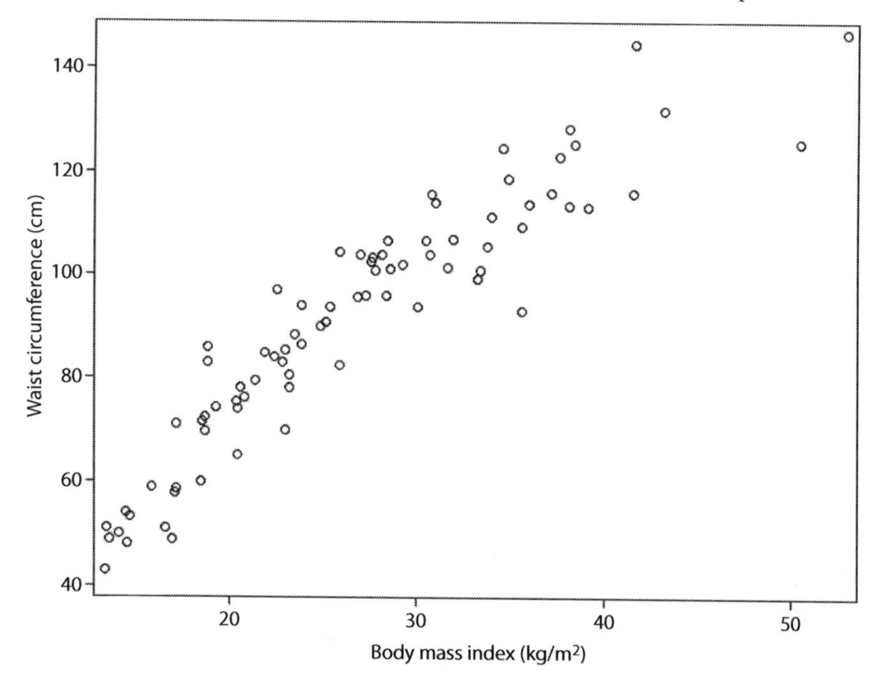

Figure 1.8 **Two-way scatterplot of BMI by waist circumference for a random sample (*n* = 100) of non-Hispanic white and non-Hispanic black participants in the 2014 NHANES Survey.** NHANES indicates National Health and Nutrition Examination Survey. The body mass index (BMI) variable was calculated using participants' measured weight and height. The waist circumference variable is the participants' measured waist circumference in centimeters. All measures were collected by trained health professionals. (Data from the National Health and Nutrition Examination Survey, Centers for Disease Control and Prevention website, https://wwwn.cdc.gov/Nchs/Nhanes/Search/nhanes13_14.aspx, accessed February 23, 2016.)

Outliers and standard distribution rules

Outlier: An outlying value is a value x such that either of the following is true:
(1) $x >$ upper quartile + 1.5*(interquartile range) or
(2) $x <$ lower quartile – 1.5*(interquartile range)

- An extreme outlying value is a value x such that either of the following is true:
  (1) $x >$ upper quartile + 3.0*(interquartile range) or
  (2) $x <$ lower quartile – 3.0*(interquartile range)
- Outliers can influence measures of data and should be considered when presenting descriptive statistics.

Empirical Rule: The empirical rule describes a unimodal and symmetric distribution using the mean and standard deviation.

When dealing with a unimodal and symmetric distribution, the empirical rule states that

- *Mean* ± 1 *standard deviation* covers approximately 67% of observations.
- *Mean* ± 2 *standard deviation* covers approximately 95% of observations.
- *Mean* ± 3 *standard deviation* covers approximately all observations.

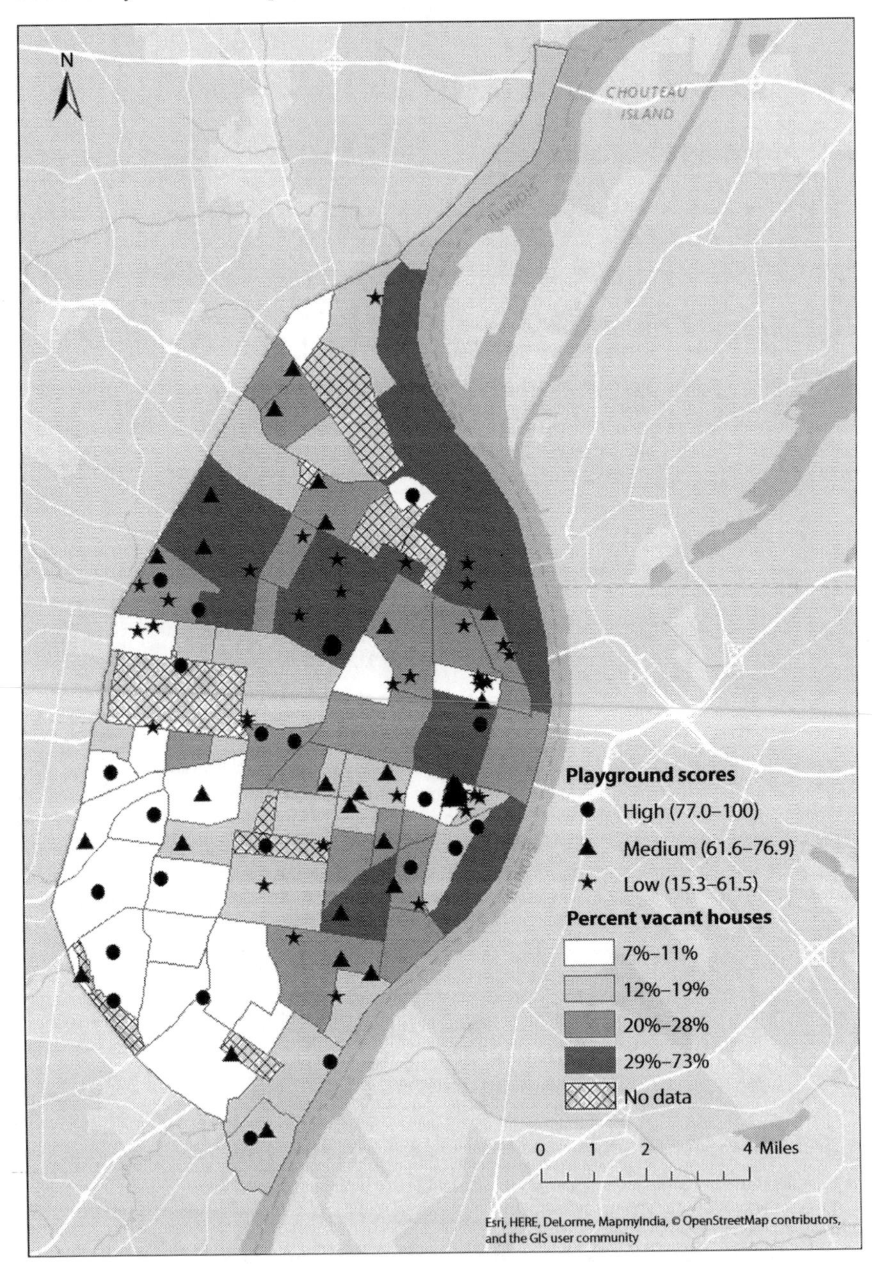

Figure 1.9 **GIS map from playground safety study in St. Louis, MO.** The graphic information system (GIS) map shows levels of playground safety in neighborhoods in St. Louis, MO, and the percent of vacant houses in each neighborhood. (Data on playground scores from Arroyo-Johnson, C., Woodward, K., Milam, L., Ackermann, N., Goodman, M. S., and Hipp, J. A., J Urban Heal., 93(4), 627-638, 2016, doi:10.1007/s11524-016-0063-8; data on percentage of vacant housing from Neighborhood Data Gateway, RISE Community Development, http://www.datagateway.org, accessed on June 15, 2015. The cartography is licensed as CC BY-SA. For more information visit http://openstreetmap.org, http://opendatacommons.org, and http://creativecommons.org.)

Table 1.2 Practice Problem 1.7 blank table

k	*Left limit*	*Right limit*	*Empirical rule, %*	*Chebyshev, %*	*Actual, %*
1					
2					
3					

Note: This table should be filled in with the appropriate values based on the data provided in Practice Problem 1.7 and Figure 1.5.

Chebyshev Inequality: The Chebyshev Inequality states that at least $1-\left(\frac{1}{k}\right)^2$ of the x observations lies within k standard deviations of the mean.

- The Chebyshev Inequality makes no assumptions about the distribution of the variable. That is, when we have a dataset that does not have a unimodal and symmetric distribution, the Chebyshev Inequality still applies, whereas the empirical rule is no longer valid.
- The Chebyshev Inequality still holds for unimodal and symmetric data but is more conservative than the empirical rule.

PRACTICE PROBLEM 1.7

Fill in Table 1.2 using the information provided.

The mean age of the study participants discussed in Figures 1.4 and 1.5 is 51.3 years with a standard deviation of 12.7 years.[3–6] Use Figure 1.5 to fill in the column of Table 1.2 with the heading *Actual*.

$$\bar{x} \pm k \times (SD)$$

PRACTICE PROBLEM 1.8

Suppose that the scale for a dataset is changed by multiplying each observation by a positive constant, c.

A What is the effect on the median?

B What is the effect on the mode?

C What is the effect on the geometric mean?

D What is the effect on the range?

E What is the effect on the arithmetic mean?

F What is the effect on the variance?

G What is the effect on the standard deviation?

PRACTICE PROBLEM 1.9

State whether each of the following observations is an example of discrete or continuous data.

A The number of Zika diagnoses in Puerto Rico during May of 2016.

B The weight of a newborn infant.

C The concentration of albumin in a sample of blood.

D The number of children injured on playgrounds in 2015.

Table 1.3 Pulse rate by shortness of breath status

Pulse rate, 60-second pulse rate	
Shortness of breath on stairs/inclines	*No shortness of breath on stairs/inclines*
76	76
76	68
72	64
62	84
74	68
82	58
70	82
80	74
80	58
64	74

Source: National Health and Nutrition Examination Survey, Centers for Disease Control and Prevention, https://wwwn.cdc.gov/Nchs/Nhanes/Search/nhanes13_14.aspx. Accessed February 23, 2016.

Note: The data are from a stratified random sample of 20 participants from the 2014 National Health and Nutrition Examination Survey. Participants over age 40 were asked, "{Have you/Has SP} had shortness of breath either when hurrying on the level or walking up a slight hill?" Respondents who answered *don't know* or who refused were excluded from this sample. In a separate setting, participants also had their pulse rate measured by a trained health technician.

Table 1.4 Practice Problem 1.10 descriptive statistics blank table

Descriptive statistics	*Shortness of breath*	*No shortness of breath*
Median		
Mean		
Range		
Interquartile range		
Standard deviation		

Note: Find the descriptive statistics named in the rows for each group named in the columns. This table should be solved using the data presented in Table 1.3.

PRACTICE PROBLEM 1.10

In Table 1.3 are data from a stratified random sample of participants in the 2014 NHANES survey.[1] The first column lists pulse rates, measured as beats per 60 seconds, for those who reported a shortness of breath while on stairs or an incline. The second column lists pulse rates for those who reported no shortness of breath while on stairs or an incline.

Fill in Table 1.4 (descriptive statistics table).

A Is the typical pulse rate per minute larger for those who experience a shortness of breath when walking up stairs or an incline or for those who do not?

B Which of the two groups has a greater amount of variability in the measurement?

References

1. National Health and Nutrition Examination Survey. Centers for Disease Control and Prevention website. https://wwwn.cdc.gov/Nchs/Nhanes/Search/nhanes13_14.aspx. Accessed February 23, 2016.
2. Behavioral Risk Factor Surveillance System (BRFSS). Centers for Disease Control and Prevention website. http://www.cdc.gov/brfss/annual_data/annual_2014.html. Published 2014. Accessed February 23, 2016.
3. Fan JH, Lyons S, Goodman MS, Blanchard MS, Kaphingst KA. Relationship between health literacy and unintentional and intentional medication nonadherence in medically underserved patients with type 2 diabetes. *Diabetes Educ.* 2016;42(2):199–208. doi:10.1177/0145721715624969.
4. Gilbert KL, Elder K, Lyons S, Kaphingst K, Blanchard M, Goodman M. Racial composition over the life course: Examining separate and unequal environments and the risk for heart disease for African American men. *Ethn Dis.* 2015;25(3):295–304. doi:10.18865/ed.25.3.295.
5. Goodman MS, Griffey RT, Carpenter CR, Blanchard M, Kaphingst KA. Do subjective measures improve the ability to identify limited health literacy in a clinical setting? *J Am Board Fam Med.* 2015;28(5):584–594. doi:10.3122/jabfm.2015.05.150037.
6. Seo J, Goodman MS, Politi M, Blanchard M, Kaphingst KA. Effect of health literacy on decision-making preferences among medically underserved patients. *Med Decis Mak.* 2016;(314):1–7. doi: 10.1177/0272989X16632197.
7. Arroyo-Johnson C, Woodward K, Milam L, Ackermann N, Goodman MS, Hipp JA. Still separate, still unequal: Social determinants of playground safety and proximity. *J Urban Heal.* 2016;93(4):627–638. doi:10.1007/s11524-016-0063-8.

Lab A: Introduction to SAS®

The basics

The choice of a statistical package is up to you. They all allow you to do the same tasks for the most part, although some packages are easier to use for certain tasks than others. However, for the purposes of the material in this book, they all work well. When deciding which package to use, think of it like learning a new language. It is more about who you want to be able to communicate with and your ability to learn new things. In this workbook, we have decided to use two programs so that you will be able to see the similarities and differences. The purpose of this lab is to introduce you to the SAS statistical software package. We are using SAS version 9.4 (SAS Institute, Cary, North Carolina) throughout this workbook.

In each chapter throughout this workbook, you will receive some SAS pointers containing the information that you need to complete the computing for that chapter. There are multiple ways to use most statistical software programs. The main options are a window-based format with pull-down menus or a command-driven format in which the user writes code and runs it. We will give some examples of both but focus on command-driven programs that the analyst can save for future use.

Getting started

You should have SAS installed on your computer. Let's open SAS. As we go through this introduction to SAS, you should be doing this on your computer to get the hands-on experience.

What is SAS?

SAS is a computer software program that allows a user to perform different procedures on data, such as analysis and manipulation. For example, SAS has many statistical procedures that can produce complex models or basic statistics, such as a mean and a standard deviation. SAS also allows a user to manipulate and clean data, such as creating new variables and changing categories of variables. We will use SAS throughout this workbook and explore a subset of what SAS can do.

SAS windowing environment

The SAS interface is divided into six windows, five of which appear when we open SAS:

1. *Editor* Window
   This is where we type syntax into SAS in order to perform statistical analyses, plot graphs, and other procedures. We can save code entered here by clicking the save button on the toolbar. This file will save with an extension of ".sas," which indicates a SAS program.
2. *Output* Window
   This is where the results of any procedure performed by SAS will appear if we have our preferences for results checked as "create listing." We can check this by going to *Tools/Options/Preferences* and clicking the *Results* tab.
3. *Results Viewer* Window
   This is where the results of any procedure performed by SAS will appear if we have "create HTML" checked. We can check this by going to *Tools/Options/Preferences* and clicking the *Results* tab. This is the only window that will not automatically appear when SAS is opened. It will open if we are in HTML mode and submit a PROC step that produces results.
4. *Explorer* Window
   In this window, we can see the contents of our current SAS environment. This window is most useful for viewing libraries and opening datasets.
5. *Log* Window
   This window is very useful. This is where we can see code that we have run and check for errors or warnings. In the log window, text appears in different colors. Black is for code that we submitted, blue is for SAS notes, green is for warnings, and red is for errors.
6. *Results* Window
   This window is different from the Results Viewer window. In this window, you will be able to see a table of contents and index of results.

SAS menus

Depending on what window we are viewing in SAS, there will be several options on the menu bar at the top of the SAS windowing environment. The following is a description of the basic SAS menus that will appear:

- *File*—Opens and saves SAS programs. Imports and exports data. Exits SAS.
- *Edit*—Cut, copy, paste, clear all, select all, and the Find tool.
- *View*—Can change which window you are viewing and open any windows if you have closed them.
- *Tools*—Can get to options and preferences here and includes various editors.
- *Run*—Submit syntax (also called code), and run procedures and data steps.
- *Solutions*—Add-ons (may not be available).
- *Window*—Controls the windows opened in SAS.
- *Help*—A good resource if we have questions about how to use SAS.

SAS programs

When we use SAS, most of our tasks will be run through SAS programs. SAS programs can contain either a DATA step or a PROC step (both of which we will go through in this lab with examples). There are several important ideas that are vital to working with SAS. As we go through examples and the rest of this lab, these will become much more apparent. Here are some of the important ideas for SAS:

- End every SAS statement with a semicolon.
- To run your code, you can highlight the selected code that you wish to run, and either click the "run" button (the little man running) on the toolbar or go to *Run/Submit.*
- Check your log window for errors and warnings every time you run code in SAS.
- Commenting throughout code is very helpful when using SAS.
  - Comments are used throughout SAS code to provide notations for what the program does so that is useful when you come back to it at a later time or if someone else needs to use your code.
  - This can be done by either starting with an asterisk (*) and ending with a semicolon (;) or starting with a slash and asterisk (/*) and ending with an asterisk and slash (*/).
  - Commented code will appear green in the program editor window and will be ignored when you tell a program to run. The following is an example of a SAS program with comments:

```
/*Merging data sets*/
DATA mylib.test_scores;
     MERGE pre_score post_score;
     BY ID;
     score_diff= post - pre;
     *Drop IDs of those who were absent;
     IF ID in (328, 504, 004, 887) THEN delete;
RUN;
```

Opening data files in SAS

For most of the computer work that we will do in this workbook, we will use data that are already in SAS format. In order to easily access this data in SAS, we will need to use libraries. A library, in SAS terms, is a way to point SAS to a specific folder on our computer where SAS datasets are stored. There are two ways to create a new library in SAS—by using the SAS menus or by using SAS code, which is the recommended way and how we will create libraries throughout this workbook.

Using SAS menus, we can create a library by clicking on *Tools/New Library*. From here, we will give our library a name and specify the folder in which our data are located in the "path" line. Using SAS code, we can specify a library via a LIBNAME statement:

```
LIBNAME mylib 'C:\Data';
```

We can replace *mylib* with what we chose to name our library, and "C:\Data" is the file path directing SAS to our data location. The data files are located on the eResources site. Save the data files in a folder on your computer, and direct SAS to use as your *mylib* library, designated by the file path. Don't forget your semicolon at the end.

Library names (also called *librefs* in SAS language) cannot be longer than eight characters, must not be one of the default SAS *librefs* (SASHELP, SASMSG, SASUSER, or WORK), must start with either a letter or an underscore, and cannot have a blank or special character (besides underscore).

Which of the following examples of a library name would not work in SAS: *_Lib*, *2_cats*, *cat%9*, *mylib2*, *lib_for_data2*?

There are two correct answers: *2_cats* and *cat%9*. The name *2_cats* cannot work as a library name because it starts with a number, and cat%9 will not work because the name includes the % symbol, which is a special character.

In addition to allowing users to make their own library, SAS has a default library called the WORK library, which is where data are automatically saved if we do not specify a *libname* before we refer to a dataset. We will go over an example of this in the PROC IMPORT code that follows in the paragraphs below.

Now that we understand what a SAS library is, we can discuss the files inside our libraries and other types of data files that can be imported into SAS. SAS data files have the extension .sas7bdat and are the type of files that can be directly used in SAS and in our libraries.

Raw text files, Excel files, and other types of files can be opened in SAS by clicking on *File/Import Data* and then using the data import wizard. Data can also be imported through the SAS procedure PROC IMPORT. Doing these procedures will turn other data files into SAS data files that are usable in SAS.

The following is an example PROC IMPORT for an Excel file:

```
PROC IMPORT DATAFILE='C:\Data\dataset1.xlsx'
     OUT=data_name DBMS=xlsx;
     SHEET='Sheet 1';
RUN;
```

The datafile= statement in the example refers to where our Excel filed titled "dataset1" is stored. The out= statement in the example refers to the SAS data file that will be created from the Excel file. The file will be saved as *data_name*, and since there is no *libref* before the dataset name, it will be stored in our work library (which stores data that we are currently using in SAS). The dbms= statement refers to the type of file that we are importing. In this case, we are importing an Excel workbook, and we refer to this by using the Excel extension ".xlsx". The sheet= is an optional statement and is used when importing Excel files with multiple sheets. We will refer to the sheet name that we want to import (in this case, 'sheet 1'). The name must be encased in single quotations.

The dataset named *er_heart.sas7bdat* contains data with the number of emergency department (ED) visits with a major diagnosis related to the heart and circulation, and the visits are listed by zip code for the St. Louis area of Missouri in 2013. These data come from the Missouri Department of Health and Senior Services, Missouri Information for Community Assessment (MICA).[1] The variable *zip* is the five-digit zip code, and the variable *visits* is the number of ED visits in 2013 with a major diagnosis related to the heart and circulation.

BOX SAS A.1 ER HEART DATASET DESCRIPTION

The *er_heart* dataset comes from the Bureau of Health Care Analysis and Data Dissemination, Missouri Department of Health and Senior Services. The data are from 2013 and contain the number of emergency department visits with a major diagnosis of heart and circulation by zip code for the St. Louis area of Missouri. The dataset includes two variables, a five-digit zip code, and the number of emergency visits with a heart or circulation diagnosis in that zip code for 2013.

Open the dataset *er_heart.sas7bdat* using a LIBNAME statement (see the following example). *Mylib* refers to what we chose to name our library. The file path in quotes refers to the location in which our data are located.

```
LIBNAME mylib 'C:\Data';
```

We can also create a library by going to *Tools/New Library.*

Run the code. Check the *Log* window to see whether the code ran. See Figure SAS A.1 for an example. In the *Explorer* window, find the library that we just created, and open it to find the dataset.

Data editor

As we have seen with creating libraries, there are also two main ways to enter and manipulate data in SAS. Using the data editor is one way, and using SAS code through DATA steps is the other. Using SAS code through DATA steps is what is more commonly used and how we will enter new data throughout this workbook.

- In the data editor, we can enter new data, make changes to the current dataset, or create new variables. Let's explore the data editor.
- Open the data editor by going to the *Explorer* window, clicking on the library, and clicking on the specified dataset.

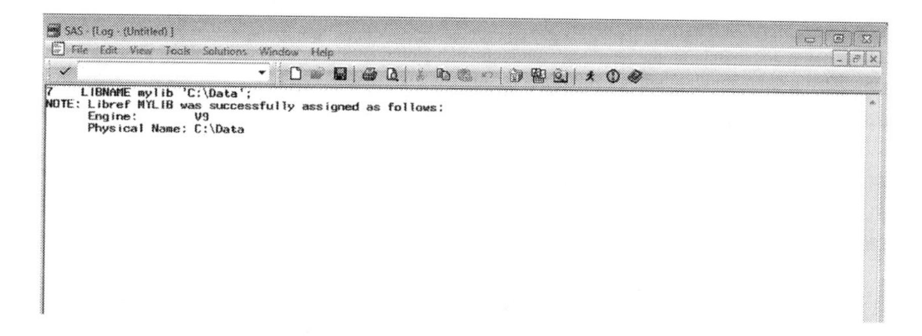

Figure SAS A.1 **Example log window after running libname statement.** The snapshot of the SAS log window shows that there were no errors or warnings when running our code. The text tells us that the MYLIB library was successfully assigned.

BOX SAS A.2 AN EXAMPLE OF A LOG WINDOW WITH ERRORS

- The log window in Figure SAS A.1 shows us what happens when everything goes right when we run SAS code, but what happens when something goes wrong? See Figure SAS A.2.
- In Figure SAS A.2, we can see that there are WARNING and ERROR messages in the SAS Log Window. The LIBNAME reference, *mylib%&jj* was not a valid name; thus, we see the errors and warnings.
- Although this book is in black and white, if we are using the *Enhanced* editor in SAS, then, by default, our warnings will appear in green, and the errors will appear in red.

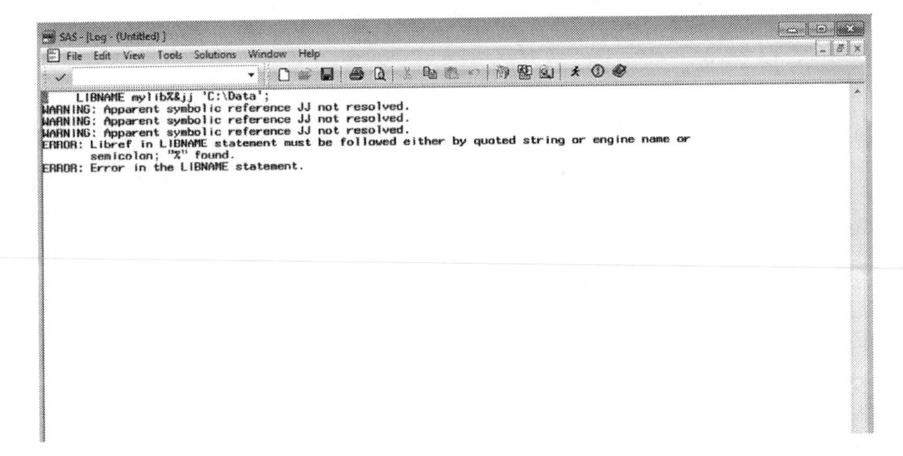

Figure SAS A.2 **Example log window after an error.** The snapshot of the SAS log window shows that there was an error when running the code and also shows a warning. Because this book is printed in black and white, we cannot see the colors from this image; however, error messages show up in red by default and warnings in green by default. The warnings tell us that the symbolic reference was not resolved because of the special character in our text that is not allowed by SAS. The error tells us more details and lets us know the % that was found.

- Notice that when the dataset is opened, the default is browse mode, where we can only look through our data.
- To make changes to our dataset, we must be in edit mode.
- To enter edit mode, go to *Edit/Edit Mode*.
- We can also change between modes by clicking the *Edit* or *Browse* buttons on the toolbar.
- Now, let's sort the data on the variable named visits. To do this, we highlight the column for visits by clicking on the variable name. Click the *Sort* button, either ascending or descending, on the SAS toolbar. Watch how the order of the observations changes. (Hint: Make sure that you are in Edit mode, or this function will not work.)

- We can also sort data using PROC SORT. See the following:

```
PROC SORT DATA=mylib.er_heart;
      BY visits;
RUN;
```

Inputting data into SAS

Refer to the data in Table SAS A.1. It contains observations of diastolic blood pressure and weight for 10 study[2] participants. We will manually input this data into SAS.

BOX SAS A.3 TABLE SAS A.1 DATA DESCRIPTION

The data in Table SAS A.1 come from the 2014 National Health and Nutrition Examination Survey (NHANES). In the survey, participants' blood pressure and weight (in kilograms) were measured by a trained health technician. Weight measurement was converted to pounds, and a random sample of 10 participants with nonmissing data is presented in Table SAS A.1.

Table SAS A.1 Diastolic blood pressure and weight for study participants

Diastolic blood pressure (mm Hg)	*Weight (pounds)*
92	221
62	136
78	175
60	159
42	108
88	175
94	324
68	135
90	185
78	159

Source: National Health and Nutrition Examination Survey, Centers for Disease Control and Prevention, National Center for Health Statistics, Hyattsville, MD, 2014, https://wwwn.cdc.gov/Nchs/Nhanes/Search/nhanes13_14.aspx. Accessed February 23, 2016.

Note: The data come from the 2014 NHANES survey and include a random sample of 10 study participants. The variables include diastolic blood pressure in mm Hg and weight in pounds.

To do this, we will use a data step and datalines. See the following syntax:

```
DATA mylib.study;
       INPUT dbp weight;
DATALINES;
92 221
62 136
78 175
60 159
42 108
88 175
94 324
68 135
90 185
78 159
;
RUN;
```

The first line in our code designates what the dataset will be named. Here, we are naming the dataset *study* and saving the dataset to the library *mylib*. The INPUT line specifies our variable names and their location in the datalines. We will name diastolic blood pressure *dbp* and type those values in the first column. We will name the participant's weight as *weight* and enter these values in the latter column. The values should be separated by a space. Next, we will enter the values for *dbp* and *weight* after we specify DATALINES (see sample code before this paragraph).

BOX SAS A.4 NOTE ON SAS VARIABLE NAMES

SAS variable names can be up to 32 characters and must start with a letter or an underscore and cannot contain blanks or special characters (except an underscore).

Make sure to put a semicolon on a separate line after the rows of data. Run this section of code. Because we specified *mylib* separated by a period before the name of the dataset, the data will be saved in the *mylib* library and placed in that folder on your computer. Find the dataset, open it, and check the data. Remember, if we had not specified *mylib* before the dataset name, the dataset would have been stored in the work library automatically. See the following shortened code for an example:

```
DATA study;
     INPUT dbp weight;
DATALINES;
92 221
62 136
;
RUN;
```

If one of the variables that we were entering was a character variable (as opposed to a numeric variable), we would have designated this by including a $ after the variable name (see the example after this paragraph). Here, we are entering *dbp* and *weight* such as in the previous example (both numeric variables) and including *sex* as a character variable (*M* for male and *F* for female).

```
DATA mylib.study;
     INPUT dbp weight sex $;
DATALINES;
92 221 M
62 136 F
78 175 F
;
RUN;
```

Labels

For the sake of clarity, we may want to give labels to our data. Labels can be given to the entire dataset or to the individual variables. This is helpful when datasets, variables, or both have abbreviated names and we want to keep a more detailed explanation of the contents of the datasets and variables. For example, we might want to label the variable *dbp* as "Diastolic Blood Pressure." To assign a label to our dataset and to our variables, we can use PROC DATASETS:

```
PROC DATASETS LIBRARY=mylib;
     MODIFY study (LABEL='Diastolic Blood Pressure and Weights of
     Study Participants');
     LABEL dbp='Diastolic Blood Pressure (mmHg)' weight='Participant
     Weight (lbs)';
RUN;
```

LIBRARY=mylib specifies the library that is the location of the dataset that we are modifying. MODIFY specifies the dataset that we are modifying. To label our dataset, we follow the dataset name with a LABEL=option and include the label that we are assigning to our dataset in quotations. In this example, we are labeling the dataset as "Diastolic Blood Pressure and Weights of Study Participants."

The second statement, LABEL, modifies labels of variables in the dataset that we specified in the previous step. To assign labels to variables, we type variablename="Label we are assigning to that variable." In our example, we are labeling both *dbp* and *weight*.

We end the procedure code with a run statement and make sure not to forget our semicolons. Now, we run this step. To do this, we can either click the *Run* button on the toolbar or go to *Run/Submit.* If we want to run only a certain part of our code and not the whole thing, we can highlight a certain section, then run. Check the log window for errors or warnings. To see the labels that we just created, we will use PROC CONTENTS:

```
PROC CONTENTS DATA=mylib.study;
RUN;
```

PROC CONTENTS will provide us with dataset and variable information, including the labels that we just assigned. Sample code for PROC contents is provided just before this paragraph. Here, we specify the dataset name in the DATA=option. Run this portion of code, check the log window for errors or warnings, and then check the results window for output.

- Are the labels that we just assigned visible?
- Check your results with the partial output presented in "Alphabetic List of Variables and Attributes":

Alphabetic List of Variables and Attributes

#	Variable	Type	Len	Label
1	dbp	Num	8	Diastolic Blood Pressure (mm Hg)
2	weight	Num	8	Participant Weight (lbs)

- Open the *er_heart.sas7bdat* dataset, and look at its thorough labeling.

BOX SAS A.5 ASSIGNING LABELS WHEN CREATING A DATASET

We can also assign labels when we are creating our dataset:

```
DATA mylib.study (LABEL='Diastolic Blood Pressure and Weights
of Study Participants');
      INPUT dbp weight;
      LABEL dbp='Diastolic Blood Pressure (mmHg)' weight=
      'Participant Weight (lbs)';
DATALINES;
92 221
62 136
78 175
;
RUN;
```

The above code is very similar to using PROC DATASETS, the difference being where we place the code. The label for the dataset goes in the DATA statement line, and the labels for the variables go on their own separate line—a procedure similar to the PROC DATASETS procedure.

Summarizing data

In this section, we will calculate some descriptive statistics. First, let's open the dataset *nhanes2014_sample.sas7bdat*, which is found on the eResources site. These data come from the 2014 National Health and Nutrition Examination Survey.[2] The dataset contains several variables, including race (1 = non-Hispanic white; 2 = non-Hispanic black), age (in years), sex (1 = males; 2 = females), urine lead level (in µg/L), and an identification number. Use a *libname* statement to open the data in SAS.

BOX SAS A.6 NHANES 2014 SAMPLE DATASET DESCRIPTION

The *nhanes2014_sample* sample dataset comes from the 2014 National Health and Nutrition Examination Survey (NHANES). The variables included in the dataset are *race*, *age*, *sex*, urine lead level (*lead*), and identification (*id*). The *id* variable was created by the administrators of NHANES. Sex was collected as male or female. Age was collected in years at the time of screening, and participants above age 80 years were recoded to age 80 (i.e., 80 years is the maximum age noted). Race was recoded by NHANES administrators to Mexican American, other Hispanic, non-Hispanic white, non-Hispanic black, and other race—including multiracial. For this sample, only those with a race of non-Hispanic white or non-Hispanic black were included. Urine lead level was measured by trained professionals and recorded in µg/L. For this example, 100 participants with nonmissing data and a race of non-Hispanic white or non-Hispanic black were randomly selected.

```
LIBNAME mylib 'C:\Data';
```

EXAMPLE PROBLEM A.1

A Navigate via the *Explorer* window to view the data in the table viewer. Describe the variables in the dataset.

The variables in the dataset include race, lead, age, sex, and identification number. Through the data editor, we can see the number values listed in the dataset for each variable.

B What is the mean urine lead level (lead) for this group?

We can use PROC MEANS or PROC UNIVARIATE for this.

```
PROC MEANS DATA=mylib.nhanes2014_sample;
VAR lead;
RUN;

PROC UNIVARIATE DATA=mylib.nhanes2014_sample;
VAR lead;
RUN;
```

In this code, we specify the dataset in question using the DATA=option. The VAR statement is where we specify which variable we want descriptive statistics for. We end our code with a RUN statement. This is the output that we should obtain from PROC MEANS:

The MEANS Procedure

Analysis Variable : lead				
N	Mean	Std Dev	Minimum	Maximum
100	0.5116000	0.5149673	0.0200000	2.7900000

From here, we can see that the mean urine lead level in the group is 0.51 μg/L. From PROC UNIVARIATE, we would have seen a table like this in our output:

The UNIVARIATE Procedure
Variable: lead

Moments			
N	100	Sum Weights	100
Mean	0.5116	Sum Observations	51.16
Std Deviation	0.51496733	Variance	0.26519135
Skewness	2.21713356	Kurtosis	5.55205811
Uncorrected SS	52.4274	Corrected SS	26.253944
Coeff Variation	100.658196	Std Error Mean	0.05149673

Basic Statistical Measures			
Location		Variability	
Mean	0.511600	Std Deviation	0.51497
Median	0.330000	Variance	0.26519
Mode	0.490000	Range	2.77000
		Interquartile Range	0.46000

Tests for Location: Mu0 = 0				
Test	Statistic		p Value	
Student's t	t	9.934611	Pr > |t|	<.0001
Sign	M	50	Pr >= |M|	<.0001
Signed Rank	S	2525	Pr >= |S|	<.0001

Quantiles (Definition 5)	
Level	Quantile
100% Max	2.790
99%	2.610
95%	1.755
90%	1.140
75% Q3	0.650
50% Median	0.330
25% Q1	0.190
10%	0.105
5%	0.065
1%	0.020
0% Min	0.020

Extreme Observations			
Lowest		Highest	
Value	Obs	Value	Obs
0.02	32	1.81	56
0.02	13	1.90	5
0.04	45	1.99	77
0.05	62	2.43	65
0.06	33	2.79	2

From here, we can also see that the mean urine lead level in the group is 0.51 μg/L.

C **What is the standard deviation of the lead variable? (Hint: We can obtain this from the SAS output provided in Example Problem A.1—Part (B).)**

The standard deviation of the urine lead level in this sample is 0.51 μg/L.

D **What is the median (50th percentile) age?**

Only PROC UNIVARIATE gives this automatically. When using PROC MEANS, we must specify MEDIAN as an option (see sample code below).

```
PROC MEANS DATA= mylib.nhanes2014_sample MEDIAN;
VAR age;
RUN;
```

The MEANS Procedure

Analysis Variable: age
Median
38.5000000

The median age in this sample is 38.5 years, as shown in our output just before this paragraph. Our code is similar to what we used in Example Problem A.1—Part (A), but we inserted MEDIAN in the first line of our PROC MEANS code. We can also add other key words in this spot to have more statistics output. For example, we could insert MEAN and STD along with median, and output would include the mean, standard deviation, and the median.

E **What is the mean age for males (male = 1, females = 2)?**

The variable *sex* contains the designation of male or female. To do this, we can use a WHERE statement in either PROC MEANS or PROC UNIVARIATE:

```
PROC MEANS DATA=mylib.nhanes2014_sample;
VAR age;
WHERE sex=1;
RUN;
```

The MEANS Procedure

Analysis Variable : age				
N	Mean	Std Dev	Minimum	Maximum
47	38.2553191	22.6816034	6.0000000	80.0000000

After running our PROC MEANS code, we can see that the mean age for males is 38.3 (see the output just before this paragraph). In the WHERE statement, we specify which variable (sex =) and which category or group we want statistics for (1). If this were a character variable, we would have put quotes around the category. For example, if males were coded as "male," instead of as 1, our statement would be read as the following:

```
WHERE sex ='male';
```

F How many girls are there in this dataset (male = 1, female = 2)?

Use PROC FREQ (shorthand for frequency) to answer this question:

```
PROC FREQ DATA=mylib.nhanes2014_sample;
TABLE sex;
RUN;
```

The FREQ Procedure

Sex	Frequency	Percent	Cumulative Frequency	Cumulative Percent
1	47	47.00	47	47.00
2	53	53.00	100	100.00

Using the SAS output above, we can conclude that there are 53 females in our sample. To get to this conclusion, we used PROC FREQ, a procedure that provides frequency tables for categorical variables. In this code, we specify the dataset in question using the DATA=option. We then use a TABLE statement to tell SAS which variables we would like frequency tables on. We end our code, as always, with a RUN statement.

G How many females in this sample have the race non-Hispanic black?

The variable race is coded as 1 = non-Hispanic white and 2 = non-Hispanic black. We will also use PROC FREQ to answer this question:

```
PROC FREQ DATA=mylib.nhanes2014_sample;
TABLE sex*race;
RUN;
```

The FREQ Procedure

Frequency Percent Row Pct Col Pct			
Table of Sex by Race			
Sex	**Race**		
	1	**2**	**Total**
1	24	23	47
	24.00	23.00	47.00
	51.06	48.94	
	44.44	50.00	
2	30	23	53
	30.00	23.00	53.00
	56.60	43.40	
	55.56	50.00	
Total	54	46	100
	54.00	46.00	100.00

There are 23 females who have the race non-Hispanic black in our sample. In the code used to answer Example Problem A.1—Part (G), we are again using PROC FREQ; however, this time, we are specifying that we want a 2 × 2 table by using the asterisk (*) between the two variables of interest. The resulting output gives us a table of sex by race.

H **List 10 observations for race and lead level using PROC PRINT:**

```
PROC PRINT DATA=mylib.nhanes2014_sample (obs=10);
VAR race lead;
RUN;
```

Obs	Race	Lead
1	2	0.83
2	2	1.70
3	1	0.49
4	1	0.11
5	1	2.79
6	2	0.19
7	2	0.75
8	2	1.81
9	2	0.49
10	1	0.34

The above code uses PROC PRINT to "print" our data. The DATA=option tells SAS the dataset that we want to print. The *obs=* option tells SAS how many observations we would like to print. If we do not specify this option, SAS automatically prints all observations in the dataset. The VAR statement tells SAS that we want to print the variables *race* and *lead*. If we do not include a VAR statement, SAS automatically prints all variables in the dataset. We end the code with a RUN statement and, of course, a semicolon.

BOX SAS A.7 A NOTE ON THE OBS= STATEMENT

- Using *obs=* in our PROC PRINT statement tells SAS how many observations we would like to be printed.
- In this example, we used obs=10, which means SAS pulls the first 10 observations.
- If we had said obs=15, then SAS would have printed the first 15 observations in the dataset.

Formats

Suppose that we wanted to format the variable *sex* in the *nhanes2014_sample* dataset to label 1 as males and 2 as females. Formatting consists of two parts. First, we must use a PROC FORMAT statement to assign the labels to the different levels. For character variables, make sure to include the dollar sign in the value line, and put the variable levels in quotation marks.

```
PROC FORMAT;
     VALUE sexfmt 1='Male' 2='Female';
     VALUE $sex2fmt 'M'='Male' 'F'='Female';
RUN;
```

Then, we can either assign formats to variables permanently or assign them on a proc-by-proc basis. To assign formats that will automatically show up in all output, write a format line into a data statement:

```
DATA mylib.nhanes2014_sample;
     SET mylib.nhanes2014_sample;
     FORMAT sex sexfmt.;
RUN;
```

To assign formats that only show up in the output from a selected proc, we can add a format line into the proc step.

```
PROC FREQ DATA=mylib.nhanes2014_sample;
     TABLE sex;
     FORMAT sex sexfmt.;
RUN;
```

If we have multiple variables that use the same format (for example, if we have three questions that all have 1 = 'Yes' 0 = 'No'), we can list the variable names and then put the format name and period only once at the end of the line (e.g., format question1 question2 question3 yesnofmt.;).

Printing SAS output

We just learned how to "print" SAS data. Now, we will discuss printing SAS output. We can print output from the session three different ways. One way is to choose *File/Print*. Another option is to copy and paste the contents of the *Results* or *Output* window to a document in a word processor and print from there. This is often a little bit neater, and it allows you to print only the relevant parts of your session. The last option is using ODS (Output Delivery System) through SAS, which is more difficult to learn, so we will just provide a brief introduction in this workbook towards the end of this section.

View the current results or output, and select a portion of text from the results. Select *Edit/Copy*. Switch to an open word processor document, place the text cursor at the target location, and choose *Edit/Paste*. Notice that the text does not necessarily have the same appearance. We can change this by highlighting the portion that we pasted and by changing the font to a fixed-width font such as Courier New.

Using ODS can be difficult to comprehend but can be very useful in printing SAS output. ODS displays SAS output in a nicer format than traditional output and can also create PDF files, HTML files, and RTF (Rich Text Format) files, among others, and create datasets from output.

For example, let's say that we want to print our output from Example Problem A.1—Part (G) to a PDF file. We could use the following code to do that:

```
ODS PDF FILE='C:\Data\ods_test.pdf';
PROC FREQ DATA=mylib.nhanes2014_sample;
                TABLE sex*race;
RUN;
ODS PDF CLOSE;
```

In this case, start ODS by using an ODS option, specifying that you want your output printed in a PDF, and specifying the file path where you want the PDF to be saved following the FILE=option. When you are finished with the code that states that you want the output printed to the PDF, close ODS by using an ODS option and by specifying what type of file you are closing—the PDF in this example. After you run the code, check your file to see the PDF that was created. The PDF will have the output from the PROC FREQ in it.

Creating new variables with formulas

Sometimes we may need to create a new variable that is a function of one or more existing variables. We will see later in the chapters why you may want to do this.

Create a new variable called *leadsq* that is the square of the urine lead level ($lead^2$). To do this, we will use a data step:

```
DATA nhanes2014_sample2;
     SET mylib.nhanes2014_sample;
     leadsq=lead**2;
RUN;
```

In this code, since we do not specify a library name before the dataset name *nhanes2014_sample2*, SAS will save the dataset to the *work* library, which is where temporary datasets are stored, but the dataset will not be saved when we exit SAS. The SET statement specifies which dataset we are copying to create the new dataset. The next line is where we create the new variable *leadsq*. The symbol that we use for exponentiation is 2 asterisks (**).

Graphs

Several SAS procedures create graphs. For this lab, we will go over a few of these examples.

EXAMPLE PROBLEM A.2

A **Using the *nhanes2014_sample* data, create a box plot for age. Are there any outliers? Does the plot give you a sense of the mean? The median? The mode?**

We will use PROC UNIVARIATE, as previously used, except that this time, we will specify the PLOT option. Look at the resulting box plot in Figure SAS A.3.

```
PROC UNIVARIATE DATA=mylib.nhanes2014_sample PLOT;
VAR age;
RUN;
```

The box plot can be seen in the resulting output, under the title of "Distribution and Probability Plot for age." The box plot is in the upper right corner of this section of graphs. From the box plot, we can tell that there are no outliers in this sample because there are no points beyond the upper or lower end of the box plot. From this box plot, we can see the mean, represented by the diamond, and the median, represented by the bar through the middle of the box. The box plot does not give us a sense of the mode.

Suppose that we had two groups for which we wanted to compare box plots on a variable such as *sex*. We could use PROC BOXPLOT to solve this problem. Unfortunately, PROC BOXPLOT does not work with just one variable. We must also have a grouping variable included; in this case, that would be *sex*. The code for PROC BOXPLOT is as follows:

```
PROC BOXPLOT DATA=mylib. nhanes2014_sample;
  PLOT age*sex;
RUN;
```

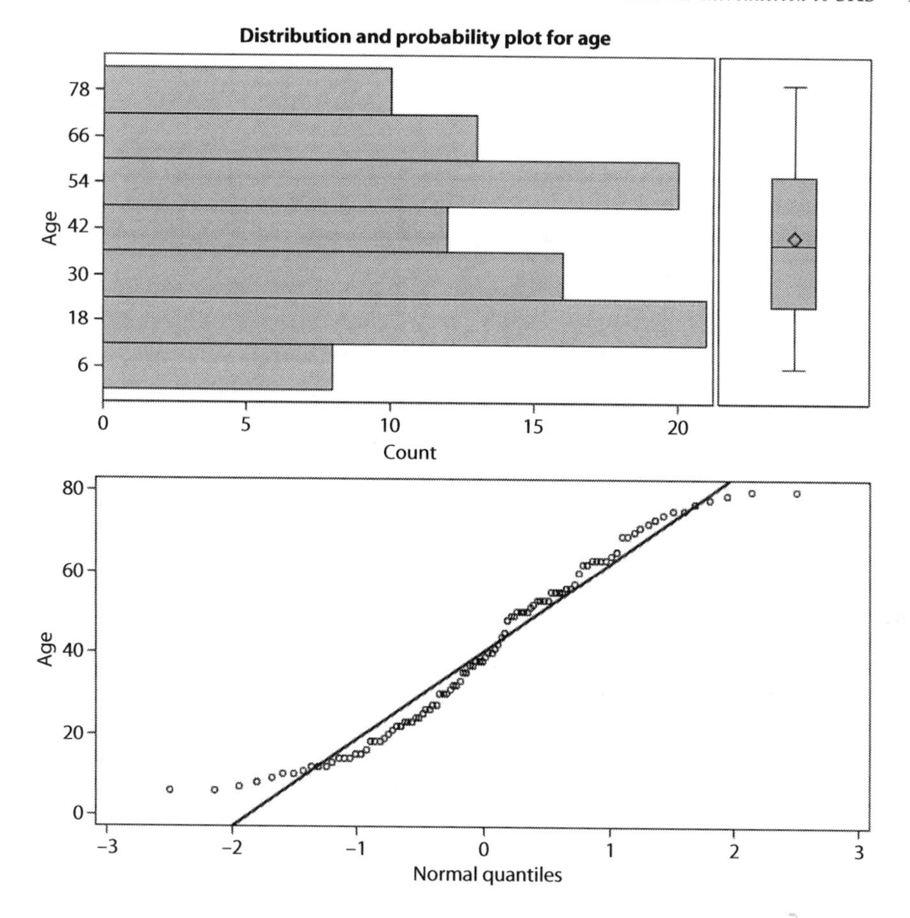

Figure SAS A.3 **SAS PROC UNIVARIATE plot output for age**. The plot output for PROC UNIVARIATE gives us a figure that contains two other plots along with a box plot for the variable *age*. We can see the box plot in the upper right corner of the figure. The diamond in the middle of the box plot represents the mean, and the line through the box represents the median.

B Construct a stem-and-leaf plot of age.

To do this, we use PROC UNIVARIATE and the plots option. The code will be the same as the code that we ran when we obtained our box plot. If we look back at our output for Example Problem A.1—Part (A), we see a different version of a stem-and-leaf plot in the upper left corner of the output (Figure SAS A.4). The reason that we could not see a stem-and-leaf plot like the one that we saw in Chapter 1 is that we have our ODS graphics option on. We must turn this off before we run our code.

```
ODS GRAPHICS OFF;
PROC UNIVARIATE DATA=mylib.nhanes2014_sample PLOT;
      VAR age;
RUN;
```

```
Stem Leaf                     #        Box Plot
   8 00                       2           |
   7 55789                    5           |
   7 01234                    5           |
   6 599                      3           |
   6 02233334                 8           |
   5 5555667                  7        +-----+
   5 0000123333              10        |     |
   4 5899                     4        |     |
   4 00124                    5        |  +  |
   3 55778889                 8        *-----*
   3 0001223                  7        |     |
   2 56677                    5        |     |
   2 012233344                9        +-----+
   1 5568889                  7           |
   1 0012223444              10           |
   0 66789                    5           |
     ----+----+----+----+
   Multiply stem. leaf by 10**+1
```

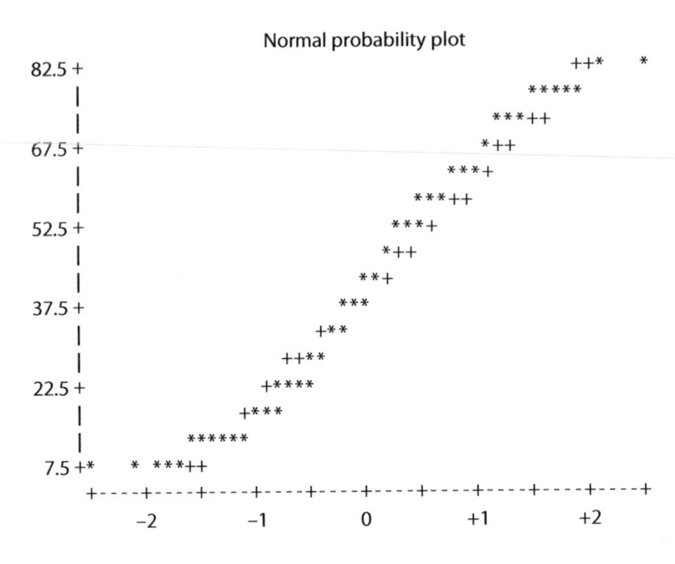

Figure SAS A.4 **Plot output for variable age from PROC UNIVARIATE including stem-and-leaf plot.** The plot output for PROC UNIVARIATE without ODS graphics on gives us a stem-and-leaf plot similar to what we learned to draw in Chapter 1, along with a box plot and normal probability plot. Notice the difference between this figure and Figure SAS A.3 when ODS graphics were on. From the stem-and-leaf plot, we can see the distribution of the variable *age*.

Our code for Example Problem A.1—Part (B) is almost the same as the code for Example Problem A.1—Part (A); however, in Example Problem A.1—Part (B), we use the ODS statement before PROC UNIVARIATE to turn graphics off and to obtain the resulting output. To turn ODS graphics back on, we use the code ODS GRAPHICS ON; thus, the graphics will reset to the default setting and will appear the next time that we run our code.

C **Create a histogram for *lead* (consider it a continuous variable). Would you describe the distribution as skewed or symmetric?**

We will also use PROC UNIVARIATE for this. However, this time, we will include a HISTOGRAM statement, and the variable name will follow.

```
ODS GRAPHICS ON;
PROC UNIVARIATE DATA=mylib.nhanes2014_sample;
        VAR lead;
        HISTOGRAM lead;
RUN;
```

After running the previous code in SAS, we obtain a histogram similar to what is presented in Figure SAS A.5. The distribution of lead is skewed to the right (positively skewed) and is not symmetric.

D **Now, create separate histograms of lead for males and females. How do the histograms differ between the two sexes?**

To do this, first we must use PROC SORT to sort our data by *sex* so that we can use a BY statement in PROC UNIVARIATE. This is a requirement in SAS. Our data must be sorted by the variable that we are using in the BY statement, or we will receive an error when we try to run the code. Remember, 1 = males and 2 = females for the *sex* variable.

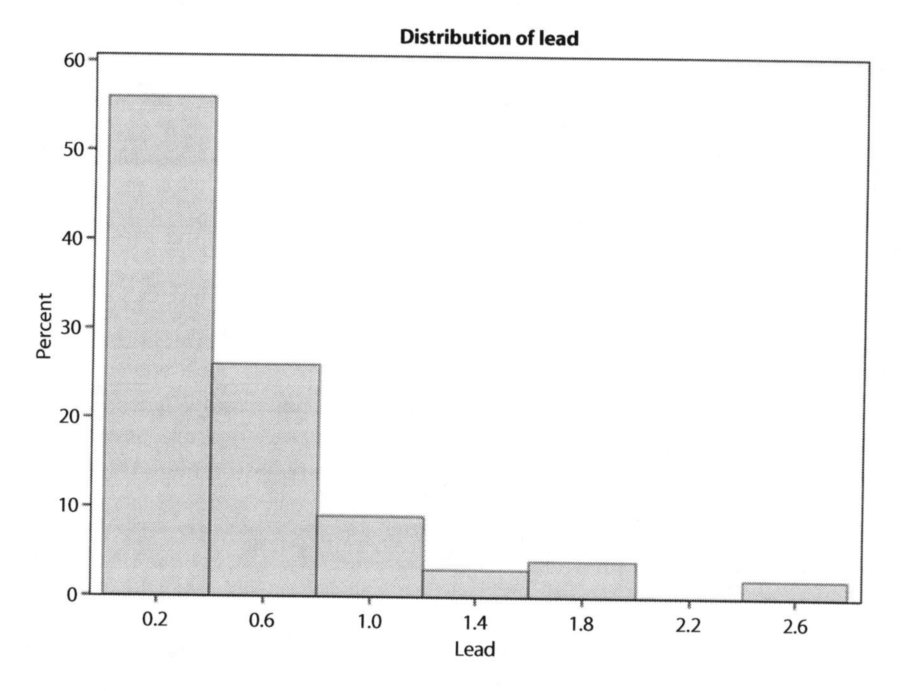

Figure SAS A.5 **Histogram of lead level.** The histogram of the variable lead shows the distribution of participants' lead levels. The distribution is skewed to the right, with a majority of the participants' lead levels being about 0.2 µg/L.

BOX SAS A.8 EXAMPLE OF ERROR LOG IF DATA ARE NOT SORTED FIRST

- Below is a snapshot of what the log window will look like if we do not sort our data by sex before using a BY statement in PROC UNIVARIATE (Figure SAS A.6).

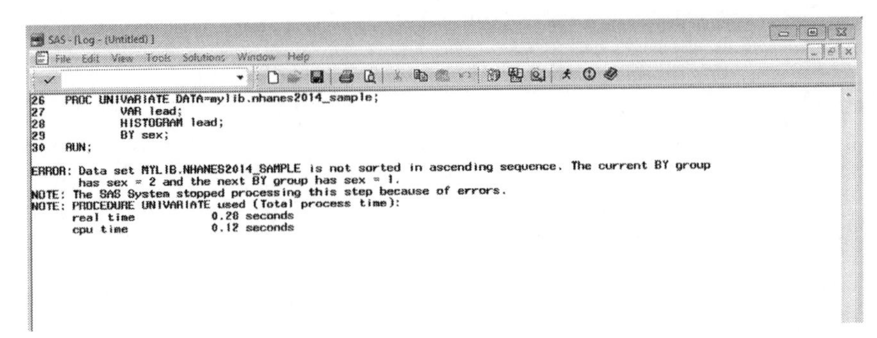

Figure SAS A.6 **Snapshot of log window if data are not sorted before using BY statement.** The snapshot of the SAS log window shows an error message that tells us the data are not sorting in ascending sequence. In order to use a BY statement in SAS, we must first sort our data. Otherwise a similar error message will appear, and we will not get the desired results.

```
PROC SORT DATA=mylib.nhanes2014_sample;
      BY sex;
RUN;

PROC UNIVARIATE DATA=mylib.nhanes2014_sample;
      VAR age;
      HISTOGRAM age;
      BY sex;
RUN;
```

The first histogram in our output is for sex = 1, or males (Figure SAS A.7). This distribution appears similar to the distribution of the group as a whole. The second histogram in our output is for sex = 2, or females (Figure SAS A.8). The distribution for females is also skewed to the right; however, it appears that most females have lead levels lower than those of the males, as we can see that the distribution is shifted toward 0.

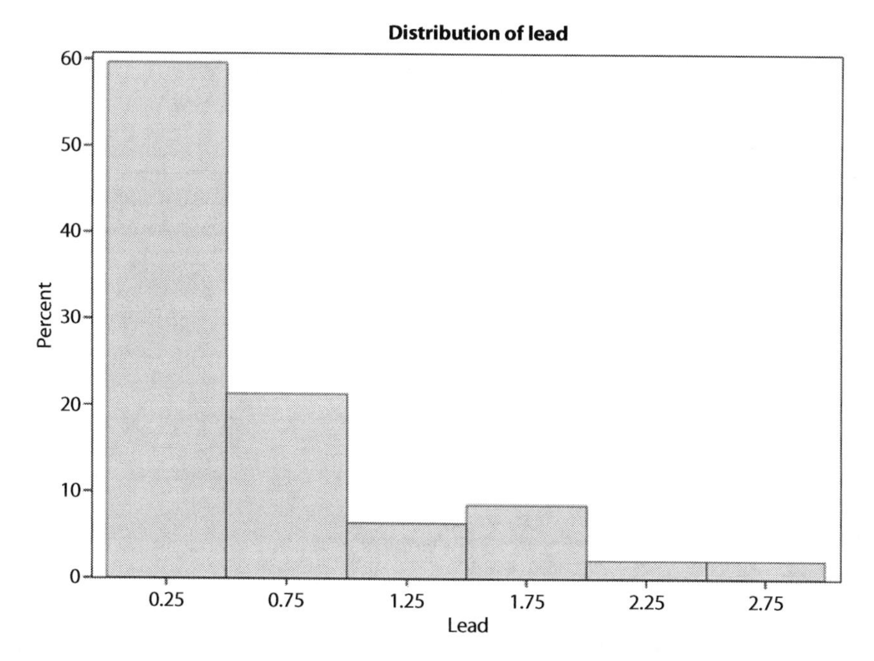

Figure SAS A.7 **Histogram of lead level for males (sex = 1).** The histogram of lead level for males show the distribution of the variable. Most participants have a lead level around 0.25 μg/L. The data are skewed to the right.

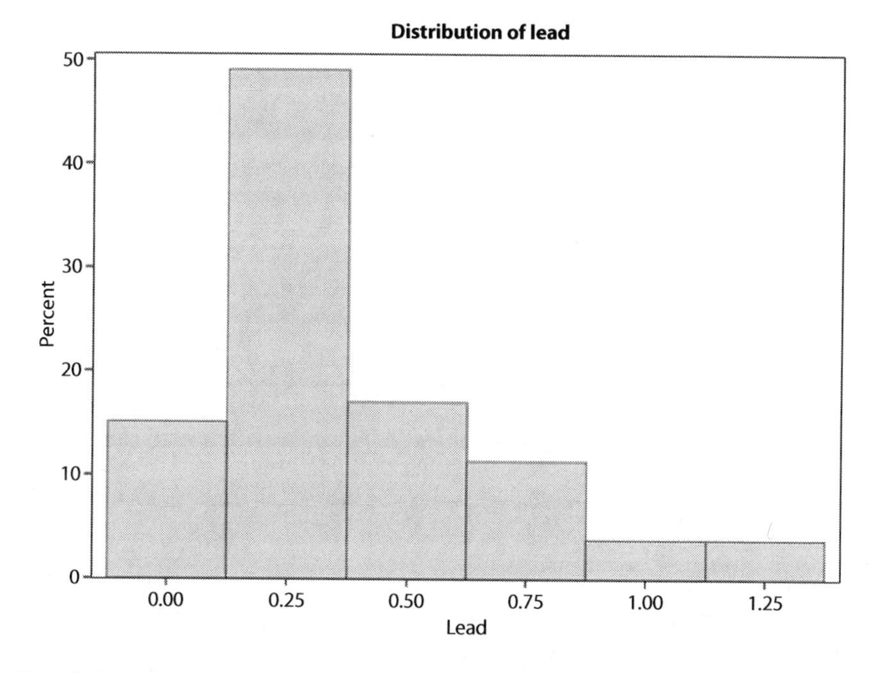

Figure SAS A.8 **Histogram of lead level for females (sex = 2).** Similar to the histogram of lead level for males, the histogram for females is also skewed to the right; however, it is less so than the males. Most female participants also have a lead level around 0.25 μg/L, but the range of values for females is not as high as the lead levels of males.

BOX SAS A.9 EXAMPLE OF USING LABELS TO MAKE A GRAPH LOOK BETTER

- Suppose that we want our graphs to have labels of "Lead Level" instead of just "lead" as seen in our previous histograms. We could use labels for this.

```
PROC UNIVARIATE DATA=mylib.nhanes2014_sample;
     VAR age;
     HISTOGRAM age;
     BY sex;
     LABEL lead= "Lead Level";
RUN;
```

- The resulting histogram for males with a labeled *x*-axis is shown in Figure SAS A.9.

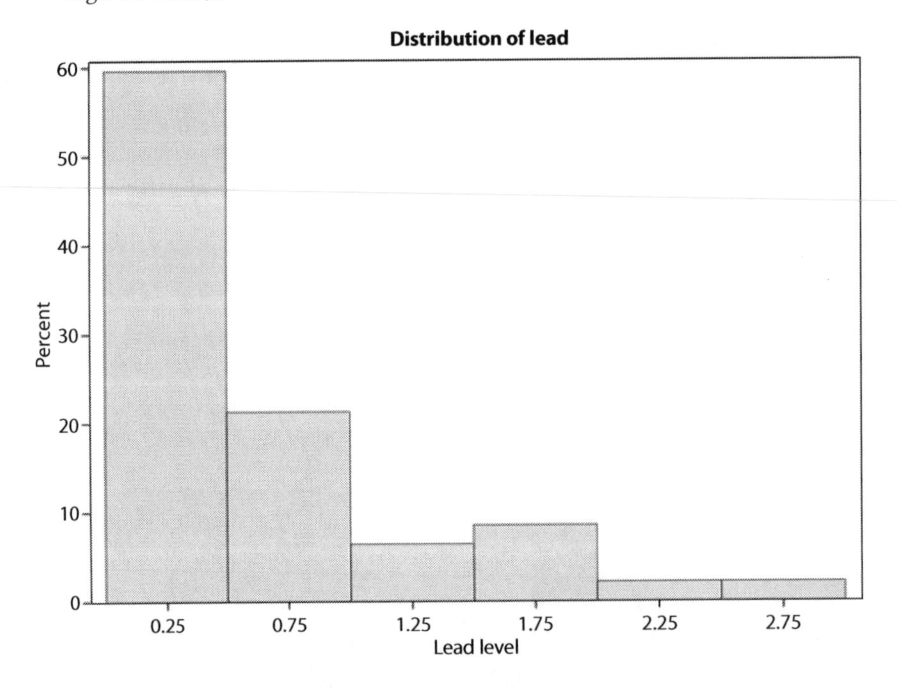

Figure SAS A.9 **Labeled histogram of lead level for males.** The histogram presented here is essentially the same as the histogram presented in Figure SAS A.7; however, this time we have used the LABEL statement to label the x-axis so that "Lead Level" will appear instead of just the variable name lead.

E Create a scatterplot of *age* vs. *lead*. Is there a relationship between the two variables?

To do this, we will use PROC SGPLOT (see the following syntax example). Here, we use the SCATTER statement, specifying *age* on our *x*-axis and *lead* on our *y*-axis.

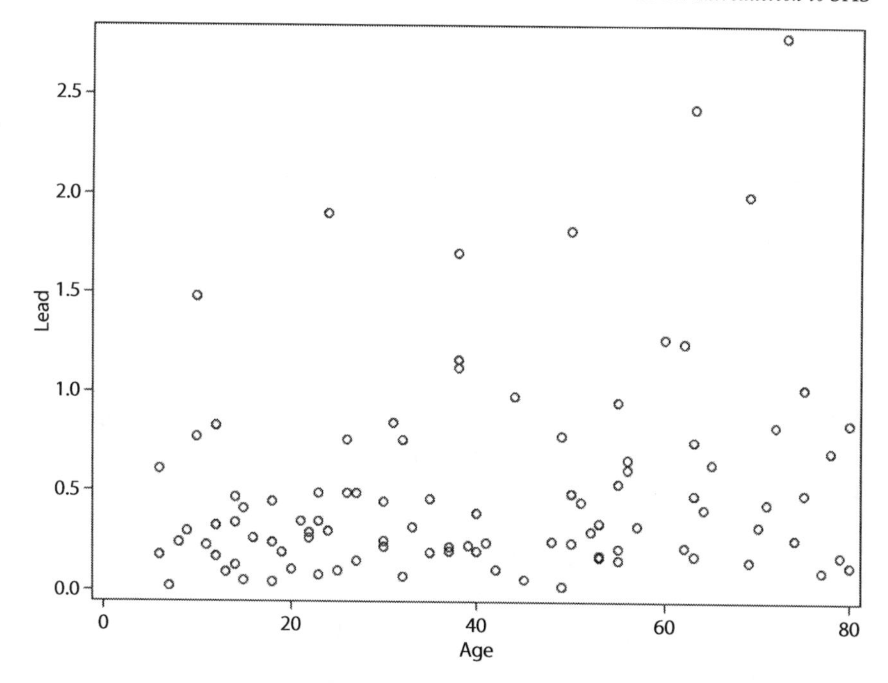

Figure SAS A.10 **Scatterplot of age and lead.** The scatterplot shows the relationship between two continuous variables, age and lead. On the x-axis, age is represented, and on the y-axis, lead is represented. Within the plot, we see points, which are representative of the data in our dataset. Each point represents a different participant. From this scatterplot, there does not appear to be a clear relationship between age and lead level.

```
PROC SGPLOT DATA=mylib.nhanes2014_sample;
   SCATTER X=age Y=lead;
   RUN;
```

When we run the previous code, we receive a resulting scatterplot of *lead* and *age* (Figure SAS A.10). In our code, we specify the dataset with the DATA=option, and, then, we use a SCATTER statement to specify that we want a scatterplot. In the SCATTER statement, we specify the variables that we would like to put into the scatterplot with the X= and Y= options. The X refers to the *x*-axis, and the Y refers to the *y*-axis. We end the procedure, like every procedure, with a RUN statement.

Saving graphs

While the results window is active, we can copy and paste graphs to a word processing program by right clicking on the graph and choosing *Copy* and then pasting it into a word processing document.

PRACTICE PROBLEM A.1

The dataset *nhanes2014_glucose* contains a sample of participants from the NHANES 2014 survey.[2] The variables include the following: whether the participant was ever told by a doctor that he or she has diabetes (*diabetes*); the participant's fasting glucose in mg/dL (*fast_glu*); the participant's two-hour glucose, also in mg/dL (*twohour_glu*); and the participant's age (*age*), sex (*sex*), race (*race*), and identification number (*id*). For the *diabetes* variable, 1 = the participant was told that he or she has diabetes and 2 = the participant was not told that he or she has diabetes. The *sex* variable is coded the same as before, 1 = males and 2 = females. For *race*, 1 = white, 2 = non-white. We want to know whether the descriptive statistics of glucose levels differ by whether a participant replied that a doctor told the participant that he or she has diabetes.

BOX SAS A.10 NHANES 2014 GLUCOSE DATASET DESCRIPTION

The *nhanes2014_glucose* dataset comes from the same survey as the *nhanes2014_sample* dataset. The *age*, *sex*, and ID variables are the same as in the previously used dataset (Box SAS A.6). For this dataset, *race* was coded as white or nonwhite, with white being those classified as non-Hispanic white and nonwhite being the other race options combined (Mexican American, other Hispanic, non-Hispanic black, and other race—including multiracial). The *diabetes* variable comes from the question "{Other than during pregnancy, {have you/has SP}} ever been told by a doctor or health professional that {you have/{he/she/SP} has} diabetes or sugar diabetes?" The response options were "Yes," "No," "Borderline," "Don't know," or they could refuse to answer the question. For this example, those who answered anything other than "Yes" or "No" to the diabetes questions were excluded. The *fast_glu* variable comes from the participants' measured glucose levels in mg/dL after participants aged 12 and older fasted for nine hours. The *twohour_glu* variable comes from the participants' measured glucose level, also in mg/dL. This measurement was taken two hours after participants drank a glucose-filled solution, which was consumed after the fasting glucose measurement was taken. For this example, a stratified random sample of 46 participants (23 who reported having diabetes and 23 who reported not having diabetes) were selected.

A What is the mean fasting glucose level for participants who had a doctor tell him or her that they have diabetes and for those who did not? What is the standard deviation? How do these compare to the mean and standard deviation of the sample as a whole?

B What are the median and interquartile range of the fasting glucose variable? What are the median and interquartile range of the two-hour glucose variable?

C What is the mean difference between fasting glucose and two-hour glucose? What is the variance of the difference? Hint: Create a variable of the difference between a participant's fasting glucose and his or her two-hour glucose. This can be done in a data step using the following code:

```
DATA nhanes2014_glucose2;
SET mylib.nhanes2014_glucose;
glucose_diff=twohour_glu-fast_glu;
RUN;
```

D Create a histogram of the *glucose_diff* variable that we just created. Describe the distribution.

E Create a scatterplot of the fasting glucose and the two-hour glucose. Is there a relationship between the two variables in this sample?

PRACTICE PROBLEM A.2

Continuing with the same dataset as in Practice Problem A.1, *nhanes2014_glucose*, we now want to look at descriptive statistics of our sample by race and sex.

A How many females are in our sample? How many non-whites are in our sample? How many non-white females are in our sample?

B Describe the fasting glucose levels in whites and non-whites. What conclusions can we make?

C Describe the fasting glucose levels in males and females. What conclusions can we make?

D Create a box plot of the fasting glucose levels for whites and nonwhites. Hint: There are two ways to do this. The first is to use a BY statement in PROC UNIVARIATE, but this will give you two separate box plots. The second is to use PROC BOXPLOT (see the code below). Note that when using PROC BOXPLOT, we must first sort our data by the categorical grouping variable—in this case *race*.

```
PROC BOXPLOT DATA=mylib.nhanes2014_glucose;
  PLOT fast_glu*race;
RUN;
```

PRACTICE PROBLEM A.3

We will use the dataset *nhanes2014_sample* for this problem. We are interested in describing lead levels by race and seeing whether there appears to be a difference in the descriptive statistics for lead levels between racial groups.

A What are the mean and standard deviation of lead level for both racial groups? Remember, 1 = non-Hispanic white and 2 = non-Hispanic black.

B What are the median and interquartile range of lead level for both racial groups?

C Do the mean and median lead level appear to be different between racial groups?

D Present the lead levels of both racial groups graphically. Describe the distribution of lead level in both groups.

E Is the mean or the median a better measure of location for lead levels in this sample? Why?

Congratulations are in order! We have successfully completed the Introduction to SAS lab. We will become even more familiar with SAS as the workbook progresses.

References

1. Emergency Room MICA. Jefferson City, MO: Bureau of Health Care Analysis & Data Dissemination, Missouri Department of Health and Senior Services. 2014. http://health.mo.gov/data/mica/EmergencyRoomMICA/. Updated August 30, 2016. Accessed June 15, 2016.
2. National Health and Nutrition Examination Survey. Hyattsville, MD: Centers for Disease Control and Prevention, National Center for Health Statistics. 2014. https://wwwn.cdc.gov/Nchs/Nhanes/Search/nhanes13_14.aspx. Accessed February 23, 2016.

Lab A: Introduction to Stata®

The basics

In this workbook, we demonstrate how to use the Stata statistical software package to complete problems, in addition to using SAS. The purpose of this workbook is to learn statistical concepts, so we have tried to make the computing aspect of this text as simple as possible. In each lab throughout the workbook, we will go over some Stata pointers, containing the information that we need to complete the computing for that chapter. We will use Stata version 14.1 (StataCorp LP, College Station, Texas) throughout this workbook, but most commands will be similar regardless of which Stata version is being used. Note that in Stata, commands that are presented in italicized text can be changed, and commands presented in nonitalicized text (the standard) should not be changed.

Getting started

Let's open Stata on our computers. Throughout the remainder of this lab, we will walk through the basics of Stata and get to know the Stata environment.

What is Stata?

Stata is a computer software program that allows a user to perform different procedures on data, such as analysis and manipulation. Stata has many statistical commands that can produce complex models or basic statistics, such as a mean and standard deviation. Stata also allows a user to manipulate and clean data, such as creating new variables and changing categories of variables. We will use Stata throughout this workbook and explore a subset of what Stata can do.

Stata Windows

The Stata interface is divided into five windows, the first four of which appear when you open Stata. (Note: If they are not all there, you can open them via the *Window* drop-down menu and pick the name of the window that you want to appear):

1 *Command* Window

    This is where we type commands into Stata in order to perform statistical analyses, plot graphs, and more. Many of the commands that we will use in this workbook are available in the *Data*, *Statistics*, and *Graphics* menus found on the toolbar at the top of the Stata screen also. We will provide commands for the analyses done throughout this workbook.

2 *Results* Window

This is where the results of any command performed by Stata will appear.

3 *Variables* Window

When we have a dataset open or if we have created a new dataset, the variable names will be listed here.

4 *Review* Window

The *Review* window is useful because as commands are sent to Stata they appear there, even if you use the *Statistics* and *Graphics* menus to perform your analyses. To learn the command-driven version of Stata, noticing the commands in the *Review* window is a good place to start. You can also call back the commands in the *Review* window by clicking on them, editing them in the *Command* window, then running them by hitting the *Enter* key.

5 *Graph* Window

This window appears when we create a graph. The resulting graph can, then, be included in a word-processed document, which we will talk about later in the Graphs section of this lab.

Stata menus

As mentioned previously, commands that you will use in this workbook are also available through the use of drop-down menus. The menus can be found on the menu bar at the top of the Stata window. The following is a description of the Stata menus:

- *File*—Opens and saves Stata data files. Opens and closes log files. Saves or prints graphs. Imports and exports data in other formats (e.g., excel, text, SAS). Exits Stata.
- *Edit*—Allows copying of output from the *Results* or *Graphs* windows to a word processor or other application.
- *Data*—Opens the Data Editor and Data Browser. Summarizes data. Labels datasets and variables. Replaces and generates data.
- *Graphics*—Contains all of Stata's graphing tools.
- *Statistics*—Includes data summaries and all statistical tests.
- *User*—Serves as storage place for any user-generated commands.
- *Window*—Controls the windows opened in Stata.
- *Help*—Serves as a good resource if you have questions about how to use Stata.

Opening existing Stata data files

For most of the computer work that we will do in this workbook, we will use already-existing Stata data files that you can access by using the following command:

```
use dataset
```

When we run the *use* command, we have to make sure that our working directory is set to the folder in which our dataset is stored. A working directory is the folder out of which the user is currently working in Stata. We can see where our working directory is set by looking at the bottom left corner of our Stata window. If we need to change our working directory, we can use the *cd* (change directions) command, followed by the file path where we want our working directory set:

```
cd "C:\Data"
```

You can find the Stata data files on the eResources site. Stata data files have the extension `.dta`. Delimited text files can be opened in Stata by using the import delimited command:

```
import delimited "C:\Data\raw.csv"
```

The syntax right before this paragraph imports a file that is comma delimited. If we have a delimiter other than a comma, we can use the *delimiters ( )* option. For example, if our data were tab delimited, we could use the following:

```
import delimited "C:\Data\raw.txt", delimiters(tab)
```

Excel files can be opened using the *import excel* command. For example, if we had an Excel spreadsheet saved in C:\Data named *TestScores* and the first row of the spreadsheet contained the variable *names*, we could use the following syntax:

```
import excel "C:\Data\TestScores.xlsx", firstrow case(lower)
```

The above code imports the *TestScores* file that has the extension .xlsx. The *firstrow case(lower)* option tells Stata that the variable names should be taken from the first row in the spreadsheet and made lowercase.

The dataset named *er_heart.dta* contains data with the number of ED visits with a major heart or circulation diagnosis by zip code for St. Louis, Missouri, in 2013. These data come from the Missouri Department of Health and Senior Services, Missouri Information for Community Assessment (MICA).[1] The variable *zip* is the five-digit zip code, and the variable visits is the number of ED visits with a major heart or circulation diagnosis for 2013.

BOX STATA A.1 ER HEART DATASET DESCRIPTION

The er_heart dataset comes from the Bureau of Health Care Analysis & Data Dissemination, Missouri Department of Health and Senior Services. The data are from 2013 and contain the number of emergency department visits with a major heart or circulation diagnosis by zip code for the St. Louis area of Missouri. The dataset includes two variables, a five-digit zip code, and the number of emergency visits with a heart or circulation diagnosis in that zip code for 2013.

Open the dataset *er_heart.dta* through a *use* command. We should see the list of variable names in the dataset appear in the variable window. See Figure Stata A.1 for an example.

```
use "C:\Data\er_heart.dta"
```

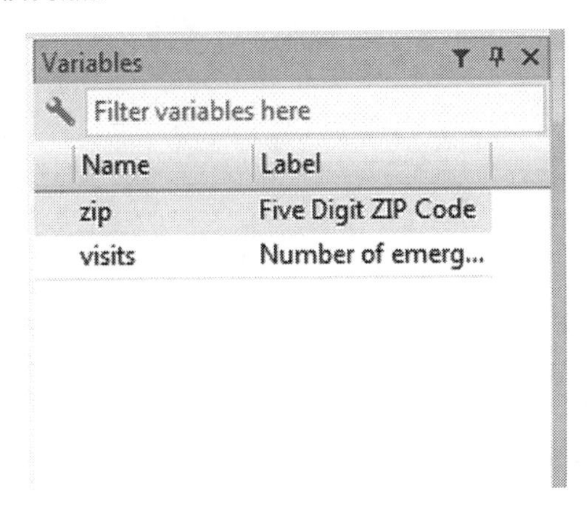

Figure Stata A.1 **Screenshot of variable window of *er_heart* dataset.** The screenshot of the variable window in Stata shows the names of the variables that we have in the dataset along with the labels of the variables. We have a variable named *zip* with the label "Five Digit ZIP Code" and a variable named *visits* with the label "Number of emerg..." If we were to stretch the label column, we could see the entire label of the variable visits.

BOX STATA A.2 A NOTE ON THE USE COMMAND AND THE WORKING DIRECTORY

In the example just before this box using the *er_heart* dataset, the *use* command includes the file path in which our *er_heart* dataset was stored.

If we had specified our working directory before running the *use* command, we could have just typed *er_heart* after our *use* command, and it would have also worked.

For example, we can set our working directory:

```
cd "C:\Data"
```

Now, we can just type the following:

```
use er_heart
```

The same results are possible with either setting a working directory or stating the file path within the *use* command.

The Do Editor

When typing commands in Stata, we might want to save the commands used in case we need to go back for reference later. The Do Editor in Stata is a good way to do this. To open a new do file type *ctrl+9*, select the *Do File* button below the menu bar (the button looks like a pen and paper) or go to *Window/Do-file Editor/New Do-file Editor*. We can also use the *do* command to run the text that is saved within the *do* file. For example, say that we had saved all of the commands that we have learned thus far in a *do* file named *LabA* saved in C:\Data. We could use the following command to run the *do* file, which would, in turn, run all the commands saved within the *do* file:

```
do "C:\Data\LabA.do"
```

We can also simply open the *do* file and copy and paste commands into our command window to run them one at a time instead of running the whole *do* file at once or highlight portions of the *do* file that you would like to execute and hit the execute button (looks like a piece of paper with a blue right arrow).

Data Editor

The Data Editor is where you can enter new data, make changes to the current dataset, or create new variables. Open the Data Editor by clicking the *Data Editor* button on the toolbar at the top of the screen. The button looks like a little spreadsheet. Alternatively, you could choose *Data/Data Editor* from the menu bar.

BOX STATA A.3 NOTE ON DATA EDITOR AND DATA BROWSER

The Data Editor is different from the Data Browser. The Data Browser allows only looking at the data and does not allow making changes to the dataset. The button for the Data Browser looks like a magnifying glass over a little spreadsheet, which is also located on the toolbar.

Sort the data on the variable visits.

- Highlight the column for visits by clicking on the variable name.
- Right click and choose *Data/Sort Data*. Keep the default settings, and click *OK*. Watch how the order of the observations changes. The default setting is to sort in ascending order.
- We can also sort our data by using the *sort* command:

```
sort visits
```

Now, try deleting data.

- We can delete a variable by highlighting the column and clicking the variable header. Then, right click, and choose *Data/Drop selected data*.
- We can delete an observation by doing the same thing but with the row highlighted.
- What happens when you close (click on "X" at top right corner) and reopen the Data Editor? Were your changes preserved?
- Now, close the Data Editor and clear out the current dataset by typing *clear* in the *Command* window. What happened in the *Variable* window?
- Note that Stata does not save any of your changes to disk until you explicitly tell it to *File/Save*, generally when exiting the program. Please, do not save your changes for this exercise.

Inputting data into Stata

Refer to the data in Table Stata A.1. It contains observations of diastolic blood pressure and weight for 10 study[2] participants. We will manually input these data into Stata.

BOX STATA A.4 TABLE STATA A.1 DATA DESCRIPTION

The data in Table Stata A.1 come from the 2014 National Health and Nutrition Examination Survey (NHANES). In the survey, participants' blood pressure and weight (in kilograms) were measured by a trained health technician. Weight was converted to pounds. A random sample of 10 participants with nonmissing data is presented in Table Stata A.1.

Open the Data Editor, and type in the values of diastolic blood pressure into the first column. Assign the variable a name by double clicking where it says "var1" in the properties box. Type *dbp* for the variable name. Enter the values for weight, and name the variable *weight*. Click on the close ("X") button on the window's upper right corner. This data file can be saved for future use by clicking *File/Save As*. Practice saving this dataset to disk, calling it *study.dta*.

BOX STATA A.5 NOTE ON STATA VARIABLE NAMES

Stata variable names need to be fewer than 32 characters, cannot start with a number, and must be made up of letters, digits, underscores, or same combination of these.

Labels

For the sake of clarity, you might want to give labels to your data. Labels can be given to the entire dataset or to the individual variables. This is helpful when you have given

Table Stata A.1 Diastolic blood pressure and weight for study participants

Diastolic blood pressure (mm Hg)	*Weight (pounds)*
92	221
62	136
78	175
60	159
42	108
88	175
94	324
68	135
90	185
78	159

Source: National Health and Nutrition Examination Survey, Centers for Disease Control and Prevention, National Center for Health Statistics, Hyattsville, MD, 2014, https://wwwn.cdc.gov/Nchs/Nhanes/Search/nhanes13_14.aspx. Accessed February 23, 2016.

Note: The data come from the 2014 NHANES survey and include a random sample of 10 study participants. The variables include diastolic blood pressure in mm Hg and weight in pounds.

abbreviated names to your dataset, variables, or both, and you want to keep a more detailed explanation of the contents of the datasets and variables. For example, you might want to label the variable *dbp* with "Diastolic Blood Pressure (mmHg)." You can assign a label to the study dataset by using the *label data* command, followed by the label that you wish to assign to the dataset in double quotation marks:

```
label data "Diastolic Blood Pressure and Weight of 10 Study
Participants"
```

Next, use the *label variable* command to label your variables (alternatively, it is also done by typing in the label column in the variables properties window when you are in the Data Editor). Type *label variable*, followed by the variable name (*dbp* in this case), and type the label that you are assigning to the variable enclosed in double quotation marks:

```
label variable dbp "Diastolic Blood Pressure (mmHg)"
```

Follow the same procedure to apply a label for the variable *weight*. These labels will appear in any tables or graphs that you make with this data.

In order to describe all of the variables in the dataset, we will use the *describe* command:

```
describe
```

You will see a table of information appear in your *Results* window. Generally, this command provides the number of observations and variables in the dataset, the storage and display type for each variable, and any special labels. There are, potentially, a label for the entire dataset, a label for each variable, and special label values used in storing a variable. Once you know that your labeled study dataset is saved, open the *er_hearts.dta* dataset, and look at its thorough labeling.

Log files

Now that we have data to work with, we will want to do some statistical analyses. The log file is where we save all the work that we do during our Stata session. Basically, as long as a log file is open, everything that appears in the *Results* window is saved in the log file (including errors). Graphs, however, are not saved to the log file.

Create a log file by using the *log* command:

```
log using "C:\Data\session1.log"
```

The *log using* command just noted creates a log file named *session1* that is saved in the C:\Data folder. We can also create a log file by clicking on the button that looks like a notebook with lines on it. Alternatively, we could pull down *File/Log/Begin*. In the window that pops up, enter a file name. For example, you could call it *session1*. Choose the .log file type, and click on *Open*. The .log extension is used so that the log file can be opened in most word processing applications.

Look at what appears in the *Results* window. Once we have opened a log file, it will record everything that we do until we suspend it or close it. We can do this by typing the appropriate command. When we want to close the log file, we type *log close*:

```
log close
```

When we close the log file, we have to open a new one before we can start recording again. However, with the *suspend* option, we can pause recording:

```
log off
```

Then, we just turn the log back on again to start recording in the same log:

```
log on
```

Once a log file is closed, no additional information can be written to that log file. However, you can suspend and resume a log file as many times as you want. You can keep adding information to a log file until you close it. You can view the current contents of the log file by going to *File/Log/View*. Leave the log file open, and go on to the next step. We will come back to saving and printing it after it has recorded something. Note, also, that you might want to just include portions of your work in a word processing document (see Printing section of this chapter).

Summarizing data

In this section, we will calculate some descriptive statistics. First, let's open the dataset *nhanes2014_sample.dta*, which is found on the eResources site. These data come from the 2014 National Health and Nutrition Examination Survey.[2] The dataset contains several variables, including *race* (1 = non-Hispanic white; 2 = non-Hispanic black), *age* (in years), *sex* (1 = males; 2 = females), urine lead level (*lead* in µg/L), and an identification (*id*) number. Make sure that your working directory is set to where the dataset is stored, and type a *use* command to open the dataset in Stata.

BOX STATA A.6 NHANES 2014 SAMPLE DATASET DESCRIPTION

The *nhanes2014_sample* dataset comes from the 2014 National Health and Nutrition Examination Survey (NHANES). The variables included in the dataset are *race*, *age*, *sex*, urine lead level (*lead*), and identification (*id*). The *id* variable was created by the administrators of NHANES. The *sex* variable was collected as male or female. The *age* variable was collected in years at the time of screening, and participants over age 80 years were recoded to age 80 (i.e., 80 years is the maximum age). The *race* variable was recoded by NHANES administrators to Mexican American, other Hispanic, non-Hispanic white, non-Hispanic black, and other race—including multiracial. For this sample, only those with a race of non-Hispanic white or non-Hispanic black were included. Urine lead level was measured by trained professionals and recorded in µg/L. For this example, 100 participants with nonmissing data and a race of non-Hispanic white or non-Hispanic black were randomly selected.

```
use nhanes2014_sample
```

EXAMPLE PROBLEM A.1

A Use the Data Editor to view the data. Describe the variables in the dataset.

The variables in the dataset include *race*, *lead*, *age*, *sex*, and *id*. Through the Data Editor, we can see the number values listed in the dataset for each variable.

B What is the mean urine lead level (*lead*) for this group?

To get the mean of lead, we can use the *mean* command:

```
mean lead
```

Using this command will give the following output:

```
Mean estimation                   Number of obs    =        100
--------------------------------------------------------------
             |       Mean   Std. Err.     [95% Conf. Interval]
-------------+------------------------------------------------
        lead |      .5116   .0514967      .4094193    .6137807
--------------------------------------------------------------
```

Also, we could have used the *means* command, which would have given us the arithmetic mean, along with the geometric mean and harmonic mean (not discussed in this book because it's not used much in clinical and public health research):

```
means lead
```

```
Variable |     Type          Obs        Mean       [95% Conf. Interval]
----------+-------------------------------------------------------------
    lead | Arithmetic        100       .5116       .4094193    .6137807
         |   Geometric       100    .3365086       .2781522    .4071081
         |    Harmonic       100    .2002655       .1537678    .2870732
------------------------------------------------------------------------
```

The mean of lead is 0.51 μg/L.

C What is the standard deviation of the *lead* variable?

To get the standard deviation of lead, we can use the *summarize* command:

```
summarize lead
```

```
    Variable |       Obs        Mean    Std. Dev.       Min        Max
-------------+--------------------------------------------------------
        lead |       100       .5116    .5149673        .02       2.79
```

The standard deviation of lead is 0.515 μg/L. As you can see from the ouput above, we could have used this command to get the mean in Example Problem A.1—Part (B).

D What is the median (50th percentile) age?

To find the median of age, we can use the *summarize* command again and add the *detail* option so that our output includes the median or 50th percentile.

```
summarize age, detail
```

The resulting output follows:

```
age
-------------------------------------------------------------
      Percentiles      Smallest
 1%            6              6
 5%          9.5              6
10%           12              7       Obs                 100
25%           22              8       Sum of Wgt.         100
50%         38.5                      Mean              40.34
                        Largest       Std. Dev.      21.56045
75%           56             78
90%         71.5             79       Variance       464.8529
95%           76             80       Skewness        .151011
99%           80             80       Kurtosis       1.841606
```

The median age is 38.5 years.

E What is the mean age for males (1 = males; 2 = females)?

To find the mean age for males, we can use a *by* command in front of our *summarize* command to obtain statistics by each category of the variable *sex*. In order to do this, we first have to sort our data by sex by using the *sort* command:

```
sort sex
```

Now, we can use the by command in front of the summarize command to obtain the mean age for males:

```
by sex : summarize age
```

We get the resulting output:

```
-----------------------------------------------------------------------
-> sex = 1
    Variable |        Obs        Mean    Std. Dev.       Min        Max
-------------+---------------------------------------------------------
         age |         47    38.25532      22.6816         6         80
-----------------------------------------------------------------------
-> sex = 2
    Variable |        Obs        Mean    Std. Dev.       Min        Max
-------------+---------------------------------------------------------
         age |         53    42.18868     20.55486         8         80
```

The mean age for males (sex = 1) is 38.3 years.

BOX STATA A.7 EXAMPLE OF ERROR MESSAGE WHEN DATA ARE NOT SORTED

What would happen if we did not sort our data before we used the *by* option in the *summarize* command, like we did in Example Problem A.1—Part (E)?

We would get an error message like the one in Figure Stata A.2. We can also see that the command is red in the *Review* window.

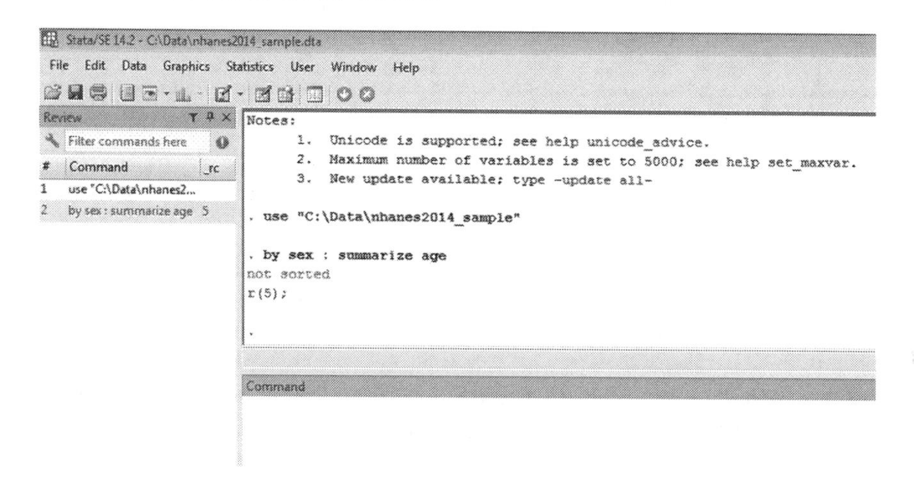

Figure Stata A.2 **Screenshot of error message when data are not sorted.** The screenshot of our Stata windowing environment after trying to run the summarize command with a by option shows an error message that says "not sorted." Because this book is printed in black and white, we cannot see the colors from this image; however, error messages show up in red by default. In the *Review* window, we also see the command show up in red.

F How many females are there in this dataset (1 = males; 2 = females)?

To get the number of females in the dataset, we want to use a tab (short for tabulate; the full word works as well) command. The *tab* command will give us a frequency table.

```
tab sex
```

```
        sex |      Freq.     Percent        Cum.
------------+-----------------------------------
          1 |         47       47.00       47.00
          2 |         53       53.00      100.00
------------+-----------------------------------
      Total |        100      100.00
```

There are 53 females in this dataset.

G How many females in this sample are recorded as non-Hispanic black for *race*?

Remember that for the *race* variable 1 = non-Hispanic white; 2 = non-Hispanic black.

To obtain the number of females that are recorded as non-Hispanic black for *race* in the dataset, we want to use a *tab* command again, but this time we will specify *sex* and *race* variables:

```
tab sex race
```

```
           |         race
       sex |         1          2 |     Total
-----------+----------------------+----------
         1 |        24         23 |        47
         2 |        30         23 |        53
-----------+----------------------+----------
     Total |        54         46 |       100
```

There are 23 females that are recorded as non-Hispanic black for *race* in the dataset.

H List 10 observations for *race* and *lead*.

To list observations in Stata, we will use the *list* command, followed by an *in* option with 1/10, which means observations 1 through 10:

```
list in 1/10
```

We obtain the resulting output:

```
     +--------------------------------------+
     | race   lead   age   sex          id |
     |--------------------------------------|
  1. |    1    .18     6     1       80346 |
  2. |    1    .48    63     1       82409 |
  3. |    2    .49    26     1       74197 |
  4. |    1    .35    23     1       82271 |
  5. |    2    .64    65     1       81820 |
     |--------------------------------------|
  6. |    2   1.48    10     1       74444 |
  7. |    1    .11    20     1       73992 |
  8. |    2    .19    35     1       77076 |
  9. |    2    1.7    38     1       73859 |
 10. |    2    .22    37     1       81219 |
     +--------------------------------------+
```

Write a command to have Stata list observation 5 through 50.

```
list in 5/50
```

You may see a blue-colored *–more* at the bottom of the *Results* window. Hit the space bar to see the additional content.

Value labels

So far, we have learned about labeling datasets and variables, but we can also label values of variables. Suppose that we wanted to format the variable *sex* in the *nhanes2014_sample* dataset to label 1 as males and 2 as females to make our output easier to interpret. We could use the following commands to do that:

```
label define sexlabel 1 "Male" 2 "Female"
label values sex sexlabel
```

The first line, *label define*, creates a label called *sexlabel* that labels values of 1 as "Male" and values of 2 as "Female." The second line, *label values*, assigns the label *sexlabel* that we just created to the variable *sex*. Now, if we run a *tab* command on the variable *sex*, we would obtain the following output:

```
tab sex
```

```
        sex |      Freq.     Percent        Cum.
------------+-----------------------------------
       Male |         47       47.00       47.00
     Female |         53       53.00      100.00
------------+-----------------------------------
      Total |        100      100.00
```

We can see that the values of *sex* are now labeled as Male and Female. Create a label for *race* variable values and assign it to the *race* variable.

Printing

We can print output from our session in two ways. One way is to choose *Print* from the *File* menu when viewing the log. The other option is to copy (pick *Copy* from the *Edit* menu after highlighting what you want to copy) and paste the contents of the log file (or the *Results* window) to a document in a word processor and print from there. This is often a little bit neater than printing from the *File* menu, and it allows you to print only the relevant parts of your session.

Here are some steps to follow:

1. View the current log snapshot (by clicking on the *Log* button), and select a portion of text from your results.
2. Select *Edit/Copy Text.*
3. Switch to an open word processing document, place the text cursor at your target location, and choose *Edit/Paste*. Notice that text does not necessarily have the same appearance.
4. Highlight the portion that you pasted, and change the font, making sure that you use a fixed-width font such as Courier New.

Creating new variables with formulas

Sometimes, we may need to create a new variable that is a function of one or more existing variables. We will see later in chapters why you might want to do this.

Create a new variable called *leadsq* that is the square of *lead* ($lead^2$). To do this, we use the *generate* command:

```
generate leadsq=lead^2
```

A caret (^) is used for exponentiation. There are many other mathematical functions that Stata can perform, some of which we will learn later in this workbook.

Graphs

Several Stata commands create graphs. For this lab, we will go over a few of these examples.

EXAMPLE PROBLEM A.2

A **Using the *nhanes2014_sample* dataset, create a box plot for age. Are there any outliers? Does the box plot give you a sense of the mean? The median? The mode?**

```
graph box age
```

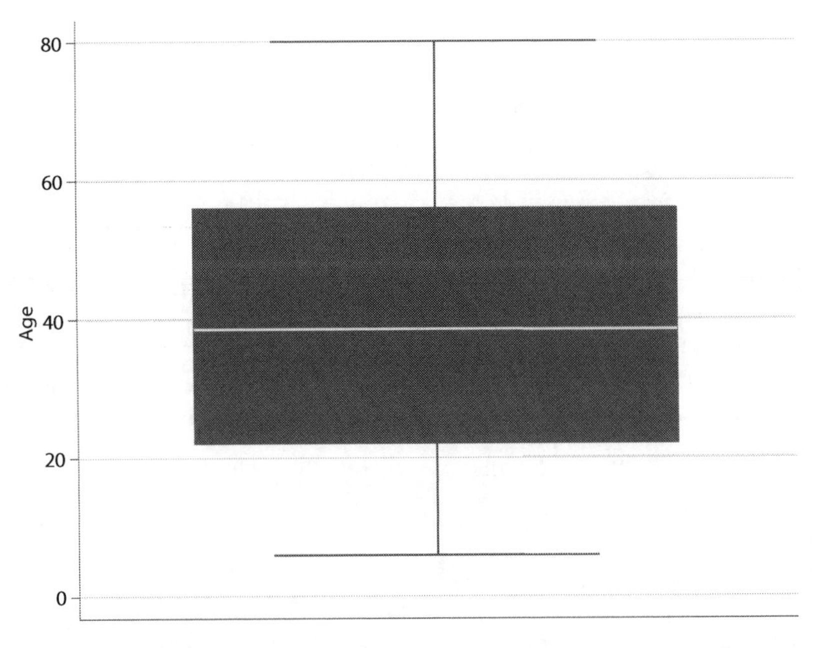

Figure Stata A.3 **Box plot of age for the NHANES 2014 sample data.** The boxplot shows the distribution of the age variable. The line through the middle of the box represents the median. When graphing boxplots in Stata, we do not get a sense of the mean, unlike other boxplots we have seen in Chapter 1 (created using SAS).

This box plot does not show any outliers. We do not get a sense of the mean or the mode in this graph. The median is represented by the bar through the middle of the box (Figure Stata A.3).

Suppose that we wanted to compare box plots across males and females. We could do this using the *graph box* command by adding a *by* option after the command. The code is as follows:

```
graph box age, by(sex)
```

B Construct a stem-and-leaf plot of age.

To create a stem-and-leaf plot in Stata, we use the *stem* command:

```
stem age
```

```
0. | 66789
1* | 0012223444
1. | 5568889
2* | 012233344
2. | 56677
3* | 0001223
3. | 55778889
4* | 00124
4. | 5899
5* | 0000123333
5. | 5555667
6* | 02233334
6. | 599
7* | 01234
7. | 55789
8* | 00
```

In this stem-and-leaf plot, Stata created two lines for most of the stems. If we wanted to see only one line per stem, we could use a *line* option to specify how many lines we would like to see:

```
stem age, lines(1)
```

C Create a histogram for *lead* (consider it a continuous variable). Would you describe the distribution as skewed or symmetric?

To create a histogram in Stata, we use the *histogram* command with a *freq* option. By default, Stata provides a density histogram. Adding the *freq* option gives a frequency histogram (Figure Stata A.4).

```
histogram lead, freq
```

D Now create separate histograms of *lead* for males and females. How do the histograms differ between the two sexes?

We, again, use the *histogram* command for this (Figure Stata A.5) but include a *by* option:

```
histogram lead, by (sex) freq
```

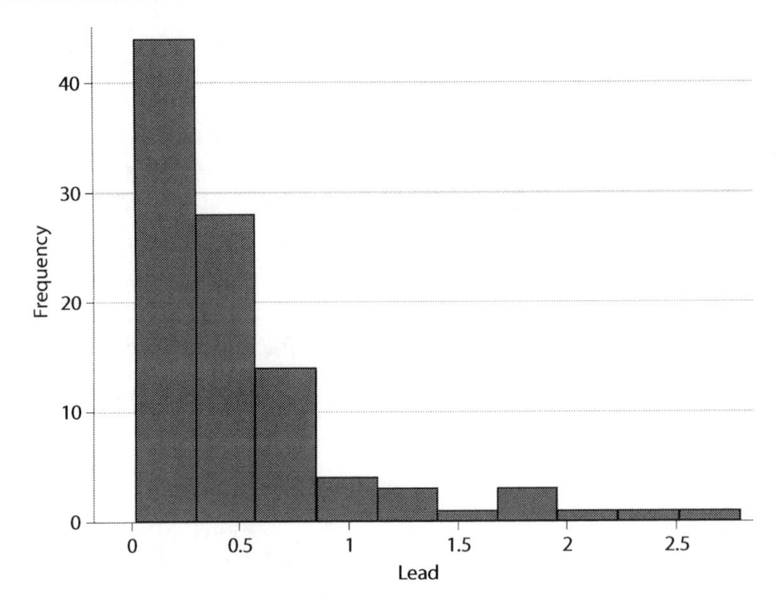

Figure Stata A.4 **Histogram of urine lead level for the NHANES 2014 sample data.** The histogram of the variable lead shows the distribution of participants' lead levels. The distribution is skewed to the right, with a majority of the participants' lead levels being between 0 and 0.5 μg/L.

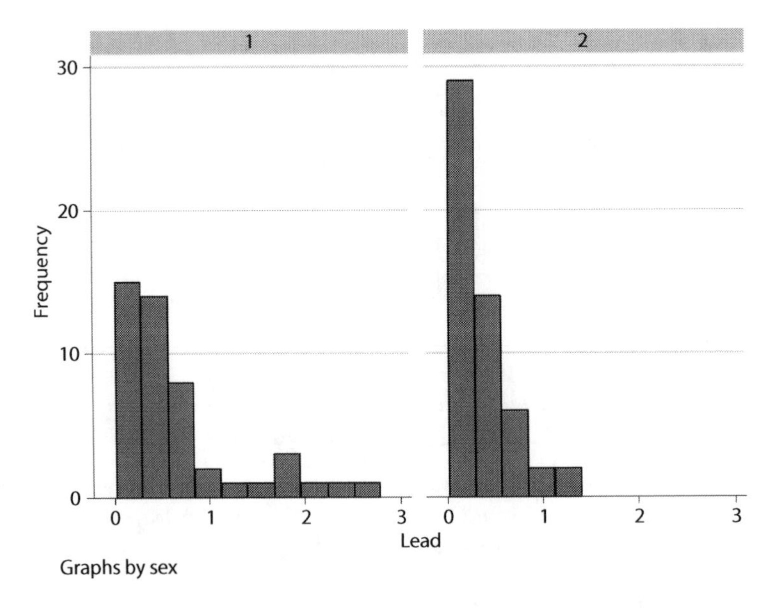

Figure Stata A.5 **Histogram of urine lead level for males and females for the NHANES 2014 sample data.** Male is indicated by 1. Female is indicated by 2. The histogram of lead level for males (sex = 1) show the distribution of the variable. The majority of participants have a lead level between 0 and 1 μg/L. The data is skewed to the right. Similar to the histogram of lead level for males, the histogram for females (sex = 2) is also skewed to the right; however, it is less so than the males. The majority of female participants also have a lead level between 0 and 1 μg/L, but the range of values for females does not go as high as for males.

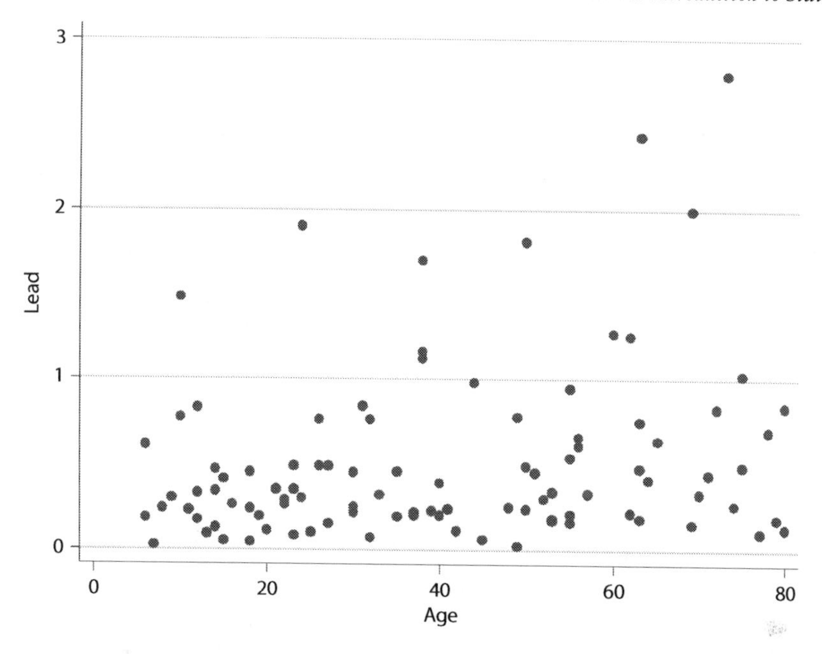

Figure Stata A.6 **Scatterplot of age by urine lead level for the NHANES 2014 sample data.** The scatterplot shows the relationship between two continuous variables, age and lead. Age is on the x-axis and lead is on the y-axis. Within the plot, we see points which are representative of the data in our dataset. Each point represents a different participant. From this scatterplot, there does not appear to be a clear relationship between age and lead level.

E Create a scatterplot of *age* vs. *lead*. Is there a relationship between the two variables?

To create a scatterplot (Figure Stata A.6), we use the *graph twoway scatter* command:

```
graph twoway scatter lead age
```

BOX STATA A.8 EXAMPLE OF USING LABELS TO MAKE A GRAPH LOOK BETTER

Suppose that we want our graphs to have labels of "Lead Level" instead of just "lead" and "Age in Years" instead of just "age" as shown in the scatterplot in Figure Stata A.6. We could use labels for this.

Previously in this lab, we learned how to use the *label* command. Let's apply that here:

```
label variable age "Age of Participant , years"
label variable lead "Urine Lead Level , micrograms/liter"
```

We labeled both variables in our scatterplot. Let's remake the scatterplot:

```
graph twoway scatter lead age
```

Now, our graph should look like Figure Stata A.7, below:

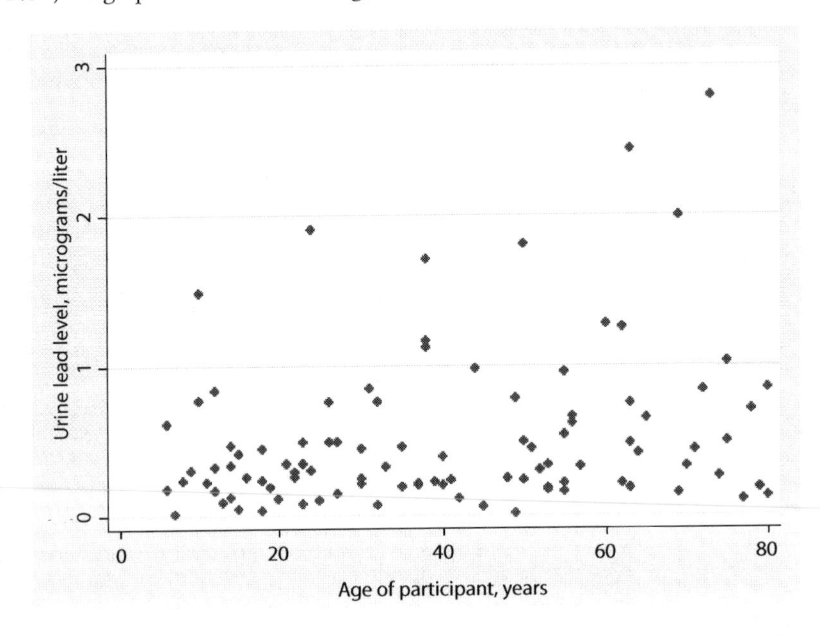

Figure Stata A.7 **Scatterplot of age by urine lead level for the NHANES 2014 sample data with labels.** The scatterplot presented here is essentially the same as the scatterplot presented in Figure Stata A.6; however, this time we have used a label option to label the *x*-axis so that "Age of Participant, years" will appear instead of just the variable name age and labeled the *y*-axis so that "Urine Lead Level, micrograms/liter" will appear instead of just the variable name lead.

There does not appear to be a relationship between age and lead.

Saving graphs

While the graph window is active, under the *File* menu you have the option to either print it or save it (you can recall the saved graphs by *File/Open* and navigating to where the graph is saved). Again, note that graphs do **not** appear in your log file. You can, therefore, copy and paste graphs to word processing programs by choosing *Copy* from the *Edit* menu while the graph window is active and then, pasting the graphs into a word processing document.

Practice cutting and pasting your scatterplot into your open word processing document.

Before exiting from Stata, close your open log file by clicking on the *Log* button and selecting *Close log file*.

Congratulations! You have successfully completed your Introduction to Stata. You will become even more familiar with Stata as the workbook progresses. Now, try some practice problems on your own.

PRACTICE PROBLEM A.1

The dataset *nhanes2014_glucose* contains a sample of participants from the NHANES 2014 survey.[2] The variables include whether a doctor or health professional ever told the participant that he or she has diabetes (*diabetes*); the participant's fasting glucose in mg/dL (*fast_glu*); the participant's two-hour glucose also in mg/dL (*twohour_glu*); and the participant's age (*age*), sex (*sex*), and ID number (*id*). For the *diabetes* variable, 1 = the participant was told by a doctor or health professional that he or she has diabetes, and 2 = the participant was not told by a doctor or health professional that he or she has diabetes. The *sex* variable is coded 1 = males, and 2 = females. For *race*, 1 = white, and 2 = nonwhite. We want to know whether the descriptive statistics of glucose levels differ by whether a participant replied that a doctor told the participant that he or she has diabetes.

BOX STATA A.9 NHANES 2014 GLUCOSE DATASET DESCRIPTION

The *nhanes2014_glucose* dataset comes from the same survey as the *nhanes2014_sample* dataset. The *age*, *sex*, and *id* variables are the same as in the previously used dataset. For this dataset, race was coded as white or nonwhite, with white being those classified as non-Hispanic white and nonwhite being the other race options combined (Mexican American, other Hispanic, non-Hispanic black, and other race—including multiracial). The *diabetes* variable comes from the question "The next questions are about specific medical conditions. {Other than during pregnancy, {have you/has SP}} ever been told by a doctor or health professional that {you have/{he/she/SP} has} diabetes or sugar diabetes?" The response options were "Yes," "No," "Borderline," "Don't know," or they could refuse to answer the question. For this example, those who answered anything other than "Yes" or "No" to the diabetes questions were excluded. The *fast_glu* variable comes from the participants' measured glucose levels in mg/dL after participants aged 12 and older fasted for nine hours. The *twohour_glu* variable comes from the participants' measured glucose level, also in mg/dL. This measurement was taken two hours after participants drank a glucose-filled solution, which was consumed after the fasting glucose measurement was taken. For this example, a stratified random sample of 46 participants (23 who reported having diabetes and 23 who reported not having diabetes) were selected.

A What is the mean fasting glucose level for those who had a doctor tell them that they have diabetes and for those who did not? What is the standard deviation? How do these compare to the mean and standard deviation of the sample as a whole?

B What are the median and interquartile range of the fasting glucose variable? What are the median and interquartile range of the two-hour glucose variable?

C What is the mean difference between fasting glucose and two-hour glucose? What is the variance of the difference? Hint: Create a variable of the difference between a participant's fasting glucose and two-hour glucose. This can be done using the following code:

```
generate glucose_diff=twohour_glu-fast_glu
```

D Create a histogram of the *glucose_diff* variable that we just created. Describe the distribution.

E Create a scatterplot of the fasting glucose and the two-hour glucose. Is there a relationship between these two variables in the sample?

PRACTICE PROBLEM A.2

Continuing with the same dataset as in Practice Problem A.1, *nhanes2014_glucose*, we now want to look at descriptive statistics of our sample by race and sex.

A How many females are in our sample? How many nonwhites are in our sample? How many nonwhite females are in our sample?

B Describe the fasting glucose levels for whites and nonwhites. What conclusions can we make?

C Describe the fasting glucose levels in males and females. What conclusions can we make?

D Create a box plot of the fasting glucose levels for whites and nonwhites.

PRACTICE PROBLEM A.3

We will use the dataset *nhanes2014_sample* for this problem. We are interested in describing lead levels by race and seeing whether there appears to be a difference in the descriptive statistics of lead levels between racial groups.

A What are the mean and standard deviation for lead for both racial groups? Remember, 1 = non-Hispanic white, and 2 = non-Hispanic black.

B What are the median and interquartile range for lead for both racial groups?

C Do the mean and median for lead level appear different between racial groups?

D Present the lead levels of both racial groups graphically. Describe the distribution of lead level in both groups.

E Is the mean or the median a better measure of location for this example? Why?

References

1. Emergency Room MICA. Jefferson City, MO: Bureau of Health Care Analysis & Data Dissemination, Missouri Department of Health and Senior Services. 2014. http://health.mo.gov/data/mica/EmergencyRoomMICA/. Updated August 30, 2016. Accessed June 15, 2016.
2. National Health and Nutrition Examination Survey. Hyattsville, MD: Centers for Disease Control and Prevention, National Center for Health Statistics. 2014. https://wwwn.cdc.gov/Nchs/Nhanes/Search/nhanes13_14.aspx. Accessed February 23, 2016.

2 Probability

This chapter will focus on the concept of probability and will include the following:

- Properties of probabilities
- Laws of probabilities

Terms

- addition law of probability
- complement
- conditional probability
- event
- exhaustive
- generalized multiplication law of probability
- intersection
- multiplication law of probability
- mutually exclusive
- probability
- relative risk
- sample space
- total probability rule
- union

Introduction

The concept of probability is vital to the core of statistics. Throughout this chapter, we will discuss the different laws and properties of probability and learn how to apply them. The remainder of this book will delve into many other topics of biostatistics, most of which are based on or incorporate the concept of probability.

Probability: The probability of an event is the relative frequency of a set of outcomes over an indefinitely large (or infinite) number of trials occurring in a particular sample space.

Event: An event is the result of an observation or experiment, or the description of some potential outcome. The symbol { } is used as shorthand for the phrase "the event."

Sample Space: The sample space is the set of all possible outcomes in which the event is contained. Omega (Ω) is used as the notation for sample space.

Example of probability in action

To further help us to understand what probability is, let's look at an example. What is the probability that at least two students in the Introduction to Biostatistics course have the same birthday (month and day)? Examine the probabilities in Table 2.1 and Figure 2.1.

Table 2.1 Birthday problem

Number of students	*Probability*
5	3%
10	12%
20	41%
23	50%
35	81%
50	97%
70	99.5%

Note: The table shows the probabilities that two students in the Introduction to Biostatistics course have the same birthday, based on the number of students in the course. As the number of students increases, the probability that two students will have the same birthday also increases.

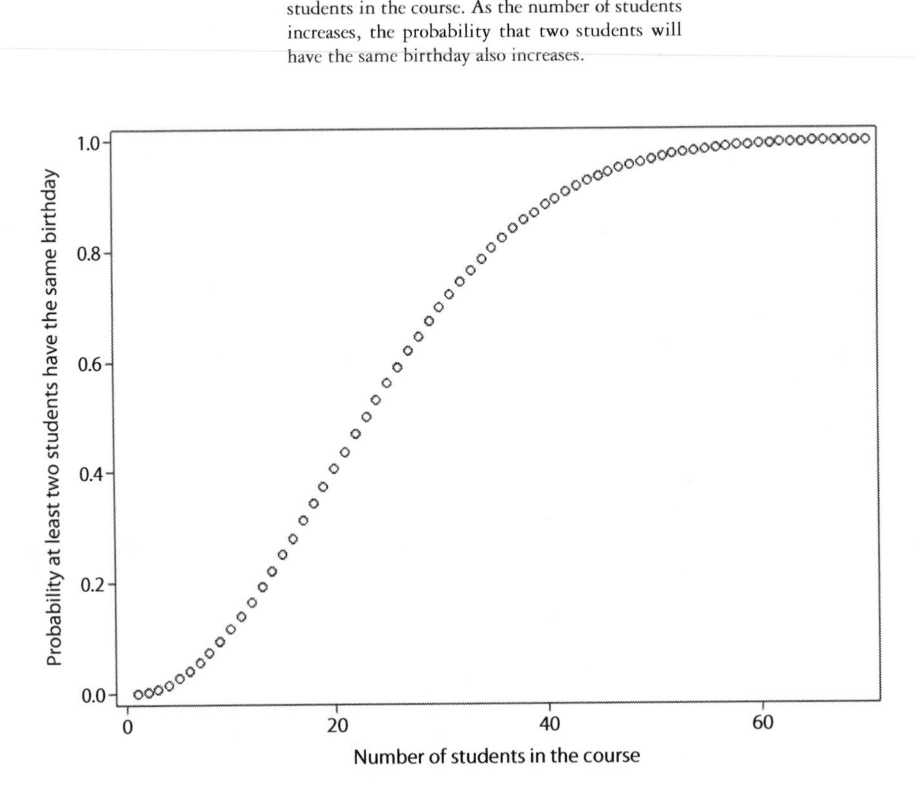

Figure 2.1 **Birthday problem.** The figure is showing the probability that at least two students have the same birthday (y-axis) by the number of students in the course (x-axis). Similar to Table 2.1, the graph shows that as the number of students in the class goes up, the probability that at least two students have the same birthday also goes up until it reaches a point that is almost to 1.

- If there were currently five people in the course, the probability that at least two people would have the same birthday would be 3% or 0.03.
- As the number of people in the course increases, the probability that two people have the same birthday also increases.
- In this example, the sample space would be all of the possible combinations of people's birthdays, and the event would be the outcomes in which at least two of the birthdays are the same.

To understand more about the concept of probability, in this chapter, we will discuss the properties, laws, and relationships that apply to probabilities.

Properties of probabilities

The probability of an event E, denoted by $P(E)$, always satisfies $0 \leq P(E) \leq 1$. That is, the probability of event E can range only between 0 and 1.

If an event has a probability of 0: There is a 0% chance the event will not occur.
If an event has a probability of 1: There is a 100% chance the event will occur.

Mutually Exclusive: Two events A and B are mutually exclusive if they cannot both happen at the same time.

Equation 2.1 shows the calculation for the probability of A or B occurring if A and B are two events that cannot happen at the same time—in other words, if A and B are mutually exclusive.

$$P(A \text{ or } B \text{ occurs}) = P(A) + P(B) \tag{2.1}$$

This equation is telling us that the probability of event A or B occurring is equal to the probability of event A occurring plus the probability of event B occurring. We can look to the Venn diagram in Figure 2.2 for a visual representation of this, with the circle around A being the sample space for event A and the circle around B being the sample space for event B.

As an example, let A be the event that a person lives to be 50, and let B be the event that a person dies before their 35th birthday. These two events are mutually exclusive because someone cannot live to be 50 and die before their 35th birthday.

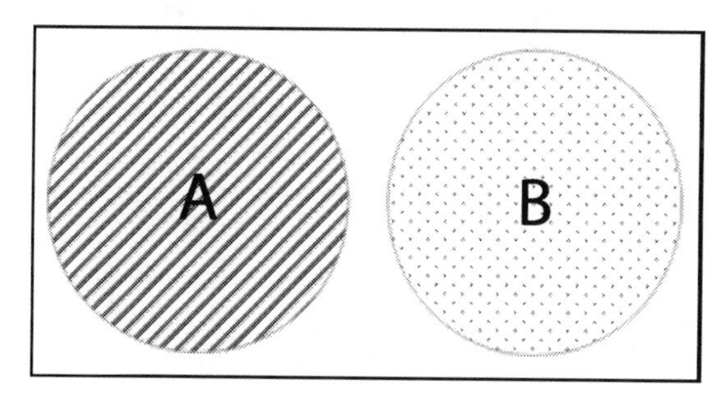

Figure 2.2 **Venn diagram for mutually exclusive events.** The Venn diagram shows a visual example of mutually exclusive events. Event A, represented by the striped circle, and event B, represented by the dotted circle, cannot occur at the same time (no overlap); thus, they are mutually exclusive events.

Null Event: A null event is an event that cannot happen and is represented by the symbol Ø.

In the example discussed previously regarding mutually exclusive events, the event of someone living to 50 and dying before their 35th birthday cannot happen; thus, it is a null event.

Complement: The complement of A is the event that A does not occur.

Equation 2.2 shows that the complement of event A is equal to 1 minus the probability of event A occurring. As we know that a probability of 1 means that there is a 100% chance of the event occurring, the probability of A occurring plus the probability that A will not occur will equal 1.

$$P(A^c) = 1 - P(A) \tag{2.2}$$

Note: The complement of an event occurring is represented by $P(A^c)$, or $P(\bar{A})$.

For a visual example of this property, we can look at the Venn diagram in Figure 2.3. Here, we see that the sample space for the complement of event A is all the space outside of the sample space for event A.

Let's think of an example to help us better understand this concept. We will say that event A is that Tom eats vegetables. The complement of event A in this example would be that Tom does not eat vegetables.

Intersection: The intersection of two events is the event in which both events occur.

- The intersection of two events is represented by $A \cap B$.
- Figure 2.4 shows us a Venn diagram example of the intersection of events A and B. Here, the intersection is where the two circles overlap.

Going back to our example with Tom, we know that Tom eats vegetables (event A). Event B is that Tom eats green foods. The intersection of events A and B would be that Tom eats green vegetables.

Equation 2.3 shows the calculation for probability of the intersection of two events (A and B), if events A and B are independent events.

$$P(A \cap B) = P(A)P(B) \tag{2.3}$$

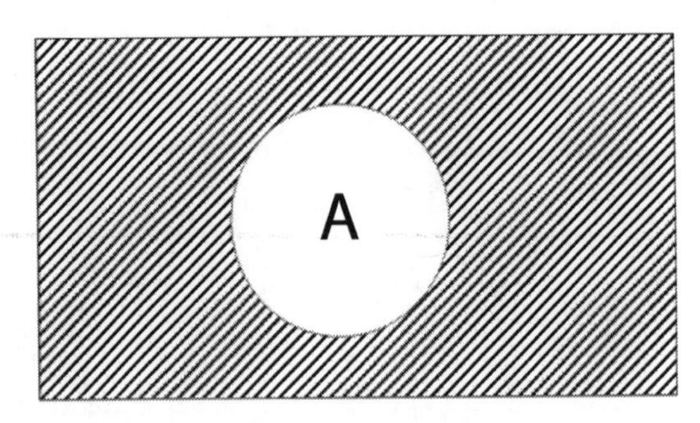

Figure 2.3 **Venn diagram for the complement of an event.** The Venn diagram shows a visual example of the complement of an event. Event A occurring is represented by the white space inside the circle, and event A not occurring, the complement of event A, is represented by the striped space outside of the circle.

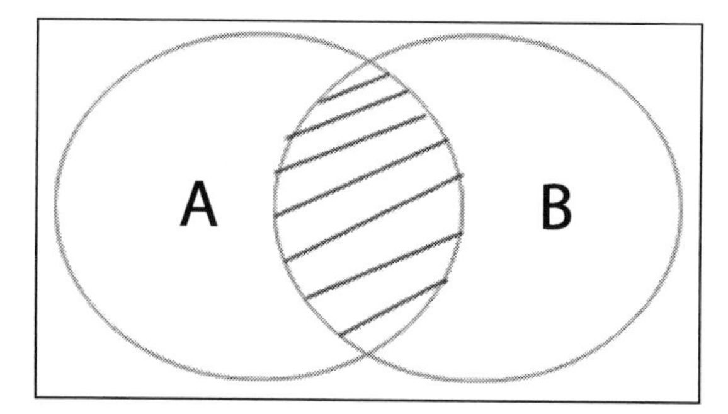

Figure 2.4 **Venn diagram for the intersection of two events.** The Venn diagram shows a visual example of the intersection of events A and B. The intersection is the section of the circles that overlap, represented by the stripes.

That is, for independent events, the probability of the intersection of events A and B occurring is the probability of event A occurring multiplied by the probability of event B occurring.

If events A and B are dependent events, the probability of the intersection of the two events is *not* equal to the multiplication of the probability of each of the events (Equation 2.4).

$$P(A \cap B) \neq P(A)P(B) \tag{2.4}$$

If two events are not independent, then they are dependent.

Union: The union of two events is the occurrence of event A or event B or both events together. We use the notation $A \cup B$ to represent the union of two events.

Figure 2.5 shows us the union of two events in Venn diagram form. Here, the sample space of the union of events A and B is in the sample space of event A, of event B, and of both simultaneously.

In our example with Tom, the union of events A and B would be that Tom eats green vegetables, green nonvegetable foods, and other nongreen vegetables.

Intersection, union, and complement can be used to describe even the most complicated situations in terms of simple events. These and other properties of probabilities presented in this section are summarized in Table 2.2 as a reference guide.

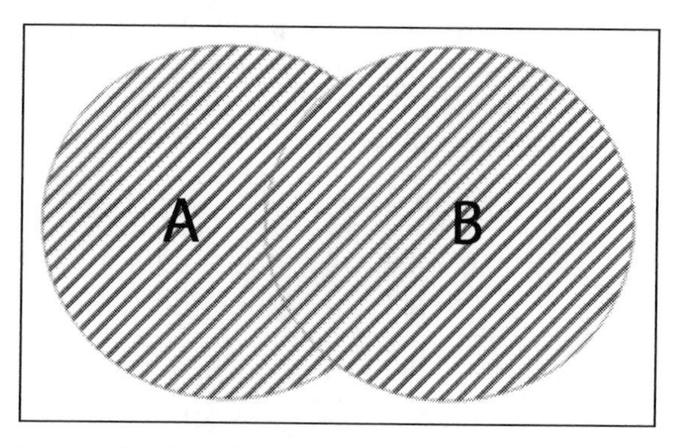

Figure 2.5 **Venn diagram for the union of two events.** The Venn diagram shows a visual example of the union of events A and B. The union is represented by the stripes and covers all space inside the circles of both A and B.

Table 2.2 Reference guide on properties of probabilities

Term	*Brief definition*	*Notation*
Probability	The relative frequency of a set of outcomes over an indefinitely large (or infinite) number of trials.	P()
Event	Result of observation or experiment.	{A}, {B}
Sample space	The set of all possible outcomes.	Ω
Mutually exclusive	*A* and *B* are mutually exclusive if they cannot happen together.	$P(A \cap B) = 0$
Complement	The complement of *A* is the event that *A* does not occur.	A^C or $\bar{A}$
Intersection	The event that both *A* and *B* occur.	$A \cap B$
Independent	*A* and *B* are independent events if the probability of one occurring is not dependent upon whether the other has already occurred.	$P(A\|B) = P(A)$ $P(B\|A) = P(B)$
Dependent	*A* and *B* are dependent events if the probability of one occurring is dependent upon whether the other has already occurred.	$P(A \cap B) \neq P(A) \times P(B)$
Union	The event that either *A* or *B* or both occur.	$A \cup B$
Null event	Cannot happen.	Ø
Exhaustive	*A* and *B* are exhaustive events if there are no other possible outcomes.	

Note: A summary of the properties of probability is provided. This table will serve as a good reference for learning notation and definitions of the different terms presented in this chapter.

Laws of probability

There are several laws of probabilities. The laws include the multiplication law, the addition law, and the total probability rule.

Multiplication Law of Probability: The multiplication law of probability tells us that if $A_1,\ldots,A_k$ are independent events, then the probability of the intersection of these events is the product of the probabilities for each individual event. Equation 2.5 shows the calculation for the multiplication law of probability.

$$P(A_1 \cap A_2 \cap \ldots \cap A_k = P(A_1) \times P(A_2) \times \ldots \times P(A_k) \quad (2.5)$$

Remember that the symbol ∩ represents the intersection of events. Let's look at an example to help us to better understand the multiplication law as it applies to independent events.

EXAMPLE PROBLEM 2.1

Suppose that we have two unrelated patients in a clinic and we want to know the probability that both patients will develop human immunodeficiency virus (HIV) after a needle stick. The Centers for Disease Control and Prevention (CDC) tells us that there is a 23 in 10,000 risk that a person will get HIV after a needle stick.[1] We can use the multiplication law for independent events to answer this.

$$\begin{aligned} &P(Patient\,1\,gets\,HIV \cap Patient\,2\,gets\,HIV) \\ &\quad = P(Patient\,1\,gets\,HIV) \times P(Patient\,2\,gets\,HIV) \\ &\quad = 0.0023 \times 0.0023 = 0.00000529 \end{aligned}$$

The probability that both patients will get HIV is 0.00000529.

Addition Law of Probability: The addition law of probability tells us that if A and B are any events, then Equation 2.6 is true:

$$P(A \cup B) = P(A) + P(B) - P(A \cap B) \tag{2.6}$$

There are a few special cases of the addition law that are important for us to note.

If events A *and* B *are mutually exclusive*, then $P(A \cap B) = 0$, and the addition law reduces to Equation 2.7:

$$P(A \cup B) = P(A) + P(B) \tag{2.7}$$

If events A *and* B *are independent*, then the addition law of probability can also be simplified. By definition, as given by the multiplication law for independent events, $P(A \cap B) = P(A) \times P(B)$; therefore, Equations 2.8 and 2.9 are resulting corollaries.

$$P(A \cup B) = P(A) + P(B) - P(A) \times P(B) \tag{2.8}$$

$$P(A \cup B) = P(A) + P(B) \times [1 - P(A)] \tag{2.9}$$

For three events, the addition law is as follows in Equation 2.10:

$$\begin{aligned} P(A \cup B \cup C) = {} & P(A) + P(B) + P(C) - P(A \cap B) - P(A \cap C) - P(B \cap C) \\ & + P(A \cap B \cap C) \end{aligned} \tag{2.10}$$

EXAMPLE PROBLEM 2.2

To help us further understand the addition law, let's go back to our HIV example. Suppose that we, again, have two unrelated patients in a clinic, but this time we want to know the probability that either patient 1, patient 2, or both patients will develop HIV after a needle stick. Based on data from the CDC, there is a 23 in 10,000 risk that a person will get HIV after a needle stick.[1] We can use the addition law for independent events to answer this question.

$$
\begin{aligned}
&P(\textit{Patient } 1 \textit{ gets HIV} \cup \textit{Patient } 2 \textit{ gets HIV})\\
&\quad = P(\textit{Patient } 1 \textit{ gets HIV}) + P(\textit{Patient } 2 \textit{ gets HIV}) \times [1 - P(\textit{Patient } 1 \textit{ gets HIV})]\\
&\quad = 0.0023 + 0.0023 \times (1 - 0.0023)\\
&\quad = 0.0023 + [0.0023 \times 0.9977]\\
&\quad = 0.0023 + 0.00229 = 0.00459
\end{aligned}
$$

The probability that either patient 1 or patient 2 or both will get HIV is 0.00459.

Conditional Probability: When describing a conditional probability, we would say that it is the probability of event B given that event A has occurred.

The conditional probability of B given A is written as $P\ (B|A)$ and defined as Equation 2.11:

$$P(B|A) = \frac{P(A \cap B)}{P(A)} \tag{2.11}$$

If A *and* B *are independent events*, then Equation 2.12 is true:

$$P(B|A) = P(B) = P(B|A^C) \tag{2.12}$$

If Events A *and* B *are dependent*, then Equation 2.13 is true:

$$P(B|A) \neq P(B) \neq P(B|\bar{A}) \textit{ and } P(A \cap B) \neq P(A) \times P(B) \tag{2.13}$$

Generalized Multiplication Law of Probability: The generalized multiplicative law of probabilities is based on conditional probabilities and expands on the multiplication law discussed previously in this chapter.

So what do we do if the events are not independent and we want to apply the multiplication law? We can apply the generalized multiplication law of probability.

If $A_1,\ldots,A_k$ is an arbitrary set of events, meaning that the events are not mutually independent, then Equation 2.14 is true:

$$
\begin{aligned}
P(A_1 \cap A_2 \cap \ldots \cap A_k) = {} & P(A_1) \times P(A_2 \mid A_1) \times P(A_3 \mid A_2 \cap A_1)\\
& \times \ldots \times P(A_k \mid A_{k-1} \cap \ldots \cap A_2 \cap A_1)
\end{aligned} \tag{2.14}
$$

Relative Risk: The relative risk is the conditional probability of event B given event A divided by the conditional probability of event B given the complement of event A. The relative risk is also referred to as the *risk ratio*.

The relative risk (RR) of B given A is represented in Equation 2.15:

$$\frac{P(B \mid A)}{P(B \mid \bar{A})} \tag{2.15}$$

Total Probability Rule: The total probability rule allows us to calculate the probability of an event based on conditional probabilities.

The total probability rule is such that for any events A and B, Equation 2.16 is true:

$$P(B) = P(B|A) \times P(A) + P(B \mid \bar{A}) \times P(\bar{A}) \quad (2.16)$$

Mutually exclusive and exhaustive

Mutually Exhaustive: A set of events $A_1,\ldots,A_k$ is exhaustive if at least one of the events must occur.

- If events $A_1,\ldots,A_k$ are mutually exclusive and exhaustive, then at least one event must occur and no two events can occur simultaneously; therefore, exactly one event must occur.
- We should note that mutually exclusive events are not necessarily exhaustive.
- Let $A_1,\ldots,A_k$ be mutually exclusive and exhaustive events. The unconditional probability of an event B, $P(B)$, can be written as a weighted average of the conditional probabilities of B given A_i, $P(B|A_i)$, as in Equation 2.17:

$$P(B) = \sum_{i=1}^{k} P(B \mid A_i) \times P(A_i) \quad (2.17)$$

Here are a few properties to note when considering mutually exclusive and exhaustive events.

- The sum of the probabilities for mutually exclusive events ≤ 1.
- The sum of the probabilities for exhaustive events ≥ 1.
- The sum of the probabilities for mutually exclusive and exhaustive events $= 1$.

EXAMPLE PROBLEM 2.3

Table 2.3 shows causes of death for infants, defined as children under the age of 1, in the United States from the years 2007 through 2013.[2] In total, there were 23,446 infant deaths.

A **Are the five causes of death mutually exclusive?**

Yes, the five causes of death are mutually exclusive because each death is classified into one of these five groups.

B **Are the five causes of death exhaustive?**

Yes, because we have a cause of death for all infant deaths that occurred, and they must be in one of the categories listed in Table 2.3.

C **For the population noted in Table 2.3, what is the probability that an infant death was caused by a disease of the respiratory system?**

$$P(\textit{disease of respiratory system}) = \frac{524}{23{,}446} = 0.0223$$

Table 2.3 Causes of infant death 2007–2013

Cause of death	*Number*	*Probability*
Disease of circulatory system	457	0.0194
Disease of respiratory system	524	0.0223
Disease of digestive system	175	0.0075
Disease of nervous system	330	0.0141
Other cause	21960	0.9366
Total	23,446	

Source: United States Department of Health and Human Services, Centers for Disease Control and Prevention, National Center for Health Statistics, Division of Vital Statistics. Linked Birth / Infant Death Records 2007–2013, as compiled from data provided by the 57 vital statistics jurisdictions through the Vital Statistics Cooperative Program, on CDC WONDER Online Database, http://wonder.cdc.gov/lbd-current.html, accessed July 7, 2016.

Note: The number and probability of infant deaths in different categories are presented. The probability of death in a certain category can be found by dividing the number of infant deaths that occurred in that category by the total number of infant deaths occurring.

D What is the probability that two randomly selected infants who died between 2007 and 2013 both died of a disease of the nervous system?

Let X = {Infant 1 died of disease of nervous system}
Let Y = {Infant 2 died of disease of nervous system}

$$P(X \cap Y) = P(X) \times P(Y) = 0.0141 \times 0.0141 = 0.0002$$

In this problem, we have the intersection of two independent events; thus, we use the multiplication law to multiply the probabilities of each event.

E Given that an infant did not die of a cause of death classified as *other* in this example, what is the probability that the infant died of a digestive system disease?

Let A = {Infant did not die of an "other" cause of death}
Let B = {Infant died of a digestive system disease}
$P(A) = 1 - 0.9366 = 0.0634$
$P(B) = 0.0075$

$$P(B|A) = \frac{P(B \cap A)}{P(A)} = \frac{0.0075}{0.0634} = 0.1183$$

We set this problem up as a conditional probability. Here, $P(B \cap A) = P(B)$ because the event that an infant did not die of an *other* cause of death AND died of digestive system disease is the event that an infant died of digestive system disease. We use the complement $1 - P(A)$ for the event "Infant did *not* die of an 'other' cause of death."

F Suppose that we have four infants who died between 2007 and 2013. What is the probability that at least one of the infants died from a disease of the respiratory system?

Let A = {Infant 1 died of disease of the respiratory system}
Let B = {Infant 2 died of disease of the respiratory system}

Let C = {Infant 3 died of disease of the respiratory system}
Let D = {Infant 4 died of disease of the respiratory system}

$$P(A \cup B \cup C \cup D) = 1 - P(\bar{A} \cap \bar{B} \cap \bar{C} \cap \bar{D})$$
$$= 1 - [(1-0.0223)(1-0.0223)(1-0.0223)(1-0.0223)] = 1 - (0.9777)^4$$
$$= 1 - 0.91374 = 0.0863$$

In this problem, we consider each of the infants dying of a disease of the respiratory system as an independent event, represented by A, B, C, and D. We can also think of the probability of at least one of the infants dying of a disease of the respiratory system as 1 – P (no infant died of a disease of the respiratory system).

PRACTICE PROBLEM 2.1

Estimates of the prevalence of diabetes (i.e., how many in the specified population have diabetes out of the total specified population) are presented for several different racial or ethnic groups (Table 2.4).[3] The prevalence rates are presented as percentages and stratified by education level.

Suppose that an unrelated non-Hispanic black person with a high school diploma, a Puerto Rican person who did not graduate from high school, and a Puerto Rican person with a bachelor's degree were selected from the community.

A What is the probability that all three of these individuals have diabetes?

B What is the probability that at least one of the Puerto Rican people has diabetes?

C What is the probability that at least one of the three people has diabetes?

D What is the probability that exactly one of the three people has diabetes?

Table 2.4 Prevalence of diabetes

Race/ethnic group	*<High school diploma (%)*	*High school diploma or GED (%)*	*>High school diploma (%)*
Non-Hispanic White	12.1	8.1	5.3
Non-Hispanic Black	16.1	9.7	8.2
Mexican/Mexican American	9.7	6.3	6.7
Puerto Rican	17.6	9.8	6.8
Cuban/Cuban American	13.4	8.2	6.0

Source: Arroyo-Johnson, C., Mincey, K. D., Ackermann, N., Milam, L., Goodman, M. S., and Colditz, G. A., *Prev Chronic Dis.*, 13(E10), 2016, doi:10.5888/pcd13.150260.

Note: The table shows the prevalence of diabetes for each racial or ethnic group by education category. The prevalence presented is the average yearly prevalence of diabetes over a 16-year period from 1997 to 2012.

E Suppose that we know that only one of the three people has diabetes, but we do not know which one. What is the conditional probability that the affected person is Puerto Rican?

F Suppose that we know that two of the three people have diabetes. What is the conditional probability that they are both Puerto Rican?

G Suppose that we know that two of the three people have diabetes. What is the conditional probability that they both have, at most, a high school education?

Suppose the probability is 0.015 that both members of a married couple who are Mexican or Mexican American and have more than a high school education will have diabetes.

H What is the conditional probability that one of the individuals in the married couple will have diabetes given that the other individual in the couple has diabetes? How does this value compare to the prevalence in the table? Why should it be the same (or different)?

I What is the probability that at least one member of the couple is affected?

Suppose that a study of diabetes is proposed in a neighborhood, where the race or ethnicity distribution is as shown in Table 2.5.

J What is the expected overall prevalence of diabetes in the community if the prevalence estimates in Table 2.5 for specific race or ethnicity and education groups hold?

K If 2000 people are in the community, then what is the expected number of cases of diabetes in the community?

Table 2.5 Race/ethnicity distribution of neighborhood

Race/ethnicity	*<High school diploma (%)*[a]	*High school diploma/ GED (%)*	*>High school diploma (%)*	*Total*
Non-Hispanic White	11	18	12	41
Non-Hispanic Black	6	9	5	20
Mexican/Mexican American	10	5	3	18
Puerto Rican	4	6	2	12
Cuban/Cuban American	3	3	3	9

Note: The hypothetical percentage of a neighborhood's total population is given by race or ethnic group and education level. Using these percentages and the prevalence of diabetes from each group given, we can calculate the expected overall prevalence of diabetes in the community.

[a] Percentage of total population.

PRACTICE PROBLEM 2.2

Probability rules

A Additive rule of probability

1. For nonmutually exclusive events:

$$P(A \textit{ and/or } B) = P(A \cup B) =$$

2. For mutually exclusive events:

$$P(A \textit{ and/or } B) = P(A \cup B) =$$

B Conditional Probability

1. What is a conditional probability?

2. For nonindependent events:

$$P(A|B) =$$

3. For independent events:

$$P(A|B) =$$

4. For mutually exclusive events:

$$P(A|B) =$$

5. Complement:

$$P(A^C|B)$$

C Multiplicative rule of probability

1. For nonindependent events:

$$P(A \textit{ and } B) = P(A \cap B) =$$

2. For independent events:

$$P(A \text{ and } B) = P(A \cap B) =$$

PRACTICE PROBLEM 2.3

Let A represent the event that a particular person has hypertension, and let B represent the event that he or she eats salty French fries.

1 What is the event $\boldsymbol{A \cap B}$?

2 What is the event $\boldsymbol{A \cup B}$?

3 What is the complement of A?

4 Are the events A and B mutually exclusive?

PRACTICE PROBLEM 2.4

Table 2.6 contains categories of the amount of time spent in an emergency department (ED) and the number and percent of patients reporting a wait time in each interval for 2011.[4]

Table 2.6 Time in emergency department, 2011

Time spent in the emergency department, hours	*People (no.)*	*People (%)*
< 1	16 198	12.3
≥ 1 but < 2	33 184	25.1
≥ 2 but < 4	47 537	36.0
≥ 4 but < 6	20 420	15.5
≥ 6 but < 10	10 487	7.9
≥ 10 but < 14	2134	1.6
≥ 14 but < 24	1340	1.0
≥ 24	794	0.6
Total	132 094	100

Source: Centers for Disease Control and Prevention, National Hospital Ambulatory Medical Care Survey: 2011 Emergency Department Summary Tables, 2011, https://www.cdc.gov/nchs/data/ahcd/nhamcs_emergency/2011_ed_web_tables.pdf.

Note: The table shows categories for amounts of time spent in the emergency department. The number of people who reported a waiting time in each category is given in the middle column, along with a percentage of the total number of people reporting in the last column. These data will be used to solve the questions in Practice Problem 2.4.

A What is the probability that the amount of time a patient spent in the ED is between two and four hours?

B What is the probability that a patient spent less than six hours in the ED?

C Given that the time spent in the ED is less than six hours, what is the probability that the wait time was between one and two hours?

PRACTICE PROBLEM 2.5

According to the CDC,[5] 68.9% of physicians were accepting new Medicaid patients in 2013.

A Suppose that a patient who has Medicaid as their insurance is looking for a new physician. The patient randomly chooses two unrelated physicians. What is the probability that both physicians will accept the new patient?

B What is the probability that both physicians will ***not*** accept the new patient?

C If five unrelated physicians are chosen from the population, what is the probability that all five will not accept the patient?

References

1. HIV Risk Behaviors. Centers for Disease Control and Prevention website. http://www.cdc.gov/hiv/risk/estimates/riskbehaviors.html. Published 2015.
2. United States Department of Health and Human Services, Centers for Disease Control and Prevention, National Center for Health Statistics, Division of Vital Statistics. Linked Birth/Infant Death Records 2007–2013, as compiled from data provided by the 57 vital statistics jurisdictions through the Vital Statistics Cooperative Program, on CDC WONDER Online Database. http://wonder.cdc.gov/lbd-current.html. Accessed July 7, 2016.
3. Arroyo-Johnson C, Mincey KD, Ackermann N, Milam L, Goodman MS, Colditz GA. Racial and ethnic heterogeneity in self-reported diabetes prevalence trends across Hispanic subgroups, National Health Interview Survey, 1997–2012. *Prev Chronic Dis*. 2016;13(E10). doi:10.5888/pcd13.150260.
4. Centers for Disease Control and Prevention. National Hospital Ambulatory Medical Care Survey: 2011 Emergency Department Summary Tables. 2011. https://www.cdc.gov/nchs/data/ahcd/nhamcs_emergency/2011_ed_web_tables.pdf.
5. Hing E, Decker SL, Jamoom E. *Acceptance of New Patients with Public and Private Insurance by Office-Based Physicians: United States, 2013*. Hyattsville, MD: National Center for Health Statistics. 2015. http://www.cdc.gov/nchs/data/databriefs/db195.pdf.

3 Diagnostic testing/screening

This chapter will focus on applying the concepts of probability to diagnostic testing and screening and will include the following:

- Diagnostic terms and concepts
- Receiver operating characteristic (ROC) curves

Terms

- Bayes theorem
- cumulative incidence
- false negative error
- false positive error
- negative predictive value (PV^-)
- positive predictive value (PV^+)
- prevalence
- ROC curve
- sensitivity
- specificity

Introduction

Probability is one of the pillars of biostatistics, and now that we have learned the basics in Chapter 2, we will apply probability to diagnostic testing and screening in this chapter.

Diagnostic terms and concepts

Positive Predictive Value of a Screening Test: The positive predictive value (PV^+) of a screening test is the probability that a person has a disease given that the test is positive: $P(\text{disease}|\text{test}^+)$.

Negative Predictive Value of a Screening Test: The negative predictive value (PV^-) of a screening test is the probability that a person does not have a disease given that the test is negative: $P(\text{no disease}|\text{test}^-)$.

Clinicians often cannot directly measure the predictive value of a set of symptoms. However, they can measure how often specific symptoms occur in healthy people and in people with disease.

Sensitivity: The sensitivity of a symptom (or set of symptoms or screening test) is the probability that the symptom is present given that the person has a disease.

Specificity: The specificity of a symptom (or set of symptoms or screening test) is the probability that the symptom is *not* present given that the person does *not* have a disease.

For a symptom or test to be effective in predicting disease, it is important that both the sensitivity and specificity are high. However, there is a trade-off between the two; as sensitivity increases, specificity decreases.

False Positive Error: A false positive error is defined as a positive test result when the person does not have the disease.

False Negative Error: A false negative error is defined as a negative test result when the person actually has the disease.

Prevalence: The prevalence of a disease is the probability of currently having the disease regardless of the duration of time one has had the disease. Prevalence is obtained by dividing the number of people who currently have the disease by the number of people in the study population.

Cumulative Incidence: The cumulative incidence of a disease is the probability that a person with no prior disease will develop a new case of the disease over some specified time period.

Table 3.1 shows the notation and definition for each of these terms.

BOX 3.1 NOTATION USED WHEN REFERRING TO DISEASES AND TESTS

D^+ = has disease	D^- = disease-free
T^+ = test positive	T^- = test negative

Table 3.1 Diagnostic testing/screening terms

Term	*Brief definition*	*Notation*
Positive predictive value	Probability of disease given a positive test result	$P(D^+ \mid T^+)$
Negative predictive value	Probability of not having disease given a negative test result	$P(D^- \mid T^-)$
Sensitivity	Probability of a positive test result given that the individual tested actually has the disease	$P(T^+ \mid D^+)$
Specificity	Probability of a negative test result given that the individual tested does not have the disease	$P(T^- \mid D^-)$
P(false positive)	Probability of a positive test result given the individual does not have the disease	$P(T^+ \mid D^-)$
P(false negative)	Probability of a negative test result given the individual does have the disease	$P(T^- \mid D^+)$
Prevalence	Proportion of individuals who have a disease at a given point in time	$P(D^+)$
Cumulative incidence	Probability that a person with no prior disease will have a new case of the disease over some specified time period	

Note: Diagnostic testing and screening terms are presented along with a definition and notation for each term. This table summarizes the main terms learned in Chapter 3 and is a good reference.

Bayes Theorem: Bayes theorem is used to calculate the conditional probability of an event on the basis of other known probabilities and is useful in diagnostic testing.

Equation 3.1 shows the Bayes theorem for two mutually exclusive and exhaustive events, A and B.

$$P(A|B) = \frac{P(A)P(B|A)}{P(A)P(B|A) + P(A^c)P(B|A^c)} \tag{3.1}$$

Previously, we mentioned that clinicians often cannot directly measure the predictive value of a set of symptoms. We can use Bayes theorem to calculate the predictive values. If A = Disease and B = Symptom, then $PV^+ = P(A|B)$. We can apply Bayes theorem here; if we know the sensitivity, specificity, and prevalence, these can be used to calculate the positive predictive value:

$$PV^+ = \frac{sensitivity \times prevalence}{sensitivity \times prevalence + (1 - specificity) \times (1 - prevalence)}$$

We can also apply Bayes theorem to find the negative predictive value:

$$PV^- = \frac{specificity \times (1 - prevalence)}{specificity \times (1 - prevalence) + (1 - sensitivity) \times prevalence}$$

Another way of representing the notation of using Bayes theorem to find the positive predictive value of a test if the prevalence, sensitivity, and specificity are known is the following:

$$P(D^+|T^+) = \frac{P(D^+)P(T^+|D^+)}{P(D^+)P(T^+|D^+) + P(D^-)P(T^+|D^-)}$$

EXAMPLE PROBLEM 3.1

Often in health research, self-reported measures of health conditions are used in place of data from medical records. In this situation, we think of the self-reported measure as the "test" and the medical record as the actual record of disease status. In one study, self-reports and medical records were available on heart disease for 493 participants.[1] Of these participants, 87 had heart disease according to their medical record, and 63 of these 87 self-reported having heart disease. According to the medical records, 406 participants did not have heart disease, and 349 of the 406 self-reported not having heart disease.

A **What is the sensitivity of the self-reported measure of heart disease?**

$$P(test + |disease+) = \frac{63}{87} = 0.724$$

B What is the specificity of the self-reported measure of heart disease?

$$P(test-|disease-)=\frac{349}{406}=0.860$$

Suppose that we ask patients in a clinic waiting room whether they have been diagnosed with heart disease. We anticipate about 15% of the patients will have heart disease.

C What is the positive predictive value of the self-reported measure of heart disease?

We can calculate the positive predictive value using Bayes theorem:

$$PV+=\frac{prevalance\times sensitivity}{prev\times sens+(1-prev)(1-spec)}=\frac{0.15\times 0.724}{0.15\times 0.724+(1-0.15)\times(1-0.860)}$$

$$=\frac{0.15\times 0.724}{0.15\times 0.724+0.85\times 0.140}=\frac{0.15\times 0.724}{0.1086+0.119}$$

$$=\frac{0.1086}{0.2276}=0.477$$

EXAMPLE PROBLEM 3.2

A study was conducted on the use of C-reactive protein (CRP) as a way to diagnose post-stroke pneumonia.[2] CRP cutoff points ranging from 14.9 to 110.5 mg/L were examined. Table 3.2 contains a few selected cutoff levels and the sensitivities and specificities of the tests corresponding to these different levels.

A As the cutoff point for the CRP level gets higher, how does the probability of a false positive result appear to change?

Table 3.2 CRP cutoff level with sensitivity and specificity

CRP level	*Sensitivity*	*Specificity*
17.2	0.939	0.407
23.5	0.848	0.556
29.5	0.788	0.704
45	0.697	0.778
59.4	0.636	0.889
77.65	0.545	0.963
105	0.394	0.963

Source: Warusevitane, A., Karunatilake, D., Sim, J., Smith, C., and Roffe, C., *PLoS ONE*, 11(3), e0150269.

Note: Selected CRP cutoff levels along with the respective sensitivity and specificity for each cutoff are presented.

Abbreviation: CRP, C-reactive protein.

As the cutoff point increases, we can see that the specificity increases. Therefore, the probability of a false positive will decrease. The probability of a false positive = 1 – specificity (see Table 3.3).

B **How does the probability of a false negative result appear to change as the cutoff increases?**

As the cutoff increases, the sensitivity decreases; therefore, the probability of a false negative (1 – sensitivity) result increases (see Table 3.4).

C **Suppose that the prevalence of pneumonia in poststroke patients is 30%. What is the probability of poststroke pneumonia among patients who have CRP levels above 59.4 mg/L? What is another name for this quantity?**

Let Pn = {poststroke pneumonia}; C = {CRP level above 59.4}

Table 3.3 CRP cutoff level with specificity and false positive

CRP level	*Specificity*	*False positive*
17.2	0.407	0.593
23.5	0.556	0.444
29.5	0.704	0.296
45	0.778	0.222
59.4	0.889	0.111
77.65	0.963	0.037
105	0.963	0.037

Source: Warusevitane, A., Karunatilake, D., Sim, J., Smith, C., and Roffe, C., *PLoS ONE*, 11(3), e0150269.

Note: Selected CRP cutoff levels along with the respective specificity values are presented. False positive values for each cutoff level are calculated by taking 1 – specificity.

Abbreviation: CRP, C-reactive protein.

Table 3.4 CRP cutoff level with sensitivity and false negative

CRP level	*Sensitivity*	*False negative*
17.2	0.939	0.061
23.5	0.848	0.152
29.5	0.788	0.212
45	0.697	0.303
59.4	0.636	0.364
77.65	0.545	0.455
105	0.394	0.606

Source: Warusevitane, A., Karunatilake, D., Sim, J., Smith, C., and Roffe, C., *PLoS ONE*, 11(3), e0150269.

Note: Selected CRP cutoff levels along with the respective sensitivity values are presented. False negative values for each cutoff level are calculated by taking 1 – sensitivity.

Abbreviation: CRP, C-reactive protein.

$P(\text{C}|\text{Pn}) = \text{sensitivity} = 0.636$

$P\left(C|\overline{Pn}\right) = 1 - P\left(\overline{C}|\overline{Pn}\right) = 1 - specificity = 1 - 0.889 = 0.111$

$P(\text{Pn}) = \text{prevalence} = 0.30$

$$P\left(Pn|C\right) = \frac{P\left(C|Pn\right)P(Pn)}{P\left(C|Pn\right)P(Pn) + P\left(C|\overline{Pn}\right)P\left(\overline{Pn}\right)} = \frac{0.636 \times 0.3}{0.636 \times 0.3 + 0.111 \times 0.7}$$

$$= \frac{0.636 \times 0.3}{0.191 + 0.078} = \frac{0.191}{0.269} = 0.71$$

The probability of poststroke pneumonia among patients who have CRP levels above 59.4 mg/L is 0.71. This is also known as the positive predictive value.

Receiver operating characteristic curves

ROC Curve: A receiver operating characteristic (ROC) curve is a plot of the sensitivity versus the false positive result (1 – specificity) of a screening test, where the different points on the curve correspond to different cutoff points used to designate a positive test.

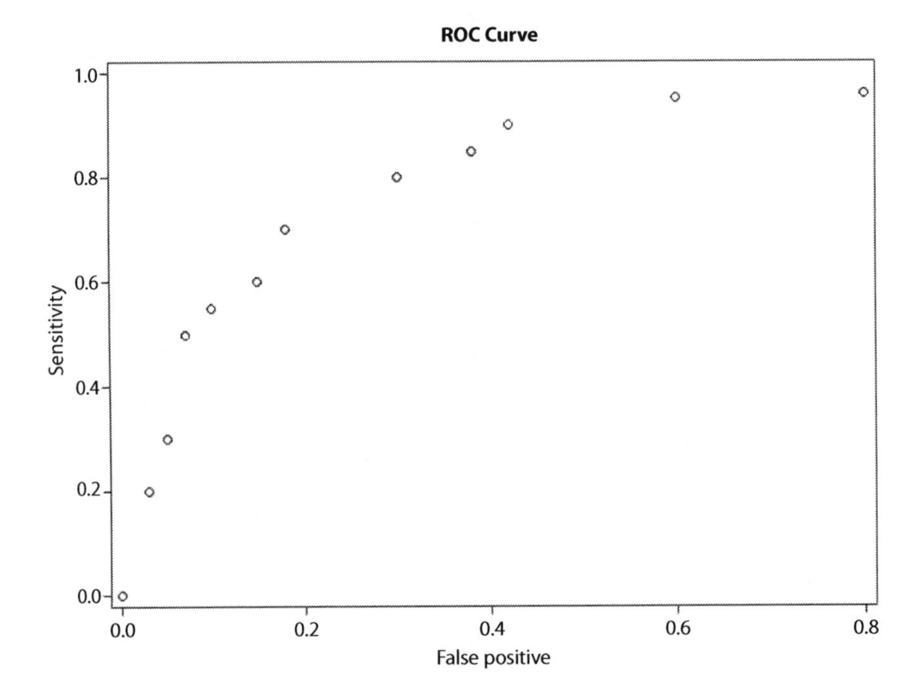

Figure 3.1 **ROC curve.** ROC indicates receiver operating characteristic. On the x-axis are the false positive values. On the y-axis are the values for sensitivity. From this ROC curve, we can see that the false positive values and sensitivity values have a positive relationship.

- The ROC curve plots *P*(true positive) versus *P*(false positive) and shows the inherent trade-off of sensitivity and specificity. There is a relationship between sensitivity and specificity, which can be seen in the ROC curve; when sensitivity is at the highest point, false positives are also high (meaning that sensitivity is low) and vice versa.
- When looking at the ROC curve, we want to choose a cutoff value in the upper left-hand corner of the graph that maximizes sensitivity and minimizes a false positive result, thus maximizing specificity. Figure 3.1 shows an example of an ROC curve.

EXAMPLE PROBLEM 3.3

The dataset *cr_protein* expands the data provided in Example Problem 3.2 and contains the full set of provided CRP cutoff levels with the sensitivities and specificities of the test corresponding to these different levels.[2] The levels of CRP are saved under the variable name *crp*, the sensitivities under *sens*, and the specificities under *spec*. The dataset is provided as both a SAS dataset and a Stata dataset (see Instructions for Problem 3.3: Parts A–D).

A How do the sensitivity and specificity change across the different CRP cutoff values?

Instructions for Example Problem 3.3: Part A

Viewing Data in SAS and Stata to Examine Sensitivity and Specificity of CRP Cutoff Values	
How to Solve in SAS	*How to Solve in Stata*

1. Open the data in SAS using a *libname* statement.
`LIBNAME mylib 'C:\Data';`
2. Explore the data using the data browser in SAS.
	1. Open the data in Stata. First, make sure that the working directory is set to the location where the *cr_protein* dataset is saved.
	2. Type the use command into Stata to open the specified dataset.
	`cd "C:\Data"`
	`use cr_protein`
	3. Explore the data in Stata using the data editor.

As the cutoff increases, sensitivity decreases and specificity increases.

B Create a variable that is the probability of a false positive result for each of the cutoff points of CRP.

Instructions for Example Problem 3.3: Part B

<table>
<tr><th colspan="2">Creating a New Variable for False Positives in SAS and Stata</th></tr>
<tr><th>How to Solve in SAS</th><th>How to Solve in Stata</th></tr>
<tr><td>1. Use a data step, and create a new variable called falsepos, which is 1 – specificity. Then, run the code.
<pre>DATA cr_protein2;
     SET mylib.cr_protein;
     falsepos = 1-spec;
RUN;</pre></td><td>1. Use a generate command, which will generate a new variable. In this example, create the variable falsepos; it is equal to 1 – specificity.
<pre>generate falsepos = 1-spec</pre></td></tr>
<tr><td>2. After running the code, check the log and dataset to verify that the new variable was created correctly.</td><td>2. After running the code, check in the data editor to verify that the new variable was created.</td></tr>
</table>

BOX 3.2 CHECKING THE CREATION OF A NEW VARIABLE IN SAS

- After running the SAS code in Part B of Example Problem 3.3, check the log and dataset to verify that a new variable was created.
- The screenshot in Figure 3.2 shows what we should see in our log. Note that there are no error or warning messages.
- Next, let's check our dataset to look for the new variable (Figure 3.3).

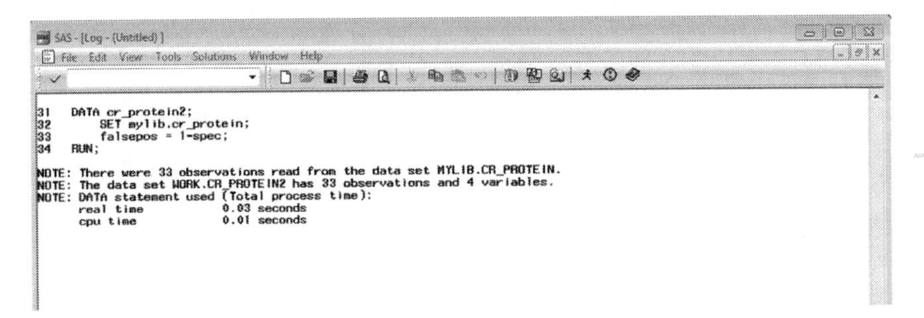

Figure 3.2 **SAS Log after creating *falsepos* variable.** The snapshot of our SAS log after running the code to create the *falsepos* variable shows no errors or warnings.

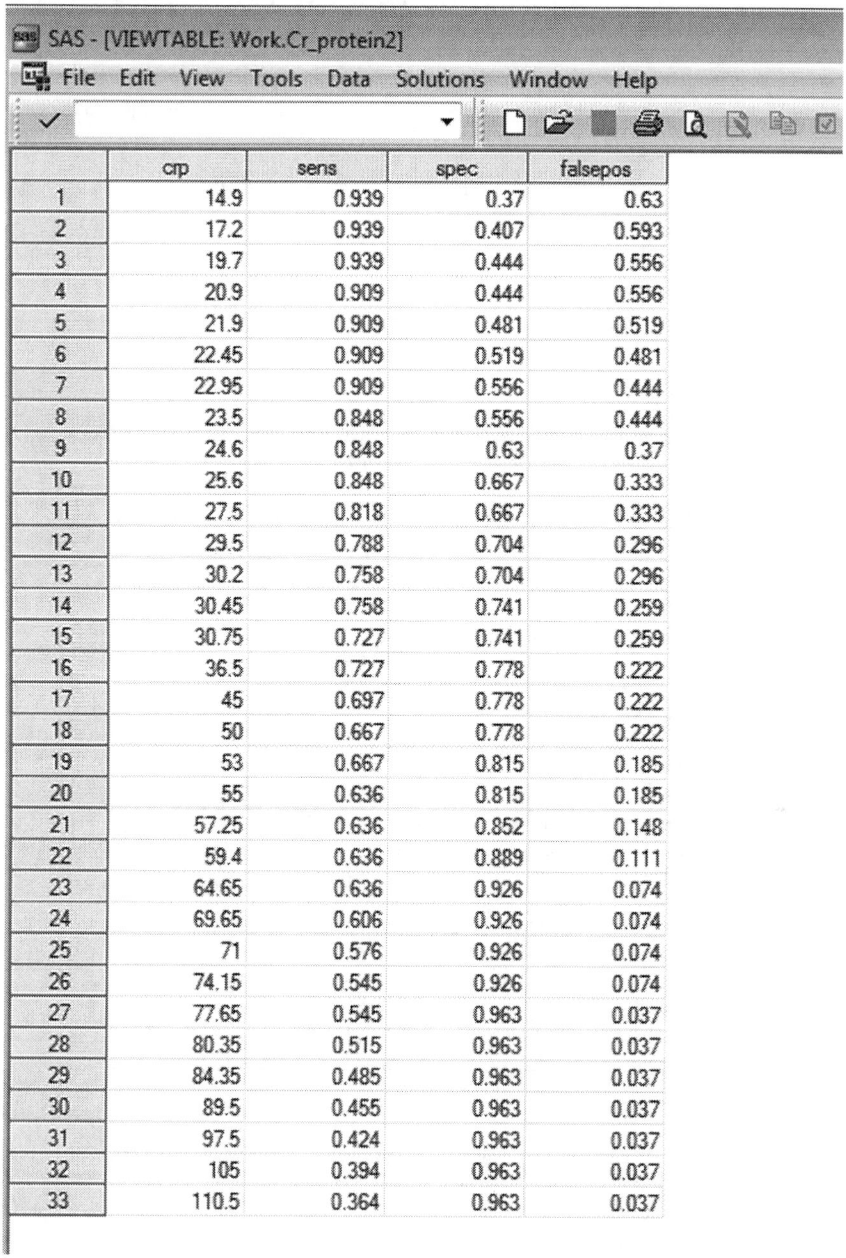

SAS - [VIEWTABLE: Work.Cr_protein2]

File Edit View Tools Data Solutions Window Help

	crp	sens	spec	falsepos
1	14.9	0.939	0.37	0.63
2	17.2	0.939	0.407	0.593
3	19.7	0.939	0.444	0.556
4	20.9	0.909	0.444	0.556
5	21.9	0.909	0.481	0.519
6	22.45	0.909	0.519	0.481
7	22.95	0.909	0.556	0.444
8	23.5	0.848	0.556	0.444
9	24.6	0.848	0.63	0.37
10	25.6	0.848	0.667	0.333
11	27.5	0.818	0.667	0.333
12	29.5	0.788	0.704	0.296
13	30.2	0.758	0.704	0.296
14	30.45	0.758	0.741	0.259
15	30.75	0.727	0.741	0.259
16	36.5	0.727	0.778	0.222
17	45	0.697	0.778	0.222
18	50	0.667	0.778	0.222
19	53	0.667	0.815	0.185
20	55	0.636	0.815	0.185
21	57.25	0.636	0.852	0.148
22	59.4	0.636	0.889	0.111
23	64.65	0.636	0.926	0.074
24	69.65	0.606	0.926	0.074
25	71	0.576	0.926	0.074
26	74.15	0.545	0.926	0.074
27	77.65	0.545	0.963	0.037
28	80.35	0.515	0.963	0.037
29	84.35	0.485	0.963	0.037
30	89.5	0.455	0.963	0.037
31	97.5	0.424	0.963	0.037
32	105	0.394	0.963	0.037
33	110.5	0.364	0.963	0.037

Figure 3.3 **SAS data view after creating *falsepos* variable.** The snapshot of our SAS data viewer shows the *falsepos* variable in the far right column. We can see that values have populated for all rows and that the values are equal to 1 – specificity.

BOX 3.3 CHECKING THE CREATION OF A NEW VARIABLE IN STATA

- After running the above Stata code in Part B of Problem 3.3, we should check our dataset to verify that a new variable was created (see Figure 3.4).
- As we can see from the dataset in our explorer window, the variable *falsepos* was created.

C Plot an ROC curve.

Instructions for Example Problem 3.3: Part C

Plotting an ROC Curve Using SAS and Stata	
How to Solve in SAS	*How to Solve in Stata*

1. Choose *falsepos* as the X variable and *sens* as the Y variable. Then, run the code.
`PROC SGPLOT DATA= cr_protein2;`
`SCATTER x = falsepos y = sens;`
`RUN;`
	1. Use a scatter command to make a scatterplot in Stata, specifying the Y variable first, *sens*, and the X variable, *falsepos*.
	`scatter sens falsepos`

2. Run the code to obtain the graph, as displayed in Figure 3.5.	2. Run the code to obtain the graph, as displayed in Figure 3.6.

Note: Remember that in SAS the results must be in HTML mode to automatically obtain the graph displayed in the Results Viewer window (if it is not displayed, go to *View/Results*, and navigate to the *sgplot* procedure that we just ran to open our graph).

D The researchers in this study concluded that a CRP level greater than 25 mg/L should prompt physicians to investigate for pneumonia, whereas a CRP level greater than 65 mg/L had the "highest diagnostic accuracy to justify consideration of this threshold as a diagnostic marker of poststroke pneumonia."[2] Should we agree with this choice? Why or why not?

Instructions for Example Problem 3.3: Part D

Displaying Cutoff Value Labels on Data Points of an ROC Curve	
How to Solve in SAS	*How to Solve in Stata*
In order to see which data points correspond to which cutoff values on our ROC curve we made using SAS, we can add a *datalabel = option* to our PROC SGPLOT code to show this. We are labeling the points with the *crp* variable (Figure 3.7).	In order to see which data points correspond to which cutoff values on our ROC curve we made using Stata, we can add an *mlabel* option to our scatter command to show this. We are labeling the points with the *crp* variable, which we put in parentheses after the *mlabel* option is specified (Figure 3.8).

`PROC SGPLOT DATA= cr_protein2;`
`SCATTER x = falsepos y = sens / datalabel=crp;`
`RUN;`
	`scatter sens falsepos, mlabel (crp)`

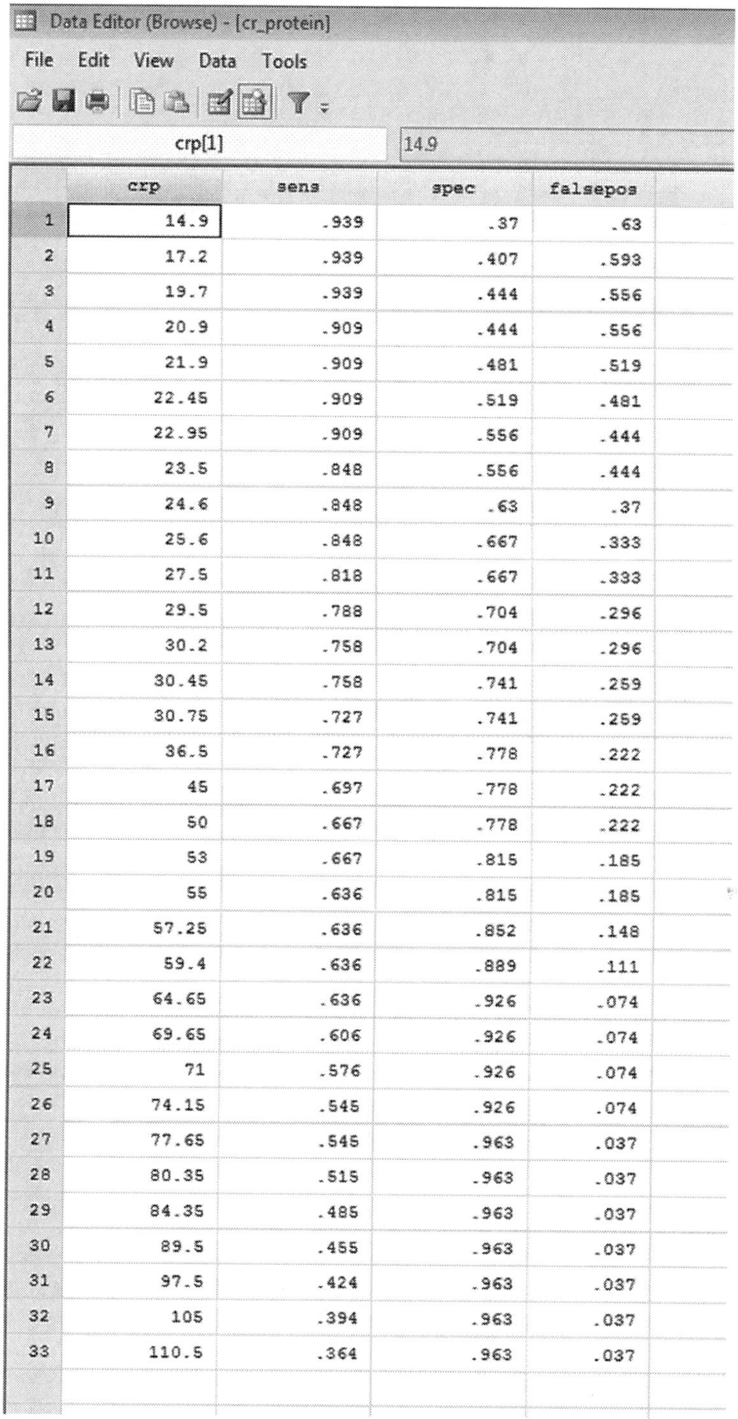

Data Editor (Browse) - [cr_protein]

File Edit View Data Tools

crp[1] 14.9

	crp	sens	spec	falsepos
1	14.9	.939	.37	.63
2	17.2	.939	.407	.593
3	19.7	.939	.444	.556
4	20.9	.909	.444	.556
5	21.9	.909	.481	.519
6	22.45	.909	.519	.481
7	22.95	.909	.556	.444
8	23.5	.848	.556	.444
9	24.6	.848	.63	.37
10	25.6	.848	.667	.333
11	27.5	.818	.667	.333
12	29.5	.788	.704	.296
13	30.2	.758	.704	.296
14	30.45	.758	.741	.259
15	30.75	.727	.741	.259
16	36.5	.727	.778	.222
17	45	.697	.778	.222
18	50	.667	.778	.222
19	53	.667	.815	.185
20	55	.636	.815	.185
21	57.25	.636	.852	.148
22	59.4	.636	.889	.111
23	64.65	.636	.926	.074
24	69.65	.606	.926	.074
25	71	.576	.926	.074
26	74.15	.545	.926	.074
27	77.65	.545	.963	.037
28	80.35	.515	.963	.037
29	84.35	.485	.963	.037
30	89.5	.455	.963	.037
31	97.5	.424	.963	.037
32	105	.394	.963	.037
33	110.5	.364	.963	.037

Figure 3.4 **Stata data view after creating *falsepos* variable.** The snapshot of our Stata data viewer shows the *falsepos* variable in the far right column. We can see that values have populated for all rows and that the values are equal to 1 – specificity.

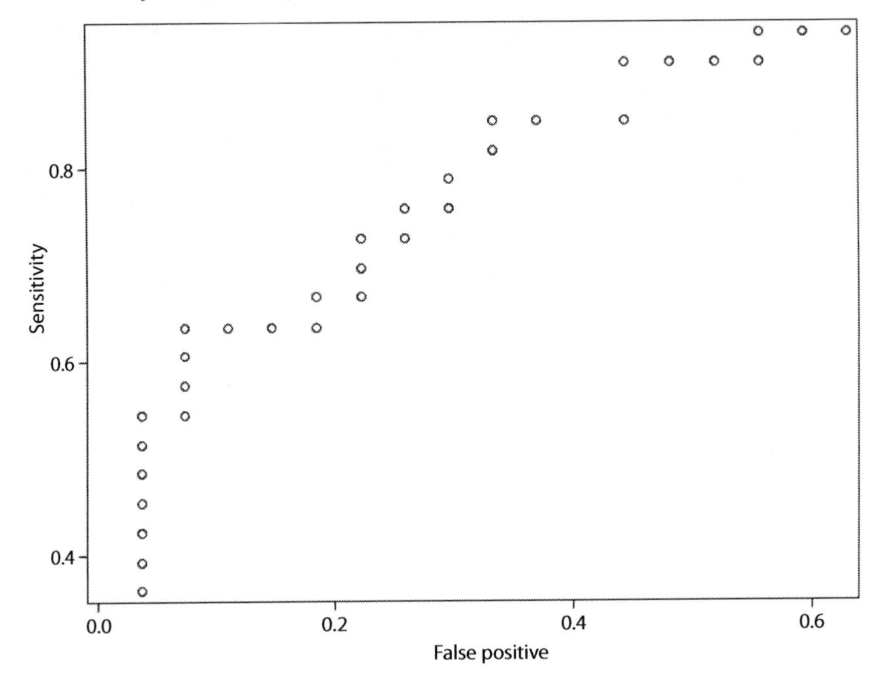

Figure 3.5 **ROC curve for CRP test for poststroke pneumonia from SAS.** The ROC curve made in SAS shows the sensitivity for the CRP test by the false positive values. The cutoff level for CRP that we would want to choose is the data point closest to the upper left-hand corner of the graph.

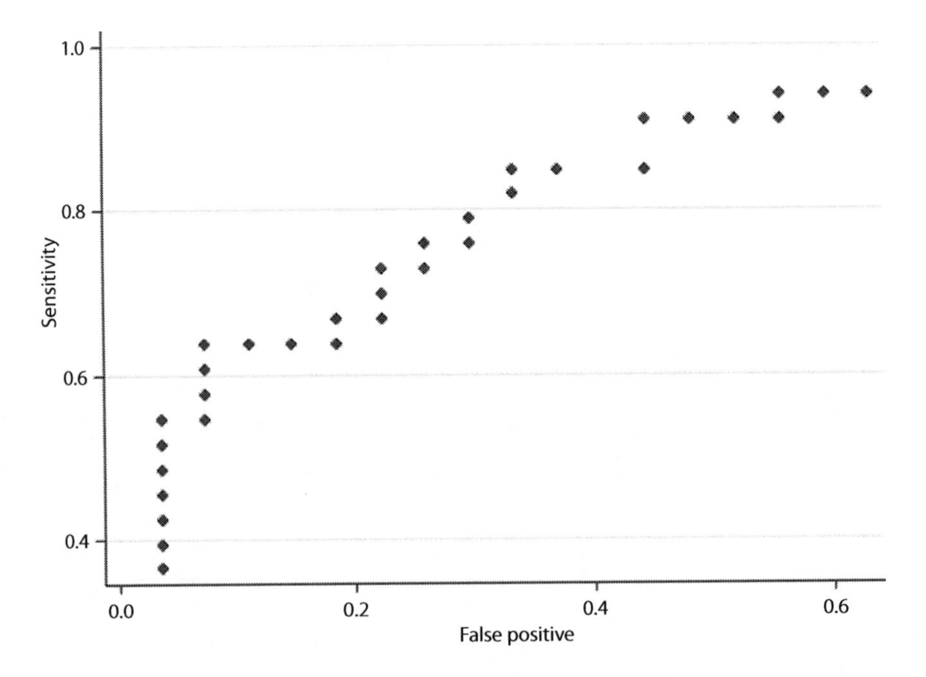

Figure 3.6 **ROC curve for CRP test for poststroke pneumonia from Stata.** The ROC curve made in Stata shows the sensitivity for the CRP test by the false positive values. The cutoff level for CRP that we would want to choose is the data point closest to the upper left-hand corner of the graph.

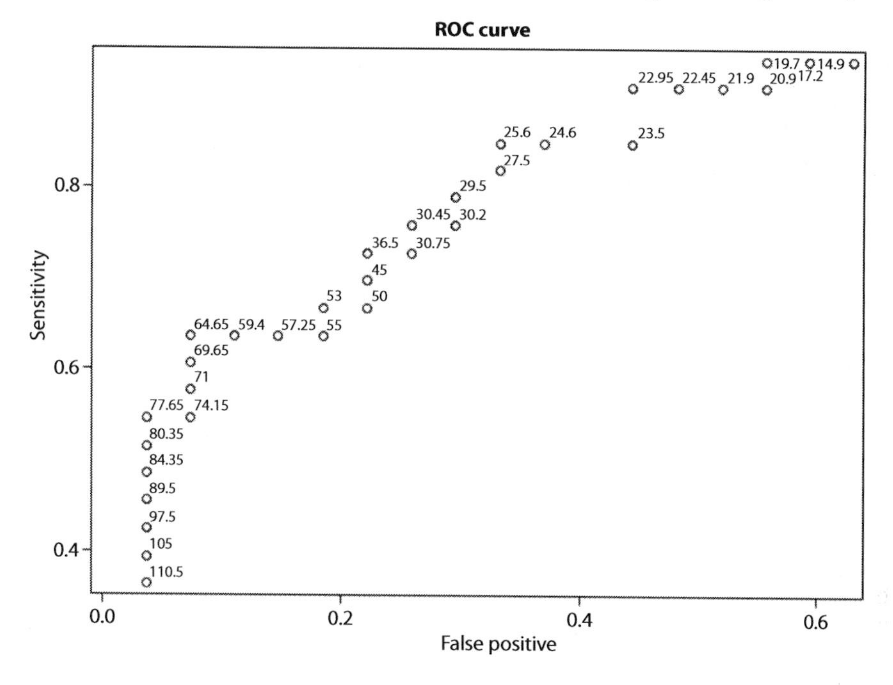

Figure 3.7 **Cutoff-labeled ROC curve for CRP test for poststroke pneumonia from SAS.** This ROC curve is the same as that presented in Figure 3.5; however, now we have data labels on our graph so that we can know which CRP cutoff value the data point is referring to.

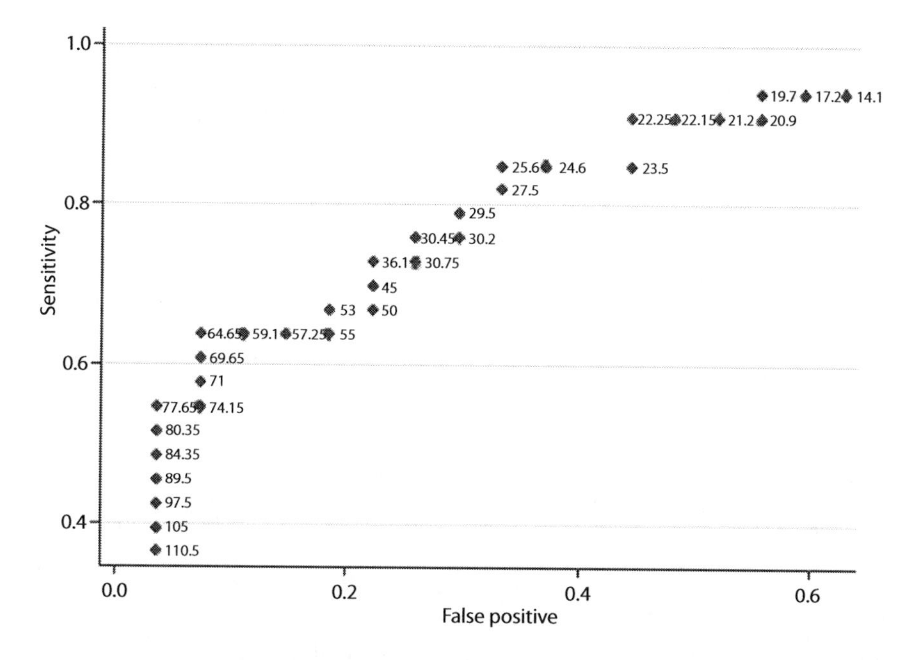

Figure 3.8 **Cutoff-labeled ROC curve for CRP test for poststroke pneumonia from Stata.** This ROC curve is the same as that presented in Figure 3.6; however, now we have data labels on our graph so that we can know which CRP cutoff value the data point is referring to.

When choosing a cutoff point, we want to choose a value that is in the upper left-hand corner of the graph that maximizes the sensitivity and minimizes the probability of a false positive result. The researchers concluded that 25 mg/L should prompt physicians to investigate for pneumonia, which makes sense in accordance with the graphs in Figure 3.7 (SAS version) and Figure 3.8 (Stata version), as the cutoff point of 25.6 mg/L maximizes sensitivity while minimizing false positives as much as possible. However, there is still a fairly high probability of false positives.

The researchers also concluded that 65 mg/L were associated with the highest diagnostic accuracy if considering CRP levels to diagnose poststroke pneumonia. Although sensitivity is not as high with 65 mg/L as it is with 25 mg/L, the probability of a false positive result is much lower.

PRACTICE PROBLEM 3.1

One study completed in Suffolk County, New York, was conducted to investigate self-reported measures of racial or ethnic neighborhood composition, as compared to census data.[3] The study showed that for Hispanic individuals who reported a "mostly white" neighborhood, the sensitivity of the measure was 0.91, and the specificity was 0.77.

A What is the probability of a false negative result?

B What is the probability of a false positive result?

In the same study, the researchers also showed that for black individuals who reported a "mostly white" neighborhood, 0.16 was the false positive rate, and 0.22 was the false negative rate.[3]

A What is the sensitivity?

B What is the specificity?

PRACTICE PROBLEM 3.2

During 2015, there was an ongoing Ebola virus disease outbreak in Sierra Leone. In order to best identify patients who had Ebola, one study proposed the Cepheid GeneXpert Ebola assay (Cepheid, Sunnyvale, California) in whole blood as a better way to test for Ebola than the standard reverse transcription polymerase chain reaction (RT-PCR) assay (also known as the Trombley assay), which was then the standard.[4] The 22 people who had Ebola according to the Trombley assay were confirmed to have the virus with the GeneXpert Ebola assay. The number of people who did not have Ebola according to the Trombley assay was 189, and of those 189, 181 tested negative for Ebola using the GeneXpert Ebola assay.[4]

A What is the sensitivity of the GeneXpert Ebola assay test?

B What is the specificity of the GeneXpert Ebola assay test?

C Suppose that the probability of having Ebola at a given time in a small village in Sierra Leone was 0.04. What is the probability that an individual in this village has Ebola given that his or her GeneXpert Ebola assay is positive?

D What is the name for the probability found in Part C?

E After the initial testing of the whole blood samples, the authors state that seven of the eight samples that had a negative result for the Trombley assay but a positive result for the Gene Xpert assay had been follow-up tests from an originally positive Trombley assay. Assuming that these seven samples should not have been included in the calculation of the specificity of the Gene Xpert assay, how does the value of specificity change from the previous value in Part B?

PRACTICE PROBLEM 3.3

Table 3.5 shows data taken from a study investigating a score for predicting individuals at risk for vitamin D deficiency. For a number of different cutoff points of the score, the observed sensitivities and specificities are given.[5]

Table 3.5 Vitamin D risk cutoff scores

Vitamin D risk score	*Sensitivity*	*Specificity*
≥12	0.03	0.99
≥11	0.07	0.99
≥10	0.12	0.97
≥9	0.27	0.88
≥8	0.38	0.81
≥7	0.61	0.66
≥6	0.74	0.50
≥5	0.82	0.36
≥4	0.93	0.20
≥3	0.98	0.10
≥2	0.99	0.08

Source: Deschasaux, M., Souberbielle, J.-C., Andreeva, V. A. et al., *Medicine (Baltimore)*, 2016;95(7).

Note: Vitamin D Risk Score cutoff levels and the sensitivity and specificity values for each level are presented. Use these values to solve Practice Problem 3.3.

A As the cutoff point for the score gets lower, how does the probability of a false positive result change?

B How does the probability of a false negative result change?

C Plot an ROC curve in SAS or Stata.

D Based on the ROC curve, what cutoff point would be good to use? Why?

PRACTICE PROBLEM 3.4

Detecting colorectal cancer early is very important. In a review on stool-based pyruvate kinase isoenzyme M2 (M2-PK) as a diagnostic tool for colorectal cancer, researchers found an average sensitivity of 0.79 and an average specificity of 0.80.[6]

A In 2013, the estimated prevalence of colorectal cancer in the USA[7,8] was 0.37%. Considering the sensitivity and specificity values of M2-PK, what is the predictive value of a positive test result?

B How does this predictive value change with a prevalence of 5%?

C How does this predictive value change with a prevalence of 10%?

D The authors of the review reported that they obtained a confidence interval of (0.73–0.83) for sensitivity and (0.73–0.86) for specificity.[6] What would the positive predictive value be if the sensitivity and specificity were at the upper ends of the confidence intervals, at (0.83 and 0.86), respectively? How does the positive predictive value compare to what we found in Part (A)? Use 0.37% as the prevalence.

E Construct a diagram illustrating the results of the diagnostic testing process. Assume that you start with a population of 1,000,000 individuals residing in the United States and that the prevalence of colorectal cancer in the United States is 0.37%.

PRACTICE PROBLEM 3.5

Prostate cancer can be detected using various medical tests. Three of these tests are the digital rectal examination (DRE), the transrectal ultrasound (TRUS), and the

Table 3.6 Results of tests of prostate cancer by test type

Test type	*People with cancer, no.*	*People without cancer, no.*	*Positive results of those with cancer, no.*	*Negative results of those without cancer, no.*
DRE	199	9320	77	8981
TRUS	200	9313	131	8606
PSA	195	9000	135	8059

Source: Mettlin, C., Murphy, G. P., Babaian, R. J. et al., *Cancer*, 77(1), 150–159, 1996.

Note: The table shows the results of three prostate cancer tests (i.e., digital rectal examination [DRE], transrectal ultrasound [TRUS], and prostate-specific antigen [PSA]) and the corresponding numbers of people with and without cancer and with positive and negative results. Use these numbers to solve Practice Problem 3.5.

prostate-specific antigen (PSA) test. The data in Table 3.6 were obtained from a study in which researchers reviewed the diagnostic properties of these tests.[9]

Suppose that researchers were trying to choose between the three tests for suspected prostate cancer on the basis of the results of this review.

A What are the sensitivity and specificity of the DRE?

B What are the sensitivity and specificity of the TRUS?

C What are the sensitivity and specificity of the PSA test?

D Which test would you consider most ideal based only on the sensitivity and specificity of each test? Why?

References

1. Lyons SA, Kaphingst KA, Goodman MS. Validating self-reported survey measures using SAS. Paper presented at SAS 2014 Global Forum; March 23–26, 2014; Nashville, TN. http://support.sas.com/resources/papers/proceedings14/1675-2014.pdf. Accessed August 4, 2016.
2. Warusevitane A, Karunatilake D, Sim J, Smith C, Roffe C. Early diagnosis of pneumonia in severe stroke: Clinical features and the diagnostic role of C-reactive protein. *PLoS One*. 2016;11(3):e0150269. doi:10.1371/journal.pone.0150269.
3. Hidalgo B, Kaphingst KA, Stafford J, Lachance C, Goodman MS. Diagnostic accuracy of self-reported racial composition of residential neighborhood. *Ann Epidemiol*. 2015;25(8):597–604. doi:10.1016/j.annepidem.2015.04.003.
4. Semper AE, Broadhurst MJ, Richards J et al. Performance of the GeneXpert Ebola assay for diagnosis of Ebola virus disease in Sierra Leone: A field evaluation study. *PLoS Med*. 2016;13(3):e1001980. doi:10.1371/journal.pmed.1001980.
5. Deschasaux M, Souberbielle J-C, Andreeva VA et al. Quick and easy screening for vitamin D insufficiency in adults: A scoring system to be implemented in daily clinical practice. *Medicine (Baltimore)*. 2016;95(7). doi:10.1097/MD.0000000000002783.
6. Uppara M, Adaba F, Askari A et al. A systematic review and meta-analysis of the diagnostic accuracy of pyruvate kinase M2 isoenzymatic assay in diagnosing colorectal cancer. *World J Surg Oncol*. 2015;13:48. doi:10.1186/s12957-015-0446-4.

7. SEER stat fact sheets: Colon and rectum cancer. National Cancer Institute website. http://seer.cancer.gov/statfacts/html/colorect.html. Accessed August 9, 2016.
8. U.S. and world population clock. United States Census Bureau website. http://www.census.gov/popclock/. Accessed August 9, 2016.
9. Mettlin C, Murphy GP, Babaian RJ et al. The results of a five-year early prostate cancer detection intervention. Investigators of the American Cancer Society National Prostate Cancer Detection Project. *Cancer*. 1996;77(1):150–159. doi:10.1002/(sici)1097-0142(19960101)77:1<150::aid-cncr25>3.0.co;2-3.

4 Discrete probability distributions

This chapter will discuss problems that can be put in a probabilistic framework, and the following topics will be discussed:

- Measures of location and spread for random variables
- Permutations and combinations
- Binomial distribution
- Poisson distribution

Terms

- Bernoulli trial (a Bernoulli random variable)
- binomial distribution
- continuous random variable
- dichotomous random variable
- discrete random variable
- factorials
- longitudinal studies
- permutations
- person-year
- Poisson distribution (distribution of rare events)
- probability mass function (probability distribution)
- random variable

Introduction

In Chapter 2, we introduced probability and some basic tools used when working with probabilities. In this chapter, we introduce some basic definitions that are essential to the understanding of statistics. These basic definitions will be incorporated throughout this chapter and will be used later in this workbook. We will introduce the concept of probability distributions with a focus on discrete probability distributions. Continuous probability distributions will be explored in Chapter 5.

Random Variable: A numeric function that assigns probabilities to different events in sample space.

Discrete Random Variable: A random variable for which there exists a discrete set of values with specified probabilities.

Examples of discrete random variables

- The number of cases of Zika virus in South America in the past five years
- The birth order of infants born in Suffolk County, New York, in 2000

Continuous Random Variable: A random variable whose possible values cannot be enumerated.

Examples of continuous random variables

- Weights of the members of a basketball team
- Annual budget (US$) for Departments of Public Health, by U.S. state

Probability Mass Function: A mathematical relationship, or rule, that assigns to any possible value r of a discrete random variable X the $P(X = r)$. This assignment is made for all values r that have positive probability. The probability mass function is sometimes called the *probability distribution*.

For any probability mass function, the probability of any particular value must be between 0 and 1.

- $0 < P(X = r) \leq 1$
- The sum of the probabilities of all values must equal exactly $1 \rightarrow \sum P(X = r) = 1$

Measures of location and spread for random variables

In Chapter 1, we talked about measures of location and spread for samples of data. Here, we take those same concepts and apply them to random variables.

The expected value of a discrete random variable is defined as

$$E(X) = \mu = \sum_{i=1}^{R} r_i \, P(X = r_i) \tag{4.1}$$

where $r_i'^s$ are the values the random variable assumes with positive probability. Remember, μ is the population mean.

The variance of a discrete random variable, denoted by $Var(X)$, is defined by

$$Var(X) = \sigma^2 = \sum_{i=1}^{R} (r_i - \mu)^2 P(X = r_i) \tag{4.2}$$

where $r_i'^s$ are the values for which the random variable takes on positive probabilities and where σ^2 is the population variance.

- The standard deviation of a random variable X, denoted by $sd(X)$ or σ, is defined by the square root of the variance.
- The cumulative distribution function (CDF) of a random variable X is denoted by $F(X)$ and, for a specific value r of X, is defined by $P(X \leq r)$.

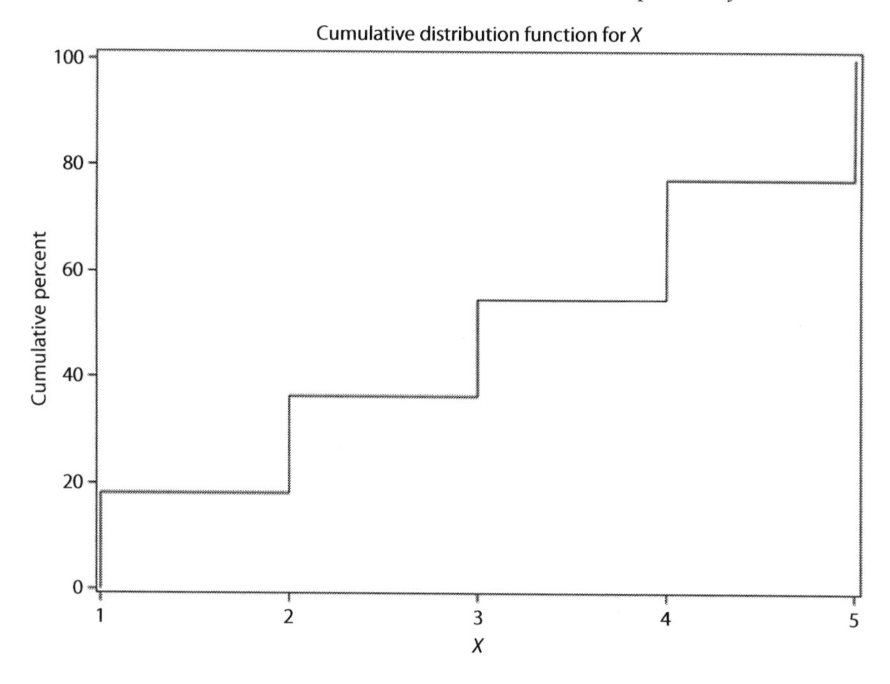

Figure 4.1 **Cumulative distribution function for a discrete random variable.** The cumulative distribution function for a discrete random variable is a step function.

- CDF is a step function for discrete random variables (Figure 4.1).
- CDF shows a smooth continuous curve for continuous random variables (Figure 4.2).

Permutations and combinations

Factorials: Represented with an exclamation point (!); n factorial would be written as $n!$ and is defined as $n \times (n-1) \times \ldots \times 2 \times 1$.

The quantity 0! has no intuitive meaning, but it is defined as 1 (0! = 1).

Permutations: The number of permutations of n things taken k at a time is ${}_nP_k = n \times (n-1) \times \ldots \times (n-k+1)$. A permutation represents the number of ways of selecting k items out of n, where the order of selection is important. Permutations can be expressed in terms of factorials as follows:

$$ {}_nP_k = \frac{n!}{(n-k)!} \tag{4.3} $$

Combinations: The number of combinations represent the number of ways of selecting k objects out of n where the order of selection does not matter. The formula for calculating n things taken k at a time is the following:

$$ {}_nC_k = \binom{n}{k} = \frac{n(n-1)\times\ldots\times(n-k+1)}{k!} \tag{4.4} $$

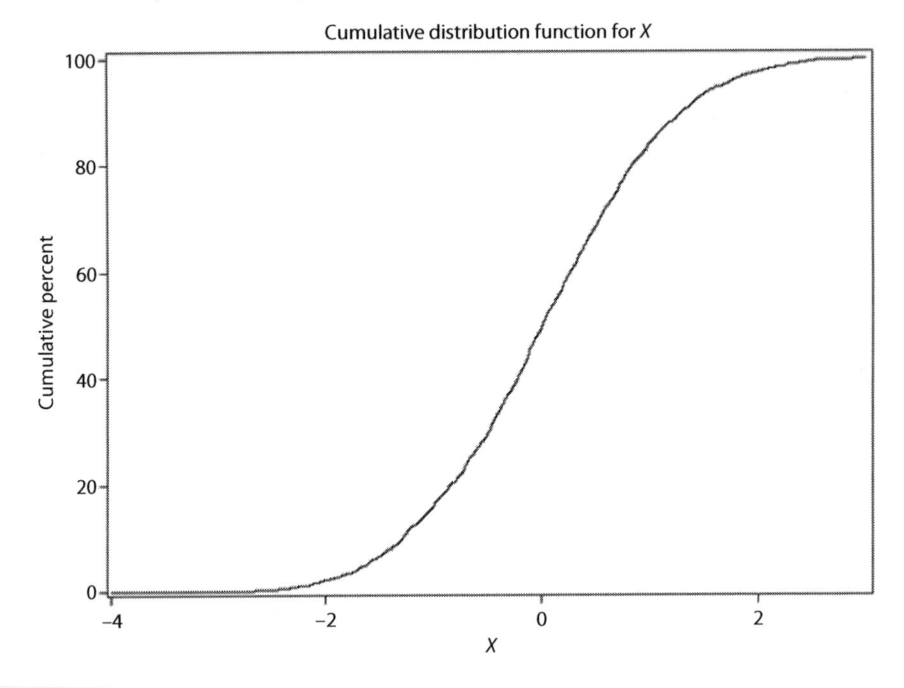

Figure 4.2 **Cumulative distribution function for a continuous random variable.** The cumulative distribution function for a continuous random variable is a smooth continuous curve.

In this workbook, we will use the more common notation for combinations $\binom{n}{k}$. In words, this is expressed as "*n* choose *k*."

Properties of combinations:

$$\binom{n}{0} = 1 \text{ for any } n$$

$$\binom{n}{k} = \binom{n}{n-k}$$

Dichotomous Random Variable: *Y* must assume one of two possible values. These mutually exclusive outcomes could represent life or death, heads or tails, adult or child, sick or healthy, and so on. For simplicity, they are commonly referred to as *failure* or *success*. A dichotomous random variable of this type is known as a *Bernoulli random variable.*[1]

Bernoulli Trial: A type of random variable that takes the value 1 with probability p and the value 0 with a probability $q = 1 - p$.

EXAMPLE PROBLEM 4.1

Suppose that we have a hospital with six trauma rooms in the ER, each with a patient inside who needs to be seen by a physician.

A In how many ways can we order when the patients are seen?

$$6! = 6 \times 5 \times 4 \times 3 \times 2 \times 1 = 720$$

B If the order in which the patients are seen is *not* important, in how many ways can we select two of the six patients in trauma rooms? What is another name for this?

The term for this is the *number of combinations*. In the following example, $n = 6$, and $k = 2$:

$${}_nC_k = \begin{pmatrix} n \\ k \end{pmatrix} = \frac{n!}{k!(n-k)!} = \frac{6!}{2!(6-2)!} = \frac{720}{2 \times 24} = 15$$

C If the order in which the patients are seen is important, in how many ways can we select two of the six patients in trauma rooms? What is another term for this?

The term for this is the *number of permutations*. Again, $n = 6$, and $k = 2$.

$${}_nP_k = \frac{n!}{(n-k)!} = \frac{6!}{(6-2)!} = \frac{720}{24} = 30$$

Binomial distribution

Binomial Distribution: The distribution of the number of successes in n statistically independent trials, where the probability of success on each trail is p. Binomial distribution has the probability mass function given by the following formula:

$$P(X = x) = \begin{pmatrix} n \\ x \end{pmatrix} p^x (1-p)^{n-x} \text{ for } x = 0,1,2 \ldots n \text{ and n} = 1,2 \ldots \tag{4.5}$$

$$P(x \textit{ successes}) = \begin{pmatrix} \# \textit{ of trials} \\ \# \textit{ of successes} \end{pmatrix} p^{\# \textit{ of successes}} (1-p)^{\# \textit{ of trials} - \# \textit{ of successes}}$$

Properties of the binomial distribution

- A sample has a fixed number of trials, n, each with one of two mutually exclusive outcomes.
- Each trial has a constant probability of success, p.
- The outcome of each trial is independent.

Parameters of binomial distribution

- p = probability of success ($0 \leq p \leq 1$).
- n = number of trials (0, 1, 2 . . ., n).
- The expected value of successes in n trials is simply the probability of success in 1 trial multiplied by n. The expected value of a binomial random variable is np.
- The variance of a binomial random variable is $np(1 - p)$.
- The binomial distribution is used with discrete random variables.
- A Bernoulli trial is a special case of the binomial random variable where $n = 1$.
- The binomial distribution is the sum of Bernoulli (dichotomous or binary) random variables that have only two mutually exclusive and exhaustive outcomes (e.g., life/death, sick/healthy, success/failure).
- The binomial distribution represents the number of successes in n trials.
- The distribution is skewed for all p, except $p = 0.5$, which has a symmetric distribution.

BOX 4.1 HELPFUL HINT FOR MUTUALLY EXCLUSIVE AND EXHAUSTIVE SETS

Use probability statement complements for mutually exclusive and exhaustive sets. For example,

$P(X > 3) = 1 - P(X < 3)$	*(continuous)*
$P(X > 3) = P(X \geq 4) = 1 - P(X \leq 3)$	*(discrete)*
$P(X \geq 3) = 1 - P(X < 3)$	*(continuous)*
$P(X \geq 3) = 1 - P(X \leq 2)$	*(discrete)*

For continuous random variables $P(X \leq 3) = P(X < 3)$ and $P(X \geq 3) = P(X > 3)$ because $P(X = x) = 0$.

EXAMPLE PROBLEM 4.2

In the United States, in accordance with the NHANES survey (2009–2012),[2] 7.6% of the population age 12 and older had depression during the survey period. The rate of depression was reported to vary by income level; 15% of the population who were living below the federal poverty line had depression, and 6.2% of the population living above the federal poverty line had depression.[2] Suppose that we have a sample of five unrelated people living below the poverty line. Let X be the random variable denoting how many of the five people living below the poverty line have depression.

A Why would the binomial distribution provide an appropriate model?

The binomial distribution would provide an appropriate model because there are two mutually exclusive outcomes (has depression or does not have depression), there are a fixed number of trials (5), the events are independent (whether one person has depression does not depend on whether others have depression), and there is a constant p of "success" (in this example, $p = 0.15$).

B What are the parameters of the distribution of the values of *X*?

$n = 5$ and $p = 0.15$

C List the possible values for X.

The possible values for *X* are 0, 1, 2, 3, 4, and 5.

D What is the mean number of people who will have depression?

$$Mean = np = 5 \times 0.15 = 0.75$$

An average, we expect $<1(0.75)$ of the 5 people to have depression

E What is the typical departure from this mean number? (The *typical departure from the mean* refers to the standard deviation.)

$$Standard\ Deviation = \sqrt{np(1-p)} = \sqrt{5 \times 0.15 \times 0.85} = \sqrt{0.6375} = 0.798$$

F In how many ways can the five people be ordered?

$$5! = 5 \times 4 \times 3 \times 2 \times 1 = 120$$

G Without regard to order, in how many ways can you select one person from this group of 5?

$$_nC_k = \binom{n}{k} = \frac{n!}{k!(n-k)!} = \frac{5!}{1!(5-1)!} = \frac{120}{1 \times 24} = 5$$

H What is the probability that exactly one person has depression? First, use the formula. Then, use the binomial probability table (Appendix Table A.1), and compare.

$$P(X = 1) = \binom{n}{x} p^x (1-p)^{n-x} = \binom{5}{1} 0.15^1 (1-0.15)^{5-1}$$

$$= 5 \times (0.15) \times (0.85)^4 = 5(0.15)(0.522) = 0.3915$$

In accordance with the binomial probabilities table found in the Appendix Table A.1, we have $n = 5$ and $x = 1$, with $p = 0.15$. In the table, we find 5 in the *n* column, 1 in the *k* column, and 0.15 across the top of the table. We see that the probability is 0.3915, the same as what we found using the formula. We can also solve Part (H) of Problem 4.2 by using SAS or Stata. Both have functions that allow us to calculate binomial probabilities using the information that we have been provided.

Instructions for Using SAS or Stata to Find a Binomial Probability

How to Solve in SAS

SAS Code

```
DATA prob4_2h;
      prob=PROBBNML(0.15,5,1) -
           PROBBNML(0.15,5,0);
RUN;
PROC PRINT DATA=prob4_2h;
RUN;
```

SAS Output

Observation	Probability
1	0.39150

The PROBBNML function in SAS gives us the probability that the number of successes is less than or equal to a specified number, under a binomial distribution with parameters n and p.

In this example, we have a probability of success (having depression) of 0.15 and an n of five people, and we want to know the probability that exactly one person will have depression. Because SAS gives us the probability of less than or equal to a number, we must use two functions and subtract the probabilities. Thus, in the above code, we are finding prob = $P(X \leq 1) - P(X \leq 0)$, which equals $P(X = 1)$.

We, then, use PROC PRINT to print our resulting probability and get the above output.

How to Solve in Stata

Stata Code

```
display binomialp(5,1,0.15)
```

Stata Output

.39150469

The *binomialp* function in Stata gives us the binomial probability that we will see a certain number of successes—in this example, one case of depression when we have n = 5 and a probability of success (having depression) of 0.15.

There is also a function binomial(n,x,p) that would give us the probability that we would see x or fewer successes, when we have our parameters n and p.

I **What is the probability that none of the people will have depression? First, use the formula. Then, use the binomial table (Appendix Table A.1), and compare.**

$$P(X=0)=\binom{n}{x}p^x(1-p)^{n-x}=\binom{5}{0}0.15^0(1-0.15)^{5-0}=1(1)(0.85)^5=0.4437$$

Using the binomial probabilities table found in the Appendix, we have n = 5 and x = 0, with p = 0.15. In the table, we find 5 in the n column, 0 in the k column, and 0.15 across the top of the table. We see that the probability is 0.4437, the same as what we found using the formula.

J What is the probability that all five of the people will have depression? First, use the formula. Then, use the binomial table (Appendix Table A.1), and compare.

$$P(X=5)=\binom{n}{x}p^{x}(1-p)^{n-x}=\binom{5}{5}0.15^{0}(1-0.15)^{5-5}=1(0.0000759)(1)=0.0001$$

In accordance with the binomial probabilities table found in the Appendix, we have $n = 5$ and $x = 5$, with $p = 0.15$. In the table, we find 5 in the n column, 5 in the k column, and 0.15 across the top of the table. We see that the probability is 0.0001, the same as what we found using the formula and rounding to four decimal places.

K What is the probability that at least three of the people have depression (use binomial table in the Appendix)?

$$P(X \geq 3) = P(X=3)+P(X=4)+P(X=5)$$
$$=0.0244+0.0022+0.0001=0.0267$$

L What is the probability that no more than one of the people has depression (use the binomial table in the Appendix)?

$$P(X \leq 1) = P(X=0)+P(X=1)=0.4437+0.3915=0.8352$$

M If we observed that all five people have depression, would we consider that such an event is rare enough to reassess the assumption of 15% probability?

Since we know that $P(X = 5) = 0.0001$ if $p = 0.15$—meaning that all five would get the disease 0.01% of the time—we should reassess the assumption of $p = 0.15$, given the reality that all five have the disease and given that the probability of that occurring with this assumption is very rare. It is likely that p would be greater than 0.15.

BOX 4.2 UNDERSTANDING PART (M) OF PROBLEM 4.2

To better understand this, let's look at two scenarios: (1) what would happen if $p = 0.25$ and (2) what would happen if $p = 0.50$.

Scenario 1: $p = 0.25$

$P(X = 5) = 0.001$ (from binomial table) → so all five would get the disease 0.1% of the time, which is higher than the 0.01% when $p = 0.15$.

Scenario 2: $p = 0.50$

$P(X = 5) = 0.0313$ (from binomial table) → so all five would get the disease 3% of the time, which is again higher than the 0.01% when $p = 0.15$ and the 0.1% when $p = 0.25$.

As p increases, the probability of all five having the disease also increases.

PRACTICE PROBLEM 4.1

In Chapter 2, we saw a table of diabetes prevalence by race or ethnicity and education level (Table 2.4).[3] Consider a group of five individuals selected from the population of non-Hispanic whites with a high school diploma or general education diploma (GED) in the United States. The number of persons in this sample who have diabetes is a binomial random variable with parameters $n = 5$ and $p = 0.081$.

A If you wish to make a list of the five persons chosen, in how many ways can they be ordered?

B Without regard to order, in how many ways can you select three individuals from this group of five?

C What is the probability that exactly three of the individuals in the sample have diabetes?

D What is the probability that two of them have diabetes?

Poisson distribution

Poisson Distribution: A discrete probability distribution commonly used with variables that represent a count or rate—for example, the number of visits to a clinic in one week.

The Poisson distribution is the second most frequently used discrete distribution after the binomial distribution. The Poisson distribution is usually associated with rare events and is also known as the *distribution of rare events*.

Poisson distribution properties

- The probability that an event occurs in the interval is proportional to the length of the interval.
- An infinite number of occurrences are possible.
- Events occur independently at rate λ.
- The probability of x events occurring in a time period t for a Poisson random variable with parameter λ is

$$P(X = x) = \frac{e^{-\lambda}\lambda^{x}}{x!}, \ldots x = 0, 1, 2, \ldots \tag{4.6}$$

where e is approximately 2.718 (Euler's number).
- For a Poisson distribution with parameter λ, the mean and variance are both equal to λ.
- If we have a dataset from a discrete distribution where the mean and variance are about the same, then we can preliminarily identify it is a Poisson distribution and use various tests to confirm this hypothesis.

- Since we are looking at a rate, there is an effect of time as well. If we look at the same town with the same population, but for 2 years rather than one, the value of λ must be doubled. Often, this is not mentioned because the length of the time of interest matches the length from the rate.
- The Poisson distribution is used with discrete random variables and represents the number of events in a specified interval/cross-section of time/space.
- The shape of the distribution can be skewed or symmetric.

Poisson distribution estimation

The following definitions will be helpful in our understanding of the estimation of the Poisson distribution:

> ***Person-Year:*** A person-year is a unit of time defined as one person being followed for one year. This unit of follow-up time is commonly used in longitudinal studies.
> ***Longitudinal Studies:*** Studies in which the same individual is followed over time.

- Let's assume the number of events X over T person-years is a Poisson distribution with parameters $\mu = \lambda T$.
- An unbiased estimator of λ is given by $\hat{\lambda} = \frac{X}{T}$, where X is the observed number of events over T person-years and λ is the incidence rate per T person-years.
- The Poisson distribution has a mean $= \lambda$, variance $= \lambda$, and standard deviation $= \sqrt{\lambda}$.
- It can take on possible values 0, 1, 2, 3, …., ∞.

EXAMPLE PROBLEM 4.3

In Missouri in 2014, there were 1067 drug overdose deaths. This equates to a rate of about 2.9 drug overdose deaths per day.[4] Let X denote the number of drug overdose deaths per day in Missouri.

A **Why would the Poisson distribution provide an appropriate model?**

The Poisson distribution would provide an appropriate model because we have independent events and a number of events over time.

B **What is the parameter of the distribution for X?**

The parameter of the distribution for X is $\lambda = 2.9$ deaths/day.

C **What are possible values of X?**

The possible values of X are 0, 1, 2, … , ∞.

D **What is the mean number of drug overdose deaths in Missouri in a one-day period?**

$Mean = \lambda = 2.9$

E What is the typical departure from this mean number?

$$\textit{Standard deviation} = \sqrt{\lambda} = \sqrt{2.9} = 1.7$$

F What is the probability that no drug overdose deaths will occur in Missouri on a given day?

$$P(X=0) = \frac{e^{-\lambda}\lambda^{x}}{x!} = \frac{e^{-2.9} \times 2.9^{0}}{0!} = \frac{0.05502 \times 1}{1} = 0.05502$$

BOX 4.3 USING POISSON PROBABILITY TABLES

Suppose that we wanted to use the Poisson probability tables (see Appendix Table A.2) to find the probability that no drug overdose deaths will occur in Missouri in a given day.

- Looking at the Poisson probabilities table, we find 0 in the *k* column, which is on the left-hand side of the table.
- We see that across the top of the table, we have only values of 2.5 and 3.
- The probabilities for those are 0.0821 and 0.0498, respectively.
- Therefore, we know the actual probability is between 0.0821 and 0.0498, closer to 0.0498 because 2.9 is closer to 3.
- Using the formula, we found the exact probability = 0.05502 (in Part F of Problem 4.4).
- The exact probability, 0.05502, is between 0.0821 and 0.0498 and closer to 0.0498 as we expect.
- If λ would have been equal to 3, then we simply would have found our probability to be 0.0498, using the Poisson table.
- Let's check this with the equation:

$$P(X=0) = \frac{e^{-\lambda}\lambda^{x}}{x!} = \frac{e^{-3} \times 3^{0}}{0!} = \frac{0.0498 \times 1}{1} = 0.0498$$

- The calculated value, 0.0498, is the same as the value we determined using the table.

G What is the probability that exactly four drug overdose deaths will occur in Missouri on a given day?

$$P(X=4)=\frac{e^{-\lambda}\lambda^{x}}{x!}=\frac{e^{-2.9}\times 2.9^{4}}{4!}=\frac{0.05502\times 70.73}{24}=0.162$$

H What is the probability that no more than four drug overdose deaths will occur in Missouri on a given day?

$$P(X\leq 4)=P(X=0)+P(X=1)+P(X=2)+P(X=3)+P(X=4)$$

$P(X=0) = 0.05502$ (from Part F)
$P(X=4) = 0.162$ (from Part G)

$$P(X=1)=\frac{e^{-2.9}\times 2.9^{1}}{1!}=\frac{0.159558}{1!}=0.159558$$

$$P(X=2)=\frac{e^{-2.9}\times 2.9^{2}}{2!}=\frac{0.4627}{2!}=0.23135$$

$$P(X=3)=\frac{e^{-2.9}\times 2.9^{3}}{3!}=\frac{1.34188}{6!}=0.22365$$

$$P(X\leq 4)=P(X=0)+P(X=1)+P(X=2)+P(X=3)+P(X=4)$$
$$=0.05502+0.159558+0.23135+0.22365+0.162=0.8316$$

Instructions for Using SAS or Stata to Find a Poisson Probability

We can also solve Example Problem 4.3—Part (H) by using SAS or Stata. Both have functions that allow us to calculate Poisson probabilities using the information we have been provided.

Using SAS

SAS Code

```
DATA prob4_4h;
     prob=POISSON(2.9,4);
RUN;
PROC PRINT DATA=prob4_4h;
RUN;
```

SAS Output

Observation	Probability
1	0.83178

The POISSON function in SAS gives us the probability that the rate is less than or equal to a specified number. Inside the parentheses of the function, we insert the mean of the Poisson distribution (in this example, 2.9) and the rate we want the probability being less than or equal to (in this example, 4).

We, then, use PROC PRINT to print our resulting probability and obtain the above output.

Using Stata

Stata Code

```
display poisson(2.9,4)
```

Stata Output

```
.83177708
```

The Poisson function in Stata gives us the probability of observing a rate of 4 or less (in this case, deaths per day) under a Poisson distribution with a mean of 2.9.

Similar to the binomial function we saw previously in this chapter, there is also a poissonp(λ,x) function that would give us the probability of observing a rate (x), under a Poisson distribution with a mean (λ).

I What is the probability that at least six drug overdose deaths will occur in Missouri on a given day?

$$P(X \geq 6) = 1 - P(X < 6) = 1 - P(X \leq 5) = 1 - \left[P(X = 5) + P(X \leq 4)\right] = 1 - \left(\left[\frac{e^{-2.9} \times 2.9^5}{5!}\right] + 0.8316\right) = 1 - 0.92564 = 0.074$$

J What is the number of drug overdose deaths such that the chance of seeing at least that many on a given day is less than 1 in 20?

We need to find r such that $P(X \leq r) < 0.05$. We already know that $P(X \geq 6) = 0.074$, which is close to 0.05, but not under.

We need to figure out what $P(X \geq 7)$ is.

$$P(X \geq 7) = 1 - P(X < 7) = 1 - P(X \leq 6) = 1 - \left[P(X = 6) + P(X = 5) + P(X \leq 4)\right] = 1 - \left(\left[\frac{e^{-2.9} \times 2.9^6}{6!}\right] + 0.9404 + 0.8316\right) = 1 - 97109 = 0.0289$$

Since $P(X \geq 7)$ is less than 0.05 and $P(X \geq 6)$ is more than 0.05, we can conclude that six is the minimum number of drug overdose deaths—such that the chance of seeing at least that many on a given day is less than 1 in 20.

RECAP

- Probability distributions show the probability associated with the possible outcomes.
- Binomial distribution is used to find the probability of x successes in n trials when the trials are independent and have the same probability.
- Poisson distribution is used to find the probability of x successes when the n is large and the p is small.

PRACTICE PROBLEM 4.2

The *New York Times* reported that there are approximately 27 gun homicides per day in the United States and approximately five gun homicides per day in Canada, after adjusting for population size differences.[5]

A What is the probability that no one will die of a gun homicide on a given day in the United States?

B What is the probability that no one will die of a gun homicide on a given day in Canada?

C What is the probability that, at most, five gun homicides will happen in Canada on a given day?

D What is the probability that seven or more gun homicides will be happen in Canada on a given day?

PRACTICE PROBLEM 4.3

Review the properties of the binomial distribution.

A What are the two parameters that characterize a binomial distribution?

B What are the possible values of the two parameters named in Practice Problem 4.3—Part (A)?

C What are the assumptions of the binomial distribution?

D What are the mean, variance, and standard deviation of the binomial distribution?

PRACTICE PROBLEM 4.4

According to the National Institutes of Health (NIH),[6] in 2014, about 71% of people aged 18 and older reported that they drank alcohol in the past year.

A Suppose that you select nine individuals from this population. In how many ways can these nine persons be ordered?

B If order was important, in how many ways can you select three individuals from this group of nine?

C What is the probability that exactly four of the nine persons have consumed alcohol in the past year?

D What is the probability that at least seven of the nine persons have consumed alcohol in the past year?

E What is the probability that at most two individuals have consumed alcohol in the past year?

PRACTICE PROBLEM 4.5

Review the properties of the Poisson distribution.

A How many parameters characterize the Poisson distribution? Name the parameter(s).

B What are the assumptions of the Poisson distribution?

C What are the possible values of the Poisson distribution?

D What are the mean, variance, and standard deviation of the Poisson distribution?

PRACTICE PROBLEM 4.6

Crohn's disease is estimated to have an incidence rate of 3.1 to 14.6 cases per 100,000 person-years.[7]

Suppose that we suspect the incidence of Crohn's disease is on the lower end of the estimate at exactly 3.1 cases per 100,000 person-years.

A What is λ?

B What is the probability that no Crohn's disease cases will occur per 100,000 person-years?

C What is the probability that three or fewer Crohn's disease cases will occur per 100,000 person-years?

Suppose that we suspect the incidence of Crohn's disease is near the upper end of the estimate at 14.5 cases per 100,000 person-years.

D What is λ?

E What is the probability that no Crohn's disease cases will occur per 100,000 person-years?

F What is the probability that eight or more Crohn's disease cases will occur per 100,000 person-years (use the Poisson probability table in Appendix Table A.2)?

References

1. Pagano M, Gauvreau K. *Principles of Biostatistics*. Vol 2. Pacific Grove, CA: Duxbury. 2000.
2. Pratt LA, Brody DJ. *Depression in the U.S. Household Population, 2009–2012*. Hyattsville, MD: National Center for Health Statistics. 2014. NCHS Data Brief 172.
3. Arroyo-Johnson C, Mincey KD, Ackermann N, Milam L, Goodman MS, Colditz GA. Racial and ethnic heterogeneity in self-reported diabetes prevalence trends across Hispanic subgroups, National Health Interview Survey, 1997–2012. *Prev Chronic Dis*. 2016;13(E10). doi:10.5888/pcd13.150260.
4. Injury Prevention & Control: Opioid Overdose: State Data. Centers for Disease Control and Prevention, National Center for Injury Prevention and Control, Division of Unintentional Injury Prevention. http://www.cdc.gov/drugoverdose/data/statedeaths.html. Published 2016. Accessed April 2, 2017.
5. Quealy K, Sanger-Katz M. Compare these gun death rates: The U.S. is in a different world. *New York Times*. June 13, 2016. http://www.nytimes.com/2016/06/14/upshot/compare-these-gun-death-rates-the-us-is-in-a-different-world.html?_r=0. Accessed August 16, 2016.

6. Alcohol Facts and Statistics. National Institute on Alcohol Abuse and Alcoholism. https://www.niaaa.nih.gov/alcohol-health/overview-alcohol-consumption/alcohol-facts-and-statistics. Published 2016. Accessed April 2, 2017.
7. Epidemiology of the IBD. National Center for Chronic Disease Prevention and Health Promotion, Centers for Disease Control and Prevention. http://www.cdc.gov/ibd/ibd-epidemiology.htm. Published 2015.

5 Continuous probability distributions

This chapter will focus on probability distributions for continuous random variables and will include the following:

- Continuous probability distributions
- Standard normal distribution

Terms

- cumulative distribution function
- inverse normal function
- normal distribution
- probability density function
- standard normal distribution

Introduction

Throughout this chapter, we will expand on what we learned in Chapter 4 and discuss continuous probability distributions, specifically the normal distribution. We will then learn how a specific normal distribution—the standard normal distribution—can be adapted and used to solve problems.

Distribution functions

The probability density function (PDF) of the random variable X is a function such that the area under the density–function curve between any two points a and b is equal to the probability that the random variable X falls between a and b. Figure 5.1 shows the area that represents the probability.

- Thus, the total area under the density function curve over the entire range of possible values for the random variable is 1.
- The cumulative distribution function (CDF) for the random variable X evaluated at point a is defined as the probability that X will take on values $\leq a$. It is represented by the area under the PDF to the left of a. Figure 5.2 shows the area that represents the probability.

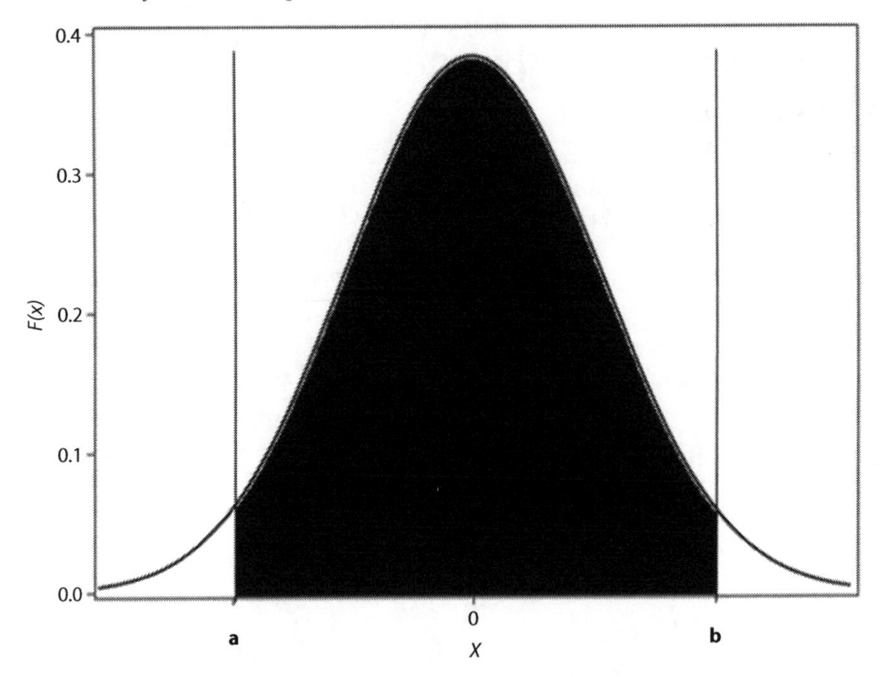

Figure 5.1 **Probability density function of random variable X.** The area between points *a* and *b*, represented by the shaded area in the figure, is equal to the probability that the random variable X falls between points *a* and *b*.

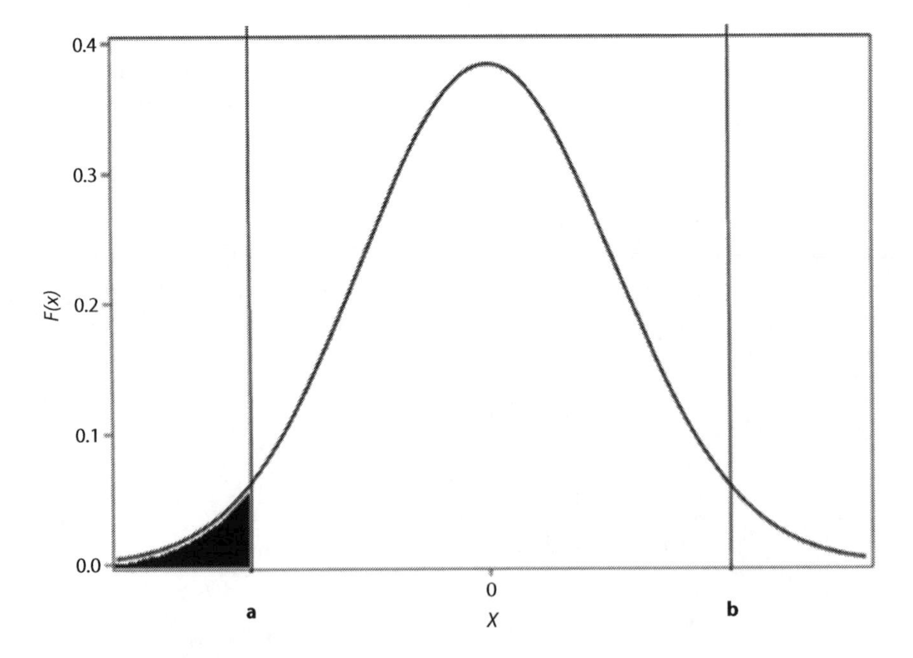

Figure 5.2 **Cumulative distribution function of random variable X.** The area to the left of *a*, represented by the shaded area in the figure, is the probability that X will take on values $\leq a$.

Normal distribution

Normal Distribution: The normal distribution is the most widely used distribution in statistics. Normal distribution (also referred to as Gaussian or *bell-shaped* distribution) is the cornerstone of most methods of estimation and hypothesis testing. It is defined by its PDF, which is given as

$$f(x) = \frac{1}{\sqrt{2\pi\sigma}} e^{\left(-\frac{(x-\mu)^2}{2\sigma^2}\right)} \text{ where } -\infty < x < \infty \tag{5.1}$$

for parameters μ (mean), σ (standard deviation), where σ > 0. Figure 5.3 shows the normal curve.

- Many distributions that are not themselves normal can be made approximately normal by transforming the data onto a different scale.
- The normal density function follows a bell-shaped curve, with the mode at μ and the most frequently occurring values around μ.
- The curve is symmetric about μ.
- The area under the normal density function is equal to 1.
- A normal distribution with mean μ and variance σ^2 will be referred to as a $N(\mu, \sigma^2)$ distribution.

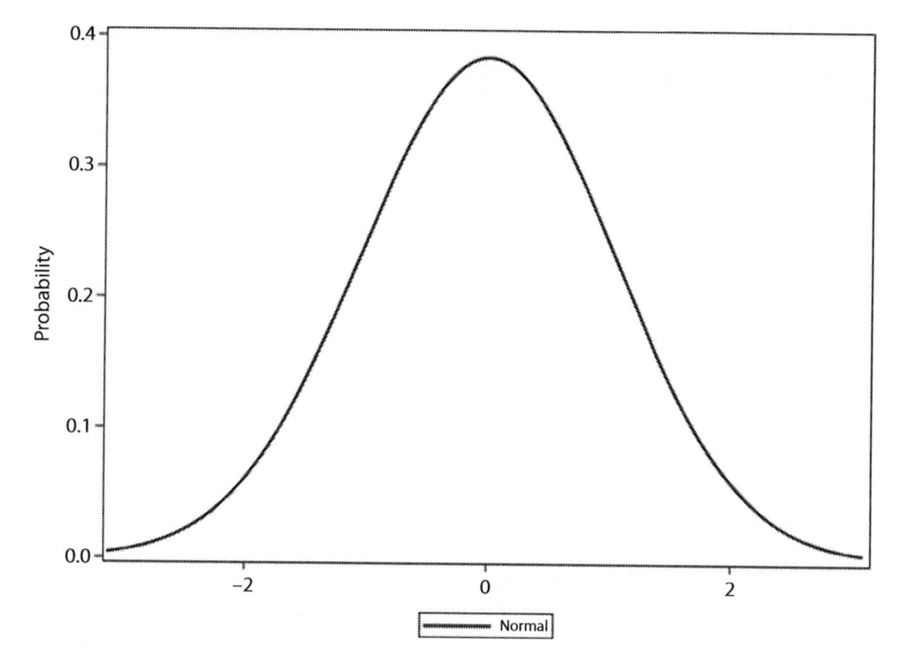

Figure 5.3 **Normal distribution curve.** The normal distribution curve is a continuous curve that takes on a "bell" shape. In this curve, μ would be at 0.

Standard normal distribution

- A normal distribution with mean 0 and variance 1, $N(0,1)$, is called a *standard normal distribution.*
- The CDF for the standard normal distribution is denoted by $\Phi(x) = P(X \leq r)$ where X follows an $N(0,1)$ distribution.
    - The CDF of the normal distribution is often used for power calculations (discussed in Chapter 7).
- The symbol ~ is used as shorthand for the phrase "is distributed as."
- Thus, $X \sim N(0,1)$ means that the random variable X is distributed as a $N(0,1)$ distribution.
- The (100u)th percentile of a standard normal distribution is denoted by Z_u. It is defined by the relationship $P(X<Z_u) = u$ where $X \sim N(0,1)$ and $0 \leq \mu \leq 1$. The function Z_u is sometimes referred to as the *inverse normal function.*
- Remember, the distribution of values is symmetric and unimodal in the standard normal distribution. Therefore, the empirical rule (see Chapter 1) is valid. The "empirical rule" states: approximately 67% of observations will lie within one standard deviation of the mean, approximately 95% of observations will lie within two standard deviations of the mean, and almost all observations will lie within three standard deviations of the mean.

Standardization of a normal variable

$$\text{If } X \sim N(\mu, \sigma^2) \text{ and } Z = \frac{X-\mu}{\sigma}, \text{ then } Z \sim N(0,1).$$

If a variable is normally distributed and we need to find a probability, the first step is to convert to the standard normal (see Figure 5.4):

- We will need to slide left or right (horizontal) to line up at 0 (i.e., subtract mean).
- We will also need to stretch or squish (vertically) to obtain a spread (standard deviation) of 1 (i.e., divide by standard deviation).

Why use the standard normal?

- We use the standard normal distribution because it has been tabulated.
- All other normal distributions can be adjusted by sliding and stretching to fit the standard normal. Then, tables from the standard normal distribution can be used.
- We use the standard normal tables to obtain probabilities instead of the probability distribution formula (i.e., we transform an arbitrary normal random variable to a standard normal random variable, usually denoted by Z). These tables can be found in the Appendix (Appendix Table A.3). Besides, no one wants to use that formula (Equation 5.1)!
- When looking at the standard normal distribution table (Appendix Table A.3), we can see that there are only positive numbers. Why is this so? Remember that the normal curve is symmetric, so $P(Z > 1.96) = P(Z < -1.96) = 0.025$.
- It is helpful to draw out the distribution when calculating normal probabilities. Visualization helps and will be useful for future concepts. See Figure 5.5 for an example.

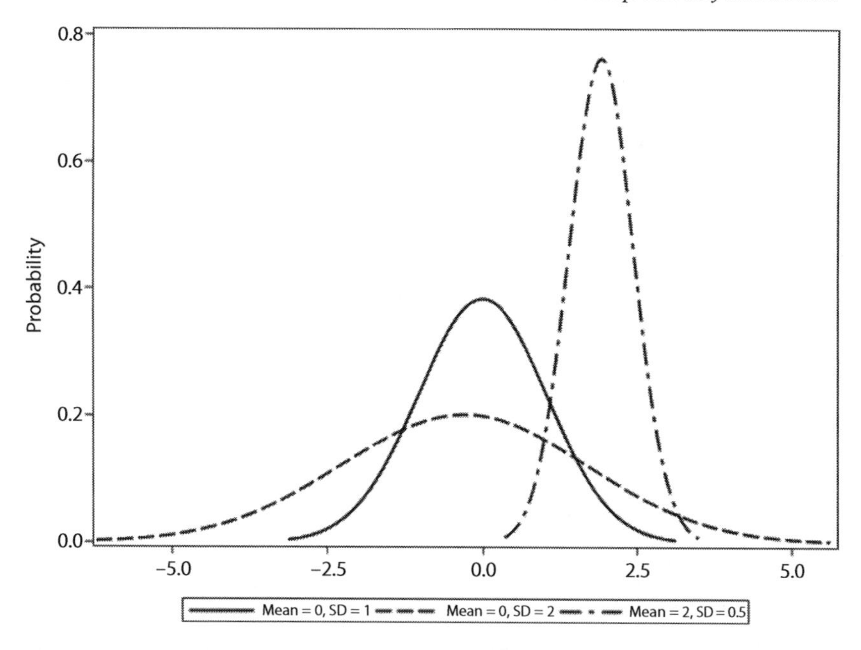

Figure 5.4 **Variation of normal distribution curves.** Several variations of the normal distribution curves are represented. The solid line represents a distribution with a mean of 0 and a standard deviation of 1. This curve is similar to the one presented in Figure 5.3. The dashed line represents a distribution with a mean of 0 and a standard deviation of 2. We can see that with an increase in standard deviation, the curve becomes wider. The dash-dot line represents a distribution with a mean of 2 and a standard deviation of 0.5. We can see that with an increase in the mean, the curve shifts and with a decrease in the standard deviation, the curve becomes narrower.

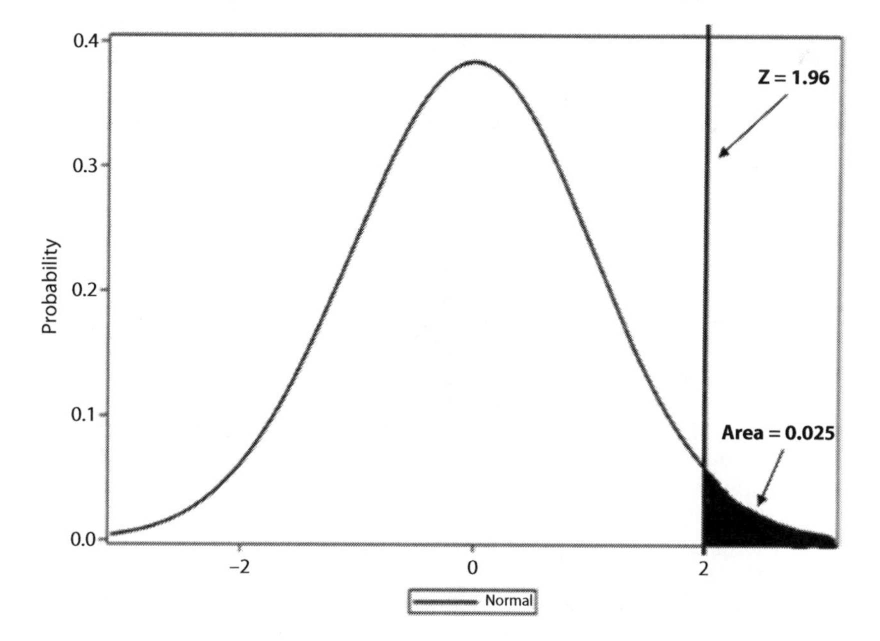

Figure 5.5 **Standard normal distribution.** The figure shows where the *z*-score is on the standard normal curve and the area of which (shaded) define, the probability.

EXAMPLE PROBLEM 5.1

Using the NHANES 2014 data,[1] a representative sample of the U. S. population, we find that the diastolic blood pressure of individuals aged 18 and over is approximately normally distributed, with a mean of 69.7 mm Hg and a standard deviation of 15.5 mm Hg.

> **BOX 5.1 EXAMPLE PROBLEM 5.1 DATA EXPLAINED**
>
> The 2014 National Health and Nutrition Examination Survey (NHANES) measured participants' blood pressures after participants were seated for 5 minutes. The measurements were taken 3 times consecutively by trained personnel. Both diastolic and systolic blood pressures were recorded in millimeters of mercury (mm Hg). For the mean and standard deviation presented in this problem, the first reading of diastolic blood pressure was used. Data were excluded for those who were under the age of 18.

Suppose that we want to know the probability that a randomly selected individual has a diastolic blood pressure less than 75 mm Hg.

A **Draw a normal curve representing this scenario.**

In Figure 5.6, we have the mean of 69.7 mm Hg and the value of 75 mm Hg to the right of the mean. We want to know the probability that the blood pressure is less than 75 mm Hg, which is represented by the shaded section to the left of the value.

B **Find the probability that a randomly selected individual has a diastolic blood pressure less than 75 mm Hg.**

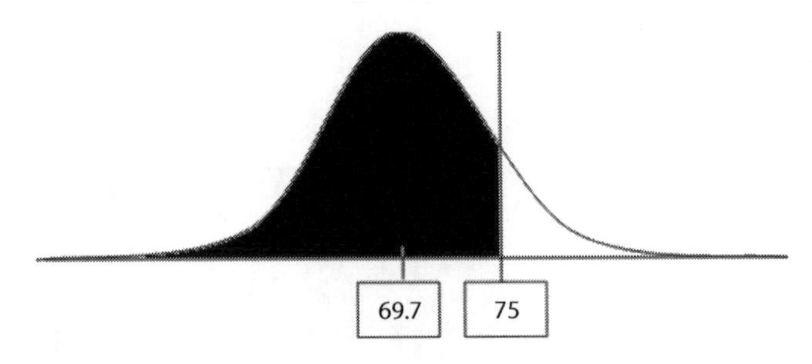

Figure 5.6 **Example Problem 5.1 Part (A).** To solve the first section of Example Problem 5.1, it can be helpful to draw a normal curve with the mean and value we are considering. Then, on the basis of the problem, we can shade in the area of the probability we are wanting to obtain, in this case the area to the left of 75 because we want to find the probability that a randomly selected individual has a diastolic blood pressure less than 75 mm Hg.

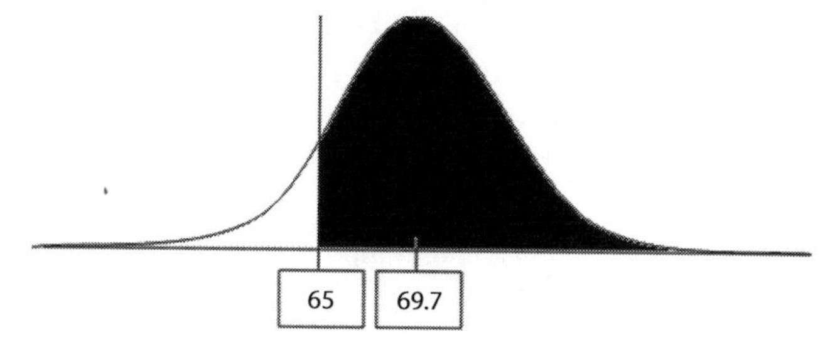

Figure 5.7 **Example Problem 5.1 Part (C).** To solve the second section of Example Problem 5.1, it can be helpful to draw a normal curve with the mean and value we are considering. Then, on the basis of the problem, we can shade in the area of the probability we are wanting to obtain, in this case the area to the right of 65 because we want to find the probability that a randomly selected individual has a diastolic blood pressure greater than 65 mm Hg.

$$P(X < 75) = P\left(Z < \frac{75 - 69.7}{15.5}\right) = P(Z < 0.341) = 1 - 0.367 = 0.633$$

Use the standardization equation to find a z-score. Then, use the standard normal distribution table to find 0.3 (the tenths place) in the z column and 0.04 (the hundredths place) across the top. The values across the top represent the hundredths place in the z-score. Because we want the area that is less than our z-score of 0.341, we subtract 0.367 from 1 to get the probability. Table A.3 provides areas in the upper tail of the standard normal distribution.

C **Suppose that we want to know the probability that a randomly selected individual has a diastolic blood pressure greater than 65 mm Hg. Draw a normal curve representing this scenario.**

In Figure 5.7, we have the mean of 69.7 mm Hg and the value of 65 mm Hg to the left of the mean. We want to know the probability that the blood pressure is greater than 65 mm Hg, which is represented by the shaded section to the right of the value.

D **Find the probability that a randomly selected individual has a diastolic blood pressure greater than 65 mm Hg.**

$$P(X > 65) = P\left(Z > \frac{65 - 69.7}{15.5}\right) = P(Z > -0.3032)$$

$$= P(Z < 0.3032) = 1 - 0.382 = 0.618$$

BOX 5.2 USING SAS OR STATA TO FIND A STANDARD NORMAL PROBABILITY

We can also solve Part (D) of Example Problem 5.1 by using SAS or Stata. Both have functions that allow us to calculate standard normal probabilities once we have calculated a Z value.

Using SAS

SAS Code:

```
DATA prob5_2d;
  prob=PROBNORM(0.3032);
RUN;
PROC PRINT DATA=prob5_2d;
RUN;
```

SAS Output:

Observation	Probability
1	0.61913

The PROBNORM function in SAS gives us the probability that Z is less than or equal to 0.3032, under a standard normal distribution.

We, then, use PROC PRINT to print our resulting probability and get the above output.

Using Stata

Stata Code:

```
display normal(0.3032)
```

Stata Output:

```
.61913128
```

The normal function in Stata gives us the probability that Z is less than or equal to 0.3032, under a standard normal distribution.

The values we obtained from SAS and Stata are the same; however, the value is slightly different from the one we obtained by hand because of the more precise calculation that is done in SAS and Stata and the need to round Z to 2 decimal places when using the standard normal Table (Appendix Table A.3).

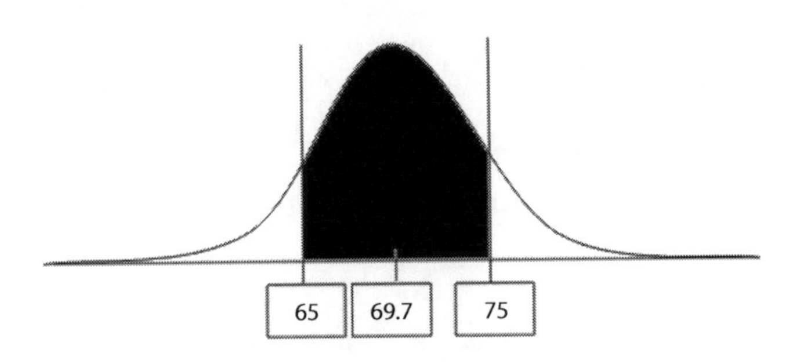

Figure 5.8 **Example Problem 5.1 Part (E).** To solve the third section of Example Problem 5.1, it can be helpful to draw a normal curve with the mean and values we are considering. Then, on the basis of the problem, we can shade in the area of the probability we are wanting to obtain, in this case the area in between 65 and 75 because we want to find the probability that a randomly selected individual has a diastolic blood pressure between 65 mm Hg and 75 mm Hg.

We use the standardization equation to find a z-score. Then, we use the standard normal distribution table to find 0.3 in the z column and 0.00 across the top. Since we have only positive values in our table, we switch the sign on our z-score, thus *greater than* becomes *less than*. Because we want the area that is less than our z-score of 0.3032, we subtract 0.382 from 1 to get the probability.

E **Suppose that we want to know the probability that a randomly selected individual has a diastolic blood pressure between 65 mm Hg and 75 mm Hg. Draw a normal curve representing this scenario (see Figure 5.8).**

F **Find the probability that a randomly selected individual has a diastolic blood pressure between 65 mm Hg and 75 mm Hg.**

$$P(65 < X < 75) = P(-0.3032 < X < 0.3419) = 1 - 0.382 - 0.367 = 0.251$$

We calculated the shaded area by subtracting the unshaded areas from 1.

G **What diastolic blood pressure would be the 90th percentile?**

Being in the 90th percentile means that the tail area of our curve would be 0.10. We want to find Z such that $P(Z < z) = 0.90$ or $P(Z > z) = 0.10$, where capital Z represents the random variable Z and lowercase z represents the z-score. To do this, we look for 0.10 in the body of the standard normal distribution table. We see that 0.10 is represented in the body of the table with a z-score of 1.28.

$$1.28 = \frac{x - 69.7}{15.5} \rightarrow 1.28 \times 15.5 = 19.84 = x - 69.7$$

$$\rightarrow 19.84 + 69.7 = x = 89.5\,mm\,Hg$$

We use the standardization equation to solve for x and find that the 90th percentile would be 89.5 mm Hg (see Figure 5.9).

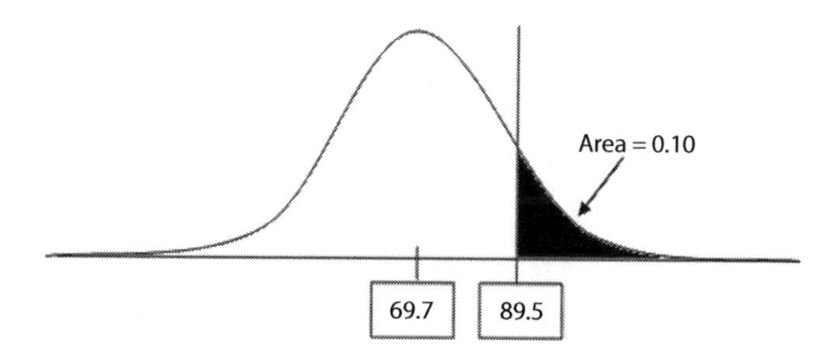

Figure 5.9 **Example Problem 5.1 Part (G).** To solve Part (G) of Example Problem 5.1, it can be helpful to draw a normal curve representing the area of the curve that corresponds to the value we want to obtain. In this case, we are looking for the 90th percentile, which corresponds to the tail area of our curve being 0.10. We mark the area that would be 0.10 by shading and marking the place where the value we are looking for would be. In solving the problem, we find that our value is 89.5 mm Hg.

H What is the probability that among five individuals selected at random from this population, exactly one will have a diastolic blood pressure between 65 mm Hg and 75 mm Hg?

X~binomial ($n = 5, p = 0.251$). We know that $p = 0.251$ from Example Problem 5.1—Part (F).

$$P(X=1) = \binom{5}{1}(0.251)^1(1-0.251)^{5-1} = \binom{5}{1}(0.251)^1(0.749)^4$$

$$= 5 \times 0.251 \times 0.315 = 0.395$$

EXAMPLE PROBLEM 5.2

Using the same NHANES data[1] from Example Problem 5.1, we find that the 60-second pulse of individuals aged 18 and over is approximately normally distributed, with a mean of 72.8 beats and a standard deviation of 35.9 beats.

BOX 5.3 EXAMPLE PROBLEM 5.2 DATA EXPLAINED

In the 2014 NHANES survey, a trained health technician also measured participants' pulse rates during the same examination as when the participants' blood pressure was measured. The 60-second pulse rate was calculated by multiplying a 30-second pulse rate by 2. For this example, if participants were under the age of 18, their data were excluded from the mean and standard deviation calculation.

A What 60-second pulse would be the 97th percentile?

As in Example Problem 5.1—Part (G), we are looking for a specific percentile here. The 97th percentile means that the tail area of our curve would be 0.03. We look for 0.03 in the body of the standard normal distribution table and use that value in the standardization equation to solve for x.

$$1.88 = \frac{x - 72.8}{35.9} \rightarrow 1.88 \times 35.9 = 67.492 = x - 72.8 \rightarrow 67.492$$

$$+72.8 = x = 140.3\,beats$$

The 97th percentile would be 140.3 beats.

B What is the probability that a randomly selected individual has a 60-second pulse between 70 beats and 75 beats?

$$P(70 < X < 75) = P\left(\frac{70-72.8}{35.9} < Z < \frac{75-72.8}{35.9}\right)$$

$$= P(-0.08 < Z < 0.06) = 1 - 0.468 - 0.476 = 0.056$$

The probability that a randomly selected individual has a 60-second pulse between 70 beats and 75 beats is 0.056.

C **What is the probability that a randomly selected individual has a 60-second pulse of 50 beats or fewer?**

$$P(X < 50) = P\left(Z < \frac{50 - 72.8}{35.9}\right) = P(Z < -0.64) = P(Z > 0.64) = 0.261$$

The probability that a randomly selected individual has a 60-second pulse of 50 beats or fewer is 0.261.

D **How would a lower standard deviation in this population affect the probability that we found in Example Problem 5.2—Part (C)? What about if the standard deviation were higher?**

If the standard deviation were lower, the *z*-score would be higher. Thus, the probability would be lower. If the standard deviation were higher, the *z*-score would be lower. Thus, the probability would be higher.

Review of probability distributions

We have covered the binomial, Poisson, and normal distributions so far in this workbook. As a review and summary, Table 5.1 contains key information for each of the distributions.

What are the relationships among all the probability distributions?

- Looking at Figure 5.10, we can see that there are relationships among the probability distributions that we have discussed in this workbook.
- First, the normal distribution can be used to approximate the binomial when $np \geq 5$ and $n(1 - p) \geq 5$.
- The binomial can be approximated by Poisson when n is large and p is small—the conservative rule says when $n \geq 100$ and $p \leq 0.01$.
- The normal distribution can be used to approximate Poisson when $\lambda \geq 10$.

RECAP OF PROBABILITY DISTRIBUTIONS

- Binomial and Poisson distributions start to look normally distributed (large *n*).
- Almost all kinds of data start to look normally distributed (large *n*).
- Tables of probabilities exist for binomial, Poisson, and standard normal (mean of 0, sd of 1) distributions.
- Probabilities can be obtained by converting from general normal to standard normal.

Table 5.1 Probability distribution review table

	Binomial	*Poisson*	*Normal*
Type of random variable	Discrete	Discrete	Continuous
Parameters	n & p	λ	μ & σ
Possible values	0, 1, 2, … , n	0, 1, 2, … , ∞	-∞ to ∞
Mean	np	λ	μ
Standard deviation	$\sqrt{np(1-p)}$	$\sqrt{\lambda}$	σ
Shape of the distribution	Skewed or symmetric (when p = 0.5)	Skewed or symmetric	Symmetric about the mean, unimodal bell curve
Assumptions	Fixed number (n) of independent trials with two mutually exclusive and exhaustive outcomes and a constant probability of success (p)	The probability an event that occurs in the interval is proportional to the length of the interval, an infinite number of occurrences are possible, and events occur independently at rate λ	Independence

Note: A review of the three types of probability distributions covered in this book are contained in this table, including features of the distributions such as parameters, assumptions, and shape of the distributions.

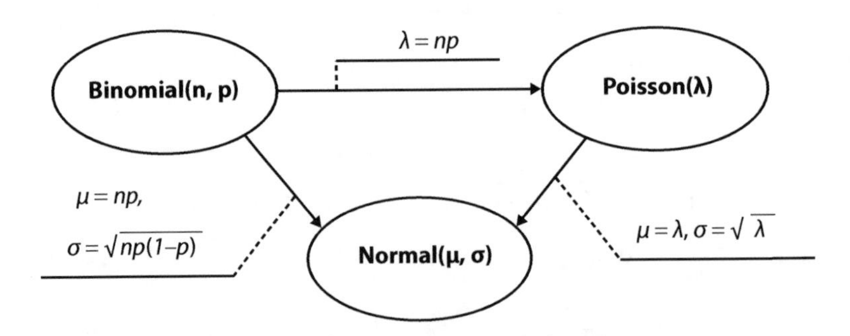

Figure 5.10 **Probability distribution relationships.** The normal distribution can be used to approximate both the binomial distribution and Poisson distribution. The Poisson can also be used to approximate the binomial. The parameter estimates for each approximation are shown.

PRACTICE PROBLEM 5.1

Review the standard normal distribution.

A What are the parameters that characterize the standard normal distribution?

B What kinds of random variables can be used with the standard normal distribution?

C What is the shape of the standard normal distribution?

D What are the possible values for the standard normal distribution?

PRACTICE PROBLEM 5.2

Using the representative sample of the U. S. population from the 2014 NHANES data,[1] we find that the weight of individuals aged 18 and over is approximately normally distributed, with a mean of 82.6 kg and a standard deviation of 34.4 kg.

BOX 5.4 PRACTICE PROBLEM 5.2 DATA EXPLAINED

In the 2014 NHANES survey, a trained health technician measured participants' weight. Body weight was measured in kilograms (kg). For this example, if participants were under the age of 18, their data were excluded from the mean and standard deviation calculation.

Suppose that we want to know the probability that a randomly selected individual has a weight greater than 85 kg.

A Draw a normal curve representing this scenario.

B Find the probability that a randomly selected individual has a weight greater than 85 kg.

C Suppose that we want to know the probability that a randomly selected individual has a weight less than 60 kg. Draw a normal curve representing this scenario.

D Find the probability that a randomly selected individual has a weight less than 60 kg.

E What is the probability that a randomly selected individual has a weight between 60 kg and 85 kg?

F What weight would be the 95th percentile?

G What is the probability that among three individuals selected at random from this population, exactly one will have a weight between 60 kg and 85 kg?

PRACTICE PROBLEM 5.3

Using a representative sample of the U. S. population from the 2014 NHANES data,[1] we find that for individuals aged 18 and over with diabetes, the age when they were first told they had diabetes is approximately normally distributed, with a mean of 48.1 years and a standard deviation of 10.9 years.

BOX 5.5 PRACTICE PROBLEM 5.3 DATA EXPLAINED

In the NHANES survey, participants who have diabetes were asked "How old {were you/was SP} when a doctor or other health professional first told {you/him/her} that {you/he/she} had diabetes or sugar diabetes?" The response was in age, with the possible answers being 1 to 79 years, with 80 and over responses coded as 80. Responses less than 1 year were recoded to 1. Data for participants who refused to answer or who responded that they did not know were excluded from the calculation, along with data for those under the age of 18 at the time of the NHANES survey.

A What is the probability that a randomly selected individual was older than 65 years when first told that he or she had diabetes?

B What is the 90th percentile of age when first told of having diabetes?

C If six individuals were randomly selected from this population, what is the probability that two of them were older than 65 years when they were first told they had diabetes?

PRACTICE PROBLEM 5.4

In a study of the playground conditions in the neighborhoods of St. Louis, Missouri,[2] researchers found the neighborhoods to have an overall playground safety score that was approximately normally distributed, with a mean of 67.0 and a standard deviation of 15.7.

A What is the probability that a neighborhood has a playground safety score between 80 and 90 in this population of neighborhoods?

B What is the probability that a neighborhood has a playground safety score between 60 and 70 in this population of neighborhoods?

C Suppose that we are considering moving to one of six randomly selected neighborhoods in St. Louis, Missouri. What is the probability that the playground safety score will be between 80 and 90?

D What is the probability that the safety score will be between 60 and 70?

PRACTICE PROBLEM 5.5

For each of the example scenarios, state which distribution (binomial, Poisson, or normal) would be the best to apply. Why?

A We know the probability of developing hypertension in a certain population is 0.15. We have randomly selected ten individuals from this population and want to know the probability that five of them have hypertension.

B We know the mean and standard deviation of the birth weight in a population, and we want to know the probability that a randomly selected infant has a birth weight within a certain range.

C We know the probability that an individual is ambidextrous in a certain population. Specifically, we want to know the probability that at least two individuals are ambidextrous among eight randomly selected individuals.

D We know the rate per year of a rare disease and want to know the probability that no cases of the disease will occur in a given year.

PRACTICE PROBLEM 5.6

In Chapter 4, Practice Problem 4.2, we used the Poisson distribution to answer questions regarding the probability of gun homicides occurring in the United States and Canada. The rate of gun homicides in the United States was reported to be 27 per day.[3]

A Could we use another distribution (besides Poisson) to estimate probabilities? If we can, which distribution could we use and why?

B Using the distribution specified in Practice Problem 5.6—Part (A), what are the parameters characterizing the distribution?

C Using the distribution specified in Practice Problem—Parts (A) and (B), what is the probability that more than 20 people will die of a gun homicide in a given day in the United States?

References

1. National Health and Nutrition Examination Survey. Hyattsville, MD: Centers for Disease Control and Prevention, National Center for Health Statistics. https://wwwn.cdc.gov/Nchs/Nhanes/Search/nhanes13_14.aspx. Published 2014. Accessed February 23, 2016.
2. Arroyo-Johnson C, Woodward K, Milam L, Ackermann N, Goodman MS, Hipp JA. Still separate, still unequal: Social determinants of playground safety and proximity. *J Urban Heal*. 2016;93(4):627–638. doi:10.1007/s11524-016-0063-8.
3. Quealy K, Sanger-Katz M. Compare these gun death rates: The U.S. is in a different world. *New York Times*. June 13, 2016. http://www.nytimes.com/2016/06/14/upshot/compare-these-gun-death-rates-the-us-is-in-a-different-world.html?_r=0. Accessed August 16, 2016.

Lab B: Probability distributions

To recap the binomial, Poisson, and normal distributions, fill in Table B.1.

PRACTICE PROBLEM B.1

Let X be a random variable that represents the number of infants in a group of 2000 who are exclusively breastfed at 6 months. According to the World Health Organization, in the United States the probability that a child is exclusively breastfed at 6 months is 0.19.[1]

A What is the mean number of U.S. infants who would be exclusively breastfed in a group of this size?

B What is the standard deviation of X?

C What is the probability that a maximum of 300 infants out of 2000 are exclusively breastfed at 6 months of age?

D What is the probability that between 350 and 400 infants are exclusively breastfed at 6 months?

PRACTICE PROBLEM B.2

The number of cases of rubella reported monthly in 2013 in the United States[2] follow a Poisson distribution with parameter $\lambda = 0.75$.

A What is the mean number of cases of rubella reported each month?

B What is the standard deviation?

Table B.1 Probability distributions

	Binomial	*Poisson*	*Normal*
Parameters			
Possible values			
Mean			
Standard deviation			

C What is the probability that no cases of rubella will be reported during a given month?

D What is the probability that a maximum of one case will be reported?

E What is the probability that two or more cases of rubella will be reported?

PRACTICE PROBLEM B.3

The distribution of weights among women in the United States from 2013 through 2014 is approximately normal with a mean of 168 pounds and standard deviation of 48 pounds.[3]

A What is the z-score corresponding to the 95th percentile of weight?

B What is the weight value corresponding to the 95th percentile of weight from 2013 through 2014?

C What is the probability that a randomly selected woman weighs more than 190 pounds?

D What is the probability that a randomly selected woman weighs less than 130 pounds?

E What is the probability that among five women selected at random from the population, at least one will weigh either less than 130 pounds or more than 190 pounds?

References

1. World Health Organization. Global Health Observatory Data Repository: Exclusive breastfeeding under 6 months. http://apps.who.int/gho/data/node.main.1100?lang=en. Updated April 2, 2015. Accessed September 29, 2016.
2. Adams D, Fullerton K, Jajosky R et al. Summary of notifiable infectious diseases and conditions—United States, 2013. *MMWR Morb Mortal Wkly Rep*. 2015;62(53):1–122. doi:10.15585/mmwr.mm6253a1.
3. National Health and Nutrition Examination Survey. Hyattsville, MD: Centers for Disease Control and Prevention, National Center for Health Statistics. 2014. https://wwwn.cdc.gov/Nchs/Nhanes/Search/nhanes13_14.aspx. Accessed February 23, 2016.

6 Estimation

This chapter will focus on estimation for means and proportions and will include the following:

- Statistical inference
- Sampling
- Randomized clinical trial
- Sampling distribution of the mean
- Central limit theorem
- Confidence intervals for means
- Using SAS to construct confidence intervals for a mean
- Using Stata to construct confidence intervals for a mean
- The *t*-distribution
- Obtaining critical values in SAS and Stata
- Sampling distribution for proportions
- Confidence intervals for proportions
- Using SAS to obtain confidence intervals for proportions
- Using Stata to obtain confidence intervals for proportions

Terms

- central limit theorem
- double-blinded clinical trial
- estimation
- hypothesis testing
- interval estimation
- point estimates
- population mean
- population proportion
- population standard deviation
- population variance
- random sample
- randomization
- randomized clinical trial
- reference (also target or study population)
- sample mean
- sample proportion
- sample standard deviation
- sample variance
- sampling distribution of $\overline{x}$
- simple random sample
- single-blinded clinical trial
- standard error of the mean (standard error)
- statistical inference
- *t*-distribution
- triple-blinded clinical trial
- unbiased estimator
- unblinded clinical trial

Introduction

The problem discussed in this chapter and the rest of this book is the basic problem of statistics: we have a dataset (data sample), and we want to infer properties about the underlying distribution (i.e., population) from this dataset. This inference usually involves inductive reasoning. A variety of probability models must be explored to see which model best "fits" the data. In this chapter, we will explore some key terms and methods for statistical inference.

Statistical inference

Statistical Inference: The theory and methods used to make judgments about the characteristics of a population, distribution of variables, and relationships between variables based on sample data. Statistical inference can be divided into two main areas: Estimation and hypothesis testing.

Estimation: The act of approximating the values of specific population parameters.

Hypothesis Testing: The act of assessing whether the value of a population parameter is equal to some specific value.

When we are interested in obtaining specific values as estimates of our parameters, these values are often referred to as *point estimates*. However, sometimes we want to specify a range within which the parameter values are likely to fall. If this range is narrow, then we may feel that our point estimate is better than if the range is wide. This type of problem involves *interval estimation*.

Point Estimates: Specific values as estimates of parameters.

Interval Estimation: Specifies a range of values for which the parameter is likely to be inside.

Sampling

Sampling consists of selecting part of a population to observe so that one may estimate the characteristics of that entire population. A good sample is a miniature of the population, which has the same general characteristics of that population.

Random Sample: The selection of some members of a population such that each member is independently chosen and has a known nonzero probability of being selected.

Simple Random Sample: A random sample in which each group member has the same probability of being selected.

Reference Population: The group we want to study. The random sample is selected from the reference population (also called the target or study population).

- In practice, there is rarely an opportunity to enumerate each member of the reference population in order to select a random sample. The researcher must assume that the sample selected has all the properties of a random sample without formally being a random sample. If the members of a population cannot be formally enumerated, then the population is effectively infinite.

- For the purposes of this workbook, we will assume that all reference populations discussed are effectively infinite. Although some reference populations are finite and well defined, many are finite but very large.

Randomized clinical trials

Randomized Clinical Trial (RCT): A type of research design for comparing different treatments in which the assignment of treatments to patients is by some random mechanism.

Randomization: The process of assigning treatments to patients on a random basis. Patients can be assigned to treatment groups by using a random number table or by using computer-generated random numbers.

When the sample sizes are large, using randomization yields treatment groups in which the types of patients are approximately equivalent. However, if sample sizes are small, patient characteristics of treatment groups may not be comparable.

It is customary to present a table of characteristics of different treatment groups in RCTs to check that the randomization process is working well. Table 6.1 presents such a table from a study comparing culturally specific cognitive behavioral therapy (CBT) to standard CBT for smoking cessation among low-income African Americans.[1,2] Descriptive statistics are calculated and stratified by type of CBT. Then, the appropriate

Table 6.1 A table of characteristics of treatment groups in randomized controlled trials

	Condition			
Characteristic	*Culturally specific CBT (n = 168)*	*Standard CBT (n = 174)*	*Statistical test*	*P-value*
Demographics				
Female/male, %	39/61	48/52	$\chi^2(1, N = 340) = 2.83$	.09
Age, *M (SD)*	49.48 (9.44)	49.52 (8.73)	$t(338) = 0.04$	.97
At least high school, %	83.20	80.10	$\chi^2(7, N = 339) = 1.82$	.97
Single, %	63.50	64.20	$\chi^2(4, N = 340) = 6.14$	.19
Household income ≤ $10,000, %	61.80	59.90	$\chi^2(9, N = 337) = 4.39$	.88
Smoking history, *M (SD)*				
Cigarettes per day	18.20 (11.53)	17.88 (10.03)	$t(335) = -0.27$	.78
Years of smoking	25.83 (12.07)	26.78 (12.23)	$t(336) = -0.71$	.47
FTND score	5.42 (2.42)	5.40 (2.32)	$t(330) = -0.11$	.91
Menthol smokers, %	96	95	$\chi^2(1, N = 342) = 0.19$	.66
Intra-CBT variables, *M (SD)*				
Session attendance	6.14 (2.31)	5.91 (2.54)	$t(340) = .88$	.38
Patch use	17.18 (7.34)	16.22 (7.28)	$t(340) = 1.21$	.23

Source: Heatherton, T. F., Kozlowski, L. T., Frecker, R. C., and Fagerstrom, K. O., *Br J Addict*, 86, 1119–1127, 1991. doi:doi:10.1111/j.1360-0443.1991.tb01879.x.

Note: There were no statistically significant differences among conditions. Possible session attendance range = 0–8. Possible patch use range = 0–25.

Abbreviations: CBT, cognitive behavioral therapy; FTND, Fagerström Test for Nicotine Dependence.

statistical test is used to compare the two groups. Both the value of the test statistic and the p-value are typically shown.

Types of clinical trials

Unblinded Clinical Trial: A type of clinical trial in which both the patient and physician are aware of the treatment assignment.

Single-Blinded Clinical Trial: A type of clinical trial in which the patient is unaware of the treatment assignment, but the physician is aware.

Double-Blinded Clinical Trial: A type of clinical trial in which neither the patient nor the physician knows the treatment assignment. The gold standard of clinical research is the randomized, double-blind study.

In rare cases when there are extremely strong concerns about bias, a triple-blinded clinical trial is performed. In this type, the patient, the physician, and the person analyzing the data are unaware of the treatment assignment.

Population and sample mean

Suppose that we have a sample of patients from whom we have taken blood pressure measurements. From what we know about our sample, we would like to be able to estimate the mean and variance of blood pressure measurements for the larger population. In statistical terms, we have a specific random sample with observations $x_1, x_2, \ldots, x_n$, where n is the number of observations and where we will estimate the population mean μ and variance σ^2 of the underlying distribution.

Population Mean (μ): The average value of some random variable X for the whole population.

We are often interested in estimating the mean of a variable for a population. A natural estimator to use for estimating the population mean is the sample mean $\bar{x}$.

Sample Mean ($\bar{x}$): The average value calculated from a sample of the population. We will use $\bar{x}$ to estimate the true population mean. To get the sample mean, we use the formula

$$\bar{x} = \frac{\sum_{i=1}^{n} x_i}{n}. \qquad (6.1)$$

Sampling distribution of the mean

Sampling Distribution of $\bar{x}$: The distribution of values of $\bar{x}$ over all possible samples of size n that could have been selected from the reference population.

Unbiased estimators

- We refer to an estimator of a parameter θ as $\hat{\theta}$.

Unbiased Estimator: An estimator $\hat{\theta}$ of a parameter θ is unbiased if the expected value of the estimator is equal to the parameter: $E(\hat{\theta}) = \theta$. This means that the average value of $\hat{\theta}$ over a large number of repeated samples of size n is θ.

- Let $x_1, x_2, \ldots, x_n$ be a random sample drawn from some population with mean μ. The expected value of the sample mean, $E(\bar{X})$, is μ.
- This property of the expected value holds for any population regardless of its underlying distribution. Because of this, we refer to $\bar{X}$ as an unbiased estimator of μ.
- Although $\bar{X}$ is an unbiased estimator of μ for any sample size n, it is preferable to estimate parameters from large samples rather than from small ones. This is because the precision of $\bar{X}$ increases as the sample size increases.

Population and sample measures of spread

In order to describe a distribution, we typically use a measure of central tendency (e.g., mean) to tell us where the center of the distribution is, along with a measure of spread that tells us how much the data points depart from the center of the distribution.

Population Variance: Let $x_1, x_2, \ldots, x_n$ be a random sample drawn from some population with variance (σ^2).

Sample Variance: Denoted by s^2, an unbiased estimate of σ^2. In other words, the expected value of the sample variance is the population variance.

Population Standard Deviation: The square root of the population variance, denoted by σ.

Sample Standard Deviation: The standard deviation calculated directly from the sample of our population, denoted by s.

Standard Error of the Mean (SEM) or Standard Error (SE): A figure that represents the estimated standard deviation obtained from a set of sample means from repeated samples of size n from a population with underlying variance (σ^2). The SE is not the standard deviation of an individual observation X_i, but rather the standard deviation of the sample mean ($\bar{X}$). The SEM, or the SE, is given by

$$\text{SE(mean)} = \frac{\sigma}{\sqrt{n}} \tag{6.2}$$

and is estimated by $\frac{s}{\sqrt{n}}$.

See Table 6.2 for a summary of the symbols and terms used in this section on the sampling distribution of the mean.

EXAMPLE PROBLEM 6.1

Suppose that we take a sample of size n and calculate a sample mean ($\bar{x}_1$). Then we take a second sample and calculate that sample mean ($\bar{x}_2$). Would we expect $\bar{x}_1$ and $\bar{x}_2$ to be exactly the same? Why or why not?

Table 6.2 Key statistical symbols

Notation	*Description*	*Use*
μ	Population mean	
$\bar{x}$	Sample mean	To estimate μ
σ	Population standard deviation	
s	Sample standard deviation	To estimate σ
$\sigma/\sqrt{n}$	True standard error of the mean	
$s/\sqrt{n}$	Estimate of standard error of the mean	To estimate $\sigma/\sqrt{n}$
p	Population proportion	
$\hat{p}$	Sample proportion	To estimate p

We would not expect to find the same sample mean in both groups as long as the two samples are different. However, it is possible (although not probable) for the two sample means to be equal. For example, this would happen if everyone in the population has the same value.

Central limit theorem

If the underlying distribution is normal, then it can be shown that the sample mean is itself normally distributed with mean (μ) and variance $\frac{\sigma^2}{n}$. This is written as

$$\bar{X} \sim N\left(\mu, \frac{\sigma^2}{n}\right). \tag{6.3}$$

However, if the underlying distribution is not normal, we would still like to make some statement about the sampling distribution of the sample mean. We can do this through the use of the central limit theorem.

Central Limit Theorem (CLT): Let $X_1, \ldots, X_n$ be a random sample from some population with mean (μ) and variance (σ^2). Then, for large n, $\bar{X} \,\dot{\sim}\, N\left(\mu, \frac{\sigma^2}{n}\right)$, even if the underlying distribution of individual observations in the population is not normal.

- The symbol $\dot{\sim}$ means "approximately distributed."

The CLT is so important because many of the distributions encountered in practice are not normal. In such cases, the CLT often can be applied. This lets us perform statistical inference based on the approximate normality of the sample mean, despite the non-normality of the distribution of individual observations. In other words, even when the individuals in the sample have values that are not normally distributed, the CLT allows for inference when the sample is large enough.

EXAMPLE PROBLEM 6.2

Suppose that we take repeated samples of size n from a population with population mean μ and standard deviation σ and calculate sample means for each sample. What does the CLT say about the following:

A The mean of the distribution of sample means?

The CLT says that the mean of the distribution of the sample means will be equal to μ.

B The standard deviation of the distribution of sample means?

This is the SE of the mean, $\frac{\sigma}{\sqrt{n}}$.

C The shape of the distribution of sample means?

Provided that n is large enough, the distribution will be approximately normally distributed.

D Does this work even when we are sampling from populations that are not normally distributed?

Yes, but the further the population departs from being normally distributed, the larger the sample size n needs to be.

Confidence intervals for means

Frequently, we wish to obtain an interval estimation for the mean.

Interval Estimation (Mean): An interval of plausible estimates of the mean and the best estimate of the mean's precise value.

- Our interval estimates will hold exactly if the underlying distribution is normally distributed but approximately if the underlying distribution is not normal, as stated in the CLT.
- When the population standard deviation (σ) is known, the CLT tells us that if n is sufficiently large, the formula for a two-sided test $P\left(\bar{X} - Z_{1-\alpha/2}\frac{\sigma}{\sqrt{n}} \le \mu \le \bar{X} + Z_{1-\alpha/2}\frac{\sigma}{\sqrt{n}}\right) = 1-\alpha.$
- In this notation, $Z_{1-\alpha/2}$ is the value corresponding to the $\left(1-\alpha/2\right)^{th}$ percentile of the normal distribution (Figure 6.1). In the vast majority of cases, α is chosen to be 0.05. Thus, the corresponding Z value is 1.96.
- We can rewrite the equation to obtain the $100(1 - \alpha)\%$ confidence interval (Table 6.3).

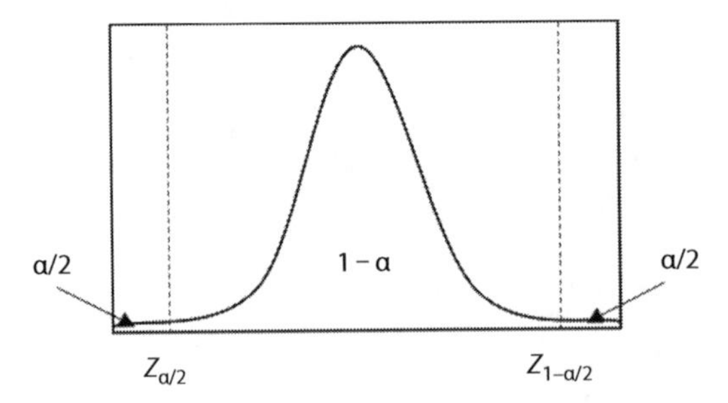

Figure 6.1 **Critical values of the standard normal distribution.** The value $Z_{1-\alpha/2}$ is the $1-\alpha/2^{\text{th}}$ percentile of the normal distribution, also expressed as the Z value, which cuts off an area of $\alpha/2$ in the upper tail of the distribution. Similarly, $Z_{\alpha/2}$, the $\alpha/2^{\text{th}}$ percentile, cuts off an area of $\alpha/2$ in the lower tail.

Table 6.3 Equations for 100(1 – α)% confidence intervals for a mean

Type of confidence interval	*σ Known*	*σ Unknown*
Two-sided	$\left(\bar{x}-Z_{1-\alpha/2}\frac{\sigma}{\sqrt{n}},\ \bar{x}+Z_{1-\alpha/2}\frac{\sigma}{\sqrt{n}}\right)$	$\left(\bar{x}-t_{n-1,\,1-\alpha/2}\frac{s}{\sqrt{n}},\ \bar{x}+t_{n-1,\,1-\alpha/2}\frac{s}{\sqrt{n}}\right)$
One-sided lower limit	$\bar{x}-Z_{1-\alpha}\frac{\sigma}{\sqrt{n}}$	$\bar{x}-t_{n-1,\,1-\alpha}\frac{s}{\sqrt{n}}$
One-sided upper limit	$\bar{x}+Z_{1-\alpha}\frac{\sigma}{\sqrt{n}}$	$\bar{x}+t_{n-1,\,1-\alpha}\frac{s}{\sqrt{n}}$

$$P\left(\bar{X}-Z_{1-\alpha/2}\frac{\sigma}{\sqrt{n}}\le\mu\le\bar{X}+Z_{1-\alpha/2}\frac{\sigma}{\sqrt{n}}\right)=1-\alpha$$
$$\rightarrow 100(1-\alpha)\ \%\ \text{confidence interval}$$
$$=\left(\bar{X}-Z_{1-\alpha/2}\frac{\sigma}{\sqrt{n}},\bar{X}+Z_{1-\alpha/2}\frac{\sigma}{\sqrt{n}}\right) \quad (6.4)$$

- For example, a 95% confidence interval takes the following form:

$$\left(\bar{X}-1.96\frac{\sigma}{\sqrt{n}},\ \bar{X}+1.96\frac{\sigma}{\sqrt{n}}\right).$$

- We interpret the confidence interval by saying, "We are 95% confident that the interval $\left(\bar{X}-1.96\frac{\sigma}{\sqrt{n}},\ \bar{X}+1.96\frac{\sigma}{\sqrt{n}}\right)$ will cover μ."

- Note that $\bar{X}$ is random, unlike μ. Remember that μ is the *unchanging* mean of the underlying population from which you draw your sample. The population mean is some unknown value.

What the confidence interval does not imply

The statement of the confidence interval does not imply that μ is a random variable that assumes a value within the interval 95% of the time. Nor does it imply that 95% of the population values lie between these limits.

What the confidence interval does imply

The meaning of the confidence interval is that if we were to select 100 random samples from the population and use these samples to calculate 100 different confidence intervals for μ, approximately 95 of the intervals would cover the true population mean, and 5 would not.

Example demonstrating the meaning of confidence interval

We took 100 random samples from a dataset containing total cholesterol levels (mg/dL).[3] Figure 6.2 shows sample mean cholesterol (indicated by dots) and the corresponding 95% confidence intervals for each of the 100 random samples. A dashed reference

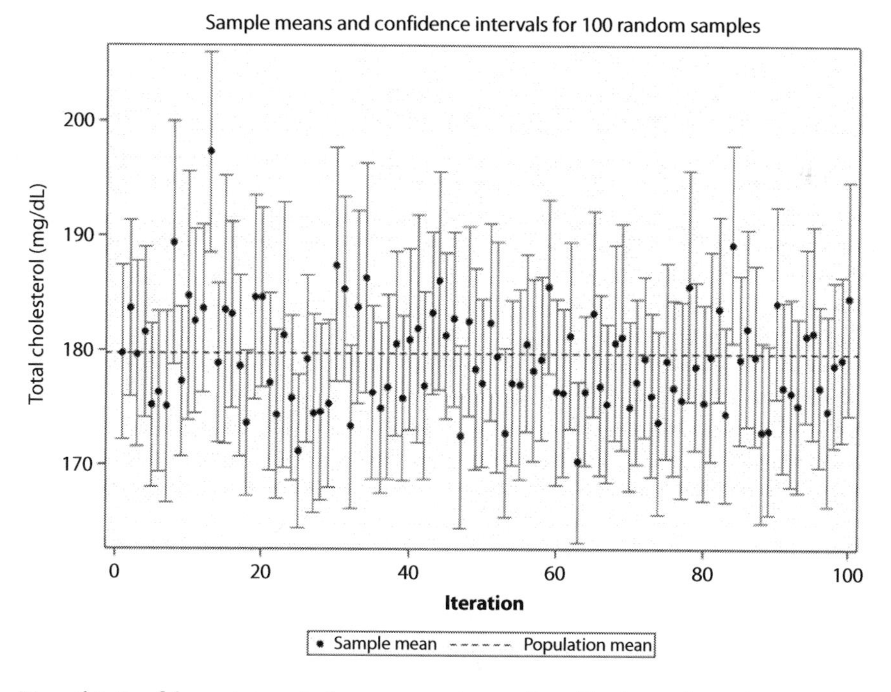

Figure 6.2 **Confidence intervals from repeated sampling.** The figure shows the variation in the 95% confidence intervals calculated using 100 random samples of 100 subjects each. Theoretically, we would expect 5 out of 100 of the 95% confidence intervals not to cover the true mean value in the population. In this example, 4 out of 100 did not cover the population mean, represented by the dashed line.

line at 179.81 mg/dL shows the true mean total cholesterol value from the population. We can see that 4 of the 100 confidence intervals do not cover the true mean value of 179.81 mg/dL.

Hand calculation of one-sided confidence interval

In some situations, we are primarily interested in determining whether a quantity is larger or smaller than some value. Thus, we are interested in only one bound (lower limit or upper limit) of a confidence interval.

- To calculate one-sided confidence intervals, we use $Z_{1-\alpha}$ for the Z value, as opposed to traditional two-sided confidence intervals, which use $Z_{1-\alpha/2}$.
- If we are interested in a one-sided lower limit, we use

$$\mu > \bar{x} - Z_{1-\alpha}\frac{\sigma}{\sqrt{n}} \tag{6.5}$$

- If the upper limit is of interest, we use

$$\mu < \bar{x} + Z_{1-\alpha}\frac{\sigma}{\sqrt{n}} \tag{6.6}$$

Width of confidence interval

The width of a confidence interval depends on a variety of factors.

- The higher the level of confidence [$100(1 - \alpha)\%$], the wider the interval.
- Increasing variability in the population (σ) will also result in a wider confidence interval.
- However, as the sample size (n) gets larger, the confidence interval narrows, as there is more information available.
- It should be noted that the size of the confidence interval does not depend on the value of the sample mean ($\bar{x}$).

Using the standard normal distribution for a mean

We can express $\bar{X}$ in standardized form by

$$Z = \frac{\bar{X} - \mu}{\sigma/\sqrt{n}} \tag{6.7}$$

where Z follows a standard normal distribution.

- Of repeated samples of size n, 95% of the Z-values will fall between -1.96 and $+1.96$ because these values correspond to the 2.5th and 97.5th percentiles from the standard normal distribution (Figure 6.3).

Using SAS to construct confidence intervals for a mean

Instead of calculating confidence intervals by hand, we can also use SAS. There are several procedures that will output confidence limits for a mean, one of which is PROC MEANS.

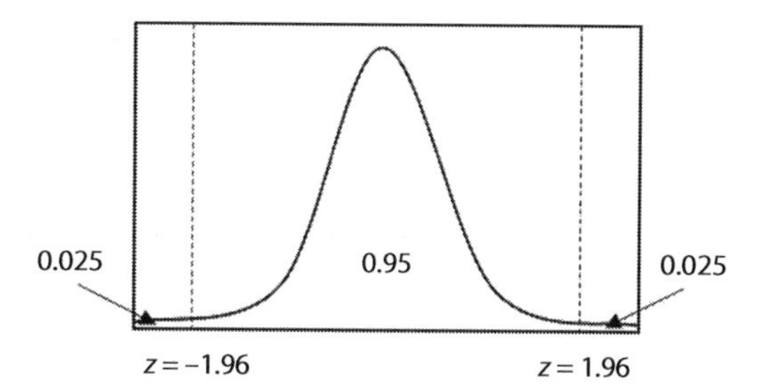

Figure 6.3 **Critical values of the standard normal distribution.** When $\alpha = 0.05$. When α is set to 0.05, the Z value that cuts off an area of $\alpha/2 = 0.025$ in the upper tail of the distribution is 1.96. The value that cuts off an area of $\alpha/2 = 0.025$ in the lower tail is −1.96.

The PROC MEANS procedure

- Specify the level of significance (ALPHA) and the continuous variable in the VAR statement.
- By default, α is 0.05 if the ALPHA option is not included. By default, the level of significance is set at 0.05, and a 95% confidence interval is produced.
- The ALPHA option can be added to change the significance level.
- The CLM option requests confidence limits, which will be given in addition to the sample size (N), sample mean (MEAN), and sample standard deviation (Std Dev).

```
PROC MEANS DATA = dataset_name N MEAN STD CLM;
     VAR continuous_variable;
RUN;
```

If a 90% confidence interval is desired instead of a 95% confidence interval, we would use the following code that adds the ALPHA option.

```
PROC MEANS DATA = dataset_name N MEAN STD CLM ALPHA = 0.10;
     VAR continuous_variable;
RUN;
```

The following box gives the output with the corresponding headings noted in parentheses: The total sample size (N), the sample mean (Mean), the sample standard deviation (Std Dev), and the lower bound (Lower 95% confidence limit for mean [CLM]) and upper bound (Upper 95% CLM) of the confidence interval.

The MEANS Procedure

Analysis Variable : continuous_variable

N	Mean	Std Dev	Lower 95% CL for Mean	Upper 95% CL for Mean
100	2.4909631	4.8883862	1.5210012	3.4609250

- If a one-sided confidence interval is desired, specify either the lower CLM (LCLM) or the upper CLM (UCLM) instead of the CLM (see sample code below).
- The output table will give the desired confidence limit.

```
PROC MEANS DATA = dataset_name UCLM;
      VAR continuous_variable;
RUN;
```

The MEANS Procedure

Analysis Variable: continuous_variable
Upper 95% CL for Mean
3.3026264

Using Stata to construct confidence intervals for a mean

In Stata, there are two options for calculating a confidence interval for a mean.

1 If we have a dataset with a continuous variable, we use the *ci* command:

```
ci means variable_name, level(1 - α)
```

where we specify the name of the continuous variable and the value of $1 - \alpha$.

2 If we have only the sample size (n), sample mean ($\bar{x}$), and sample standard deviation (s), we can use the *cii* command:

```
cii means n sample_mean s, level(1 - α)
```

where we specify the sample size, sample mean, sample standard deviation, and the value of $1 - \alpha$.

For example, if we would like the 95% confidence interval for the continuous variable named *continuous_variable* used in the SAS example, we would type one of the following two options:

```
ci means continuous_variable, level(95)
```

```
    Variable |    Obs        Mean    Std. Err.    [95% Conf. Interval]
-------------+--------------------------------------------------------
continuous~e |    100    2.490963    .4888386    1.521001    3.460925
```

Or:

```
cii means 100 2.490963 4.888386, level(95)

    Variable |        Obs        Mean    Std. Err.       [95% Conf. Interval]
-------------+---------------------------------------------------------------
             |        100    2.490963     .4888386        1.521001    3.460925
```

The output gives the sample size (Obs), sample mean (Mean), standard error (Std. Err.), and upper and lower bounds (both bounds indicated by 95% Conf. Interval). We can see that both methods produce a 95% confidence interval of (1.52, 3.46).

Requesting a one-sided confidence interval

To request a one-sided confidence interval, we use the same approach but change the value of the level option.

- In order to request a one-sided limit, multiply the α level by 2. A two-sided test with twice the desired alpha level is equivalent to a one-sided test with the desired alpha level, as $Z_{1-2\alpha/2} = Z_{1-\alpha}$.
- For example, if a 95% one-sided confidence interval is desired, specify level(90).
- For a 99% one-sided interval, specify level(98). Stata will, then, produce the correct upper or lower limit of interest.

Using either of the Stata commands, we can get the desired lower or upper bound from the output.

```
ci means variable_name, level(1 - 2α)
cii means n sample_mean s, level(1 - 2α)
```

Note that the line in the output will say "[100(1 – 2α)% Conf. Interval]" even though we are trying to get a bound for a 100(1 – α)% confidence limit, but this can be ignored. Taking one bound in the 100(1 – 2α)% interval is equivalent to the upper or lower bound of the 100(1 – α)% confidence limit.

```
    Variable |   Obs        Mean     Std. Err.       [90% Conf. Interval]
-------------+-----------------------------------------------------------
continuous~e |   100    2.490963     .4888386          1.6793    3.302626
```

In this example, the upper bound of the one-sided 95% confidence interval is 3.30.

The t-distribution

The assumption that σ is known is somewhat artificial because σ is rarely known in practice. When σ is unknown, it is reasonable to estimate σ by the sample standard deviation (s). Thus, it would seem logical to construct confidence intervals using the equation $\frac{\bar{X}-\mu}{s/\sqrt{n}}$ because we are using the same standardization formula but are replacing the unknown σ with known s. However, this quantity is no longer normally distributed.

This dilemma was first solved in 1908 by a statistician named William Gossett, who chose to identify himself by the pseudonym "student." This is why the distribution of $\frac{\bar{X}-\mu}{s/\sqrt{n}}$ is usually referred to as the "student's t-distribution."

t-distribution: A family of distributions indexed by one parameter referred to as the *degrees of freedom* (df) of the distribution. Therefore, it is not itself a unique distribution.

- The shape of the t-distribution depends on the sample size (n), with df $= n - 1$.
- The shape of the t-distribution is a symmetric bell curve (like the Z distribution) with wider tails than the normal distribution because the population standard deviation (σ) is estimated by the sample standard deviation (s).
- As the degrees of freedom increase, the t-distribution approaches the normal distribution.
- When we compare values in the standard normal table with values for infinite degrees of freedom in the t-distribution table, we see that they are very similar.
- The difference between the t-distribution and the normal distribution is greatest for small values of n ($n < 30$).
- For a sample of size n drawn from an underlying normally distributed population, we use the following notation for the t-statistic. Note the similarities and differences between this formula and the calculation of a z-score.

$$t = \frac{\bar{X}-\mu}{s/\sqrt{n}} \sim t_{n-1} \tag{6.8}$$

Obtaining critical values in SAS and Stata

Table 6.4 displays critical values for the normal distribution that correspond to commonly used levels of significance.

When working with the t-distribution, you have a choice between using the t table (Appendix Table A.4) and using SAS or Stata to calculate probabilities.

Suppose that you have a random variable, T, which follows a t-distribution with $n - 1$ degrees of freedom. You can calculate cutoffs for the t-distribution using SAS functions in a data step or by typing the Stata function into the command window. For example, in SAS, complete the following procedure:

Table 6.4 Common critical values of the standard normal distribution

α	$1-\alpha$	$Z_{1-\alpha}$	$Z_{1-\alpha/2}$
0.10	0.90	1.28	1.645
0.05	0.95	1.645	1.96
0.01	0.99	2.33	2.58

```
DATA;
   cutoff = <insert function here>;
RUN;
```

- After running the data step, simply open the dataset, and see the value for the variable "cutoff" or use PROC PRINT.

- If you want to calculate the probability that T takes on a value greater than some value k—i.e., $P(T > k)$, type

`1 - PROBT(k, df)` in SAS

or

`di ttail(df, k)` in Stata.

- If you want the probability that T is less than some value k—i.e., $P(T < k)$, then make use of the fact that $P(T < k) + P(T > k) = 1$, and use the command

`PROBT(k, df)` in SAS

or

`di 1 - (ttail(df, k))` in Stata.

- To find the value T of a t-distribution with $n - 1$ degrees of freedom that cuts off an area of p in the right tail, use

`TINV(1 - p, df)` in SAS

or

`di invttail(df, p)` in Stata.

Table 6.5 provides a summary of these commands.

- For example, to find the value of a t-distribution with $n - 1 = 11$ degrees of freedom that cuts off $p = 0.10$ to the right, you would type the following:

Using SAS	*Using Stata*

SAS Code
 	
`DATA example;`
` cutoff = TINV(0.90,11);`
`RUN;`
 	
`PROC PRINT DATA = example;`
` VAR cutoff;`
 	
`RUN;`
	Stata Code
	
	`di invttail(11, 0.10)`

SAS Output Obs: 1 — Cutoff: 1.36343	Stata Output 1.3634303

SAS Output table:

Obs	Cutoff
1	1.36343

Check that the value of 1.36 is in agreement with the cutoff value from Table A.4 in the Appendix.

Table 6.5 Software commands for calculating *t*-distribution cutoffs

Probability	*SAS*	*Stata*
$P(T > k)$	`1 - PROBT(k, df)`	`di ttail(df, k)`
$P(T < k)$	`PROBT(k, df)`	`di 1 - (ttail(df, k))`
Value that cuts off an area of p in the right-tail use	`TINV(1 - p, df)`	`di invttail(df, p)`

EXAMPLE PROBLEM 6.3

Suppose that you are interested in estimating the mean total cholesterol of the population of obese persons in the United States. Assume that the total cholesterol levels follow a normal distribution with ***unknown*** mean μ but with ***known*** standard deviation $\sigma = 39.7$ mg/dL. A random sample of 353 obese patients is selected from the underlying population.[3] The mean total cholesterol for these individuals is $\bar{x} = 189.9$ mg/dL.

E What is the point estimate for μ?

The sample mean, $\bar{x} = 189.9$ mg/dL, is the point estimate and our best guess for μ.

F Construct a 95% confidence interval for μ.

Since σ is known, we will use the normal distribution and not the *t*-distribution for the confidence interval. Because we are calculating a 95% confidence interval, we will use 1.96 as the Z value. We also know $n = 353$.

Then, we will use the formula for the two-sided 95% confidence interval for a mean, and we will substitute our values.

$$95\%\ \text{CI} = \left(\bar{x} - 1.96\frac{\sigma}{\sqrt{n}},\ \bar{x} + 1.96\frac{\sigma}{\sqrt{n}}\right) = \left(189.9 - 1.96\frac{39.7}{\sqrt{353}},\ 189.9 + 1.96\frac{39.7}{\sqrt{353}}\right)$$

$$= (185.8,\ 194.0)$$

G Interpret the confidence interval.

We are 95% confident that the interval (185.8, 194. 0 mg/dL) covers the true mean total cholesterol for the population of obese persons in the United States.

EXAMPLE PROBLEM 6.4

A genetic self-efficacy measure was administered to a sample of 192 patients at a primary care center.[4] The scale ranged from 1 (low genetic knowledge and awareness) to 5 (full ability to assess genetic risk and understand genetic issues). The genetic self-efficacy score in this sample had a mean of $\bar{x} = 3.37$ with a standard deviation $s = 1.09$.

A Calculate a 90% confidence interval for the true mean of the genetic self-efficacy score in this population.

We know that n = 192, $\bar{x}$ = 3.37, and s = 1.09. Because σ is unknown, we will use the t-distribution. We can find the critical t-value by either using the t-distribution tables or by using SAS or Stata.

Problem 6.4 *Part (A)* t-*Distribution Cutoff Calculation*

Using SAS	*Using Stata*
SAS Code	Stata Code

`DATA a;`
`cutoff = TINV(0.95,191);`
`RUN;`
 	
`PROC PRINT DATA = a;`
`RUN;`
	`di invttail(191, 0.05)`

SAS Output	Stata Output
Obs: 1 — Cutoff: 1.65287	1.6528705

Thus, the t-value when α = 0.10 with n – 1 = 192 – 1 = 191 degrees of freedom is $t_{n-1,\, 1-\alpha/2} = t_{192-1,\, 1-0.10/2} = t_{191,\, 095} = 1.65$.

$$
\begin{aligned}
90\%\ \text{CI:} & \left(\bar{x} - t_{n-1,1-\alpha/2}\frac{s}{\sqrt{n}},\ \bar{x} + t_{n-1,1-\alpha/2}\frac{s}{\sqrt{n}}\right) \\
&= \left(3.37 - 1.65\frac{1.09}{\sqrt{192}},\ 3.37 + 1.65\frac{1.09}{\sqrt{192}}\right) \\
&= (3.37 - 0.13,\ 3.37 + 0.13) = (3.24,\ 3.50)
\end{aligned}
$$

B Interpret the 90% confidence interval.

We are 90% confident that the true mean genetic self-efficacy score in this population lies in the interval (3.24, 3.50).

C Construct a 99% confidence interval for the mean.

First, we will find the t-value that corresponds to $\alpha = 0.01$ with $n - 1 = 192 - 1 = 191$ degrees of freedom.

Problem 6.4 *Part (C) t-Distribution Cutoff Calculation*	
Using SAS	*Using Stata*

SAS Code
`DATA c;`
`cutoff = TINV(0.995,191);`
`RUN;`
`PROC PRINT DATA = c;`
`RUN;`
	Stata Code
	`di invttail(191, 0.005)`

SAS Output Obs: 1, Cutoff: 2.60181	Stata Output 2.6018143

Thus, we will use the value $t_{n-1,\,1-\alpha/2} = t_{192-1,\,1-0.01/2} = t_{191,\,0.995} = 2.60$.

$$99\%\ \text{CI: } \left(\bar{x} - t_{n-1,1-\alpha/2}\frac{s}{\sqrt{n}},\ \bar{x} + t_{n-1,1-\alpha/2}\frac{s}{\sqrt{n}}\right)$$

$$= \left(3.37 - 2.60\frac{1.09}{\sqrt{192}},\ 3.37 + 2.60\frac{1.09}{\sqrt{192}}\right)$$

$$= (3.37 - 0.20,\ 3.37 + 0.20) = (3.17,\ 3.57)$$

D Interpret the 99% confidence interval.

We are 99% confident that the interval (3.17, 3.57) covers the true mean genetic self-efficacy score in this population.

E How do the 90% and 99% confidence intervals compare?

The 99% confidence interval is wider than the 90% confidence interval. The 99% confidence interval has a width of 0.40, whereas the 90% confidence interval has a width of 0.26.

PRACTICE PROBLEM 6.5

Data from the National Air Toxics Assessment (NATA) is used to calculate an environmental health hazards index for all census tracts in the United States; NATA measures potential exposure to harmful toxins in the environment.[5] The index takes into account carcinogenic, respiratory, and neurologic hazards, and indicates the national percentile rank of the census tract. The lowest value is 0, indicating maximum exposure to toxins harmful to health; the highest value is 100, indicating the best environmental quality and least exposure to toxins. There are 305 census tracts in the city of St. Louis, Missouri, but we have a sample of 210 census tracts with values of the environment health hazards index. The average score of the sample environmental health hazards index is 25.30 with a standard deviation of 12.30. Data for this problem are in the datasets *ch6_health_hazards.sas7bdat* and *ch6_health_hazards.dta*.

BOX 6.1 DESCRIPTION OF *ch6_health_hazards* DATASET

In this problem, we will use the variable *health_hazards_index*, which is a numeric variable. Each census tract has a unique identifier, called a FIPS code, which is composed of a 2-digit state code, a 3-digit county code, and a 6-digit tract code, for a total identifier length of 11 digits. This identifier variable is named *census_tract*.

A What is the point estimate for μ?

B Construct a 95% confidence interval for μ by hand.

C Interpret the interval from Practice Problem 6.1—Part (B).

D Given that the average environmental health hazards index of all census tracts in the United States is 49.49, what can we say about the level of environmental health hazards in St. Louis compared to the United States as a whole?

E Write and run the SAS or Stata code to produce a 95% confidence interval for the mean. Check that the output agrees with the hand calculation in Practice Problem 6.1—Part (B).

Sampling distribution for proportions

In Chapter 4, we introduced the binomial distribution. To recap, this distribution is used in a scenario in which we have a random variable, X, that counts the number of successes in n independent trials where each trial has probability p of success.

- The mean of the distribution is $\mu_x = np$, and the standard deviation is $\sigma_x = \sqrt{np(1-p)}$.
- We know that we can use the normal approximation to the binomial distribution when there is a large sample size.
- The rule of thumb is that the sample size is sufficiently large if both np and $n(1-p) \geq 5$. If this condition is met, then X follows an approximately normal distribution with mean np and standard deviation $\sqrt{np(1-p)}$, written $X \sim N\left(np, \sqrt{np(1-p)}\right)$.

- Using the standardized form, we have $Z = \frac{X - np}{\sqrt{np(1-p)}}$, where Z follows a standard normal distribution, $Z \sim N(0,1)$.

In many cases, we may want to estimate the true unknown population proportion or probability of outcome, p.

Population Proportion: A parameter, denoted by p, that estimates the proportion of the population with some characteristic. Similar to other population parameters, population proportions are unknown and we often want to estimate them. In order to estimate the population proportion, we use the sample proportion, $\hat{p}$.

Sample Proportion, $\hat{p}$**:** An estimate of p calculated from a random sample drawn from the population. This is similar to the case with continuous data described previously in the chapter where $\bar{x}$ is an estimate of μ.

- If we perform n number of trials and observe x successes, we have $\hat{p} = \frac{x}{n}$ for the sample.
- As a result of the CLT, we conclude that the sampling distribution of $\hat{p}$ is approximately normal with mean p and standard deviation $\sqrt{\frac{p(1-p)}{n}}$. This is often written as

$$\hat{p} \sim N\left(p, \sqrt{\frac{p(1-p)}{n}}\right). \tag{6.9}$$

Thus,

$$Z = \frac{\hat{p} - p}{\sqrt{\frac{p(1-p)}{n}}} \tag{6.10}$$

follows a standard normal distribution.

Confidence intervals for proportions

As in the continuous case, it is often desired to calculate an interval around the point estimate. We can use the application of the CLT to get an interval estimate around $\hat{p}$:

$$\left(\hat{p} \pm Z_{1-\alpha/2}\sqrt{\frac{\hat{p}(1-\hat{p})}{n}}\right). \tag{6.11}$$

We can interpret the confidence interval by saying, "We are 100(1 – α)% confident that the interval $\left(\hat{p} - Z_{1-\alpha/2}\sqrt{\frac{\hat{p}(1-\hat{p})}{n}}, \hat{p} + Z_{1-\alpha/2}\sqrt{\frac{\hat{p}(1-\hat{p})}{n}}\right)$ will cover p."

- Unlike in the estimation of the mean, estimates for proportions follow a standard normal distribution (instead of a t-distribution) since only one parameter, p, needs to be estimated from the data.

- We can also construct one-sided confidence limits (bounds) for a proportion. The interval estimator should be used only if $n\hat{p}(1 - \hat{p}) \geq 5$.
- If we assume the normal approximation to the binomial holds, then a one-sided lower limit $100(1 - \alpha)\%$ confidence interval is of the form

$$p > \hat{p} - Z_{1-\alpha}\sqrt{\frac{\hat{p}(1-\hat{p})}{n}}. \tag{6.12}$$

- The one-sided upper limit $100(1 - \alpha)\%$ confidence interval is of the form

$$p > \hat{p} + Z_{1-\alpha}\sqrt{\frac{\hat{p}(1-\hat{p})}{n}}. \tag{6.13}$$

- The formulas for both one-sided and two-sided confidence intervals for a proportion are displayed in Table 6.6.

Using SAS to obtain confidence intervals for proportions

We can use PROC FREQ to calculate confidence intervals for a proportion if we have a dataset with a binary variable that specifies whether the subject has the event of interest.

- In the TABLES statement, specify the event indicator and the level of significance (ALPHA). The default is $\alpha = 0.05$, which will produce a 95% confidence interval.
- The BINOMIAL option tells SAS that we are in a binomial (proportion) situation.
- By default, the proportion calculated will be for the first level of the one-way frequency table. If we would like to switch the proportion calculated, we use the LEVEL option after the BINOMIAL statement:

```
PROC FREQ DATA = dataset_name;
    TABLES binary_variable / BINOMIAL (LEVEL = "1") ALPHA = 0.05;
RUN;
```

- There will be multiple tables in the output, but the one with the heading "Binomial Proportion" gives the confidence interval.

Table 6.6 Equations for $100(1 - \alpha)\%$ confidence intervals for a proportion

Type of confidence interval	*Formula*
Two-sided	$\left(\hat{p} - Z_{1-\alpha/2}\sqrt{\frac{\hat{p}(1-\hat{p})}{n}}, \hat{p} + Z_{1-\alpha/2}\sqrt{\frac{\hat{p}(1-\hat{p})}{n}}\right)$
One-sided lower limit	$\hat{p} - Z_{1-\alpha}\sqrt{\frac{\hat{p}(1-\hat{p})}{n}}$
One-sided upper limit	$\hat{p} + Z_{1-\alpha}\sqrt{\frac{\hat{p}(1-\hat{p})}{n}}$

- The line "95% Lower Conf Limit" gives the lower limit, and "95% Upper Conf Limit" gives the upper limit.
- This assumes that the normal approximation is appropriate; if not, the exact confidence interval is given at the bottom of the output table.

Binomial Proportion	
binary_variable = 1	
Proportion	0.4000
ASE	0.0828
95% Lower Conf Limit	0.2377
95% Upper Conf Limit	0.5623
Exact Conf Limits	
95% Lower Conf Limit	0.2387
95% Upper Conf Limit	0.5789

- Unlike for confidence intervals around a mean, we cannot use the SIDES option if we would like a one-sided confidence interval.
- However, we can manipulate the level of significance in the ALPHA option to receive the correct limit in the output. In order to do so, let the ALPHA option be ALPHA = 2α. Then, find the corresponding lower or upper bounds in the output.
- Note that the line in the output will say "$100(1 - 2\alpha)$ % Lower Conf Limit" or "$100(1 - 2\alpha)$% Upper Conf Limit," but as long as one bound is selected it is equivalent to the upper or lower bound of the $100(1 - \alpha)$% confidence limit.

Using Stata to obtain confidence intervals for proportions

Just as for confidence intervals for means, in Stata, we can compute confidence intervals for a proportion by simply entering the parameters or by calculating from a dataset.

- If we have a dataset with a binary variable, we use the *ci* function:

```
ci proportions binary_variable, level(1 - α) Wald
```

  where we specify the name of the binary variable and the desired confidence level.
- If we have the sample size (n) and probability of success ($\hat{p}$), we use the *cii* function:

```
cii proportions n p, level(1 - α) wald
```

  where we specify the sample size (n) first, then the value of $\hat{p}$ and the desired confidence interval. You can also input x (the number of success) instead of $\hat{p}$ in the Stata command above.

- The *wald* option overrides the default option of an exact confidence interval. If we would like the exact confidence interval instead, then the *wald* option can be left out.

Mirroring the example in SAS, we want to find the 95% confidence interval for a binary variable called *binary_variable*. We know that out of 35 observations there are 14 successes. Thus, we can use either of the following two lines of code to get the same output.

```
ci proportions binary_variable, level(95) wald
```

```
                                                    -- Binomial Wald ---
    Variable |   Obs  Proportion    Std. Err.   [95% Conf. Interval]
-------------+---------------------------------------------------------
binary_var~e |    35          .4     .0828079    .2376996    .5623004
```

Or:

```
cii proportions 35 14, level(95) wald
```

```
                                                  -- Binomial Wald ---
    Variable |   Obs  Proportion   Std. Err.   [95% Conf. Interval]
-------------+-------------------------------------------------------
             |    35          .4    .0828079   .2376996    .5623004
```

We see that both approaches give a 95% confidence interval of (0.24, 0.56).

To produce a one-sided confidence interval for a proportion, we use the same approach as when calculating one-sided intervals for a mean. Let the level option be level($1 - 2\alpha$). Then, find the corresponding lower or upper bounds in the output. Note that the line in the output will say "[100($1 - 2\alpha$)% Conf. Interval]" even though we are trying to get a bound for a 100($1 - \alpha$)% confidence limit, but this can be ignored. Taking one bound in the 100($1 - 2\alpha$)% interval is equivalent to the upper or lower bound of the 100($1 - \alpha$)% confidence limit.

EXAMPLE PROBLEM 6.6

The Youth Risk Behavior Surveillance System (YRBSS) monitors health risk behaviors of 9th through 12th grade students in the United States.[6] Students who reported having at least one drink of alcohol on at least one day in the month before the survey were classified as currently drinking alcohol. In 2013, the percentage of high school students who reported that they had at least one drink of alcohol in the previous month was 34.9%. We wish to examine drinking behavior for students who reported missing school because of feeling unsafe either at school or on their way to or from school. Out of a sample of 200 high school students who reported missing school because of unsafe conditions, 90 were currently drinking alcohol. Data for the problem are in the dataset *ch6_youth_drinking*.

BOX 6.2 DESCRIPTION OF *ch6_youth_drinking* DATASET

The Youth Risk Behavior Surveillance System (YRBSS) asks each student, "During the past 30 days, on how many days did you have at least one drink of alcohol?" The response is a 7-level categorical variable, ranging from "0 days" to "All 30 days." Students reporting that they currently drank at least one drink of alcohol on at least 1 day during the 30 days before the survey were classified as current drinkers (variable *alcoholic_drink* = *1*). Those who reported not having at least one drink any day in the prior month were coded as *alcoholic_drink* = *0*. All students surveyed were asked, "During the past 30 days, on how many days did you not go to school because you felt you would be unsafe at school or on your way to or from school?" The sample in the dataset (*ch6_youth_drinking*) is limited to those students reporting at least "1 day" of missed school.

A Find a point estimate for the true proportion *p*.

$$\hat{p} = \frac{x}{n} = \frac{90}{200} = 0.45$$

B First, check that the normal approximation is appropriate, and construct a 99% confidence interval for p.

For the normal approximation to hold, we must check that $n\hat{p} \geq 5$ and $n(1-\hat{p}) \geq 5$. In this case, we have $n = 200$ and $\hat{p} = 0.45$, so $n\hat{p} = 200(0.45) = 90$ and $n(1-\hat{p}) = 200(1-0.45) = 200(0.55) = 110$. This means that the normal approximation can be used since both numbers are greater than or equal to 5.

For a two-sided 99% confidence interval, the Z value is $Z_{1-\alpha/2} = Z_{1-0.01/2} = 2.58$.

$$\left(\hat{p} - Z_{1-\alpha/2}\sqrt{\frac{\hat{p}(1-\hat{p})}{n}}, \hat{p} + Z_{1-\alpha/2}\sqrt{\frac{\hat{p}(1-\hat{p})}{n}}\right)$$

$$= \left(0.45 - 2.58\sqrt{\frac{0.45(1-0.45)}{200}},\ 0.45 + 2.58\sqrt{\frac{0.45(1-0.45)}{200}}\right)$$

$$= (0.45 - 0.09,\ 0.45 + 0.09) = (0.36,\ 0.54)$$

C Interpret the confidence interval.

We are 99% confident that the true proportion of students lies in the interval (0.36, 0.54) for those who had at least one alcoholic drink in the previous month among those who missed at least 1 day of high school in the previous month because of unsafe conditions.

D Calculate a 95% confidence interval for *p*.

For a two-sided 95% confidence interval, the Z value is $Z_{1-\alpha/2} = Z_{1-0.05/2} = 1.96$.

$$\left(\hat{p} - Z_{1-\alpha/2}\sqrt{\frac{\hat{p}(1-\hat{p})}{n}}, \hat{p} + Z_{1-\alpha/2}\sqrt{\frac{\hat{p}(1-\hat{p})}{n}}\right)$$

$$= \left(0.45 - 1.96\sqrt{\frac{0.45(1-0.45)}{200}},\ 0.45 + 1.96\sqrt{\frac{0.45(1-0.45)}{200}}\right)$$

$$= (0.045 - 0.07,\ 0.045 + 0.07) = (0.38,\ 0.52)$$

We are 95% confident that the interval (0.38, 0.52) covers p, the true proportion of students who are current drinkers among those who missed at least 1 day of high school in the previous month because of unsafe conditions.

E How do the 99% and 95% confidence intervals compare?

The 99% confidence interval is wider than the 95% confidence interval. The 99% confidence interval has a width of 0.18, whereas the 95% confidence interval has a width of 0.14.

F Write the SAS or Stata code to calculate the 99% and 95% confidence intervals. Check that the output matches the hand calculations in Example Problem 6.6—Parts (B) and (D).

In SAS, we can use PROC FREQ to find the confidence intervals. Since our indicator of youth drinking has levels 0 and 1, by default SAS will calculate the proportion of the lowest level. Using the LEVEL option, we can override the default and specify that the proportion we are interested in is the proportion of 1s rather than the proportion of 0s.

```
PROC FREQ DATA = ch6_youth_drinking;
     TABLES alcoholic_drink / BINOMIAL (LEVEL = "1")
          ALPHA = 0.01;
RUN;
```

Binomial Proportion	
alcoholic_drink = 1	
Proportion	0.4500
ASE	0.0352
99% Lower Conf Limit	0.3594
99% Upper Conf Limit	0.5406
Exact Conf Limits	
99% Lower Conf Limit	0.3590
99% Upper Conf Limit	0.5434

We can see that SAS calculates the 99% confidence interval to be (0.3594, 0.5406), and this matches the hand calculation in Example Problem 6.5—Part (B) after rounding.

```
PROC FREQ DATA = ch6_youth_drinking;
      TABLES alcoholic_drink / BINOMIAL (LEVEL = "1");
RUN;
```

Binomial Proportion	
alcoholic_drink = 1	
Proportion	0.4500
ASE	0.0352
95% Lower Conf Limit	0.3811
95% Upper Conf Limit	0.5189
Exact Conf Limits	
95% Lower Conf Limit	0.3798
95% Upper Conf Limit	0.5218

SAS calculates the 95% confidence interval to be (0.38, 0.52), and this matches the hand calculation in Example Problem 6.5—Part (D).

To perform the calculations in Stata, we use the *ci* command. We need to specify the confidence interval (99% and 95%) in the level option.

```
ci proportions alcoholic_drink, level(99) wald
                                                   -- Binomial Wald ---
    Variable |     Obs  Proportion    Std. Err.    [99% Conf. Interval]
-------------+------------------------------------------------------------
alcoholic_~k |     200          .45    .0351781    .3593872    .5406128

ci proportions alcoholic_drink, level(95) wald
                                                   -- Binomial Wald ---
    Variable |     Obs  Proportion    Std. Err.    [95% Conf. Interval]
-------------+------------------------------------------------------------
alcoholic_~k |     200          .45    .0351781    .3810522    .5189478
```

The 99% confidence interval from the output is (0.36, 0.54) and the 95% confidence interval is (0.38, 0.52). These intervals match the hand calculations in Example Problem 6.5—Parts (B) and (D).

PRACTICE PROBLEM 6.2

Consider the t-distribution with 21 degrees of freedom.

A What proportion of the curve lies to the left of $t = 2.518$?

B What proportion of the area lies to the right of $t = 1.323$?

C What proportion of the area lies between $t = -1.721$ and $t = 2.831$?

D What value of t cuts off the lower 2.5% of the distribution?

PRACTICE PROBLEM 6.3

In the United States, laws mandating seat belt use in cars resulted from findings that seat belts can significantly reduce injuries and death during car crashes. Even decades after these laws were passed, some drivers and passengers do not wear seat belts while in a vehicle. Among a sample of 459 U.S. adults, 395 reported always wearing a seat belt.[7] The dataset for this sample is *ch6_seat_belt*.

BOX 6.3 DESCRIPTION OF *ch6_seat_belt* DATASET

The Behavioral Risk Factor Surveillance System (BRFSS) asks each participant, "How often do you use seat belts when you drive or ride in a car?" Those who answered "Always" received a value of 1 for the variable *wear_seat_belt*. Those who reported "Nearly always," "Sometimes," "Seldom," or "Never" were coded as *wear_seat_belt* = *0*.

A Find the point estimate for the true proportion of U.S. adults who always use a seat belt.

B We are interested in determining the one-sided lower limit for seat belt use. To do this, construct a 99% one-sided confidence interval for p by hand.

C Interpret the interval from Practice Problem 6.3—Part (B).

D Construct a 90% two-sided confidence interval for p by hand.

E Interpret the confidence interval in Practice Problem 6.3—Part (D).

F Use a statistical software package to check the confidence intervals calculated in Practice Problem 6.3—Parts (B) and (D).

PRACTICE PROBLEM 6.4

We are interested in examining the birthweights of a sample of 247 male babies.[3] The sample mean is $\bar{x} = 7.37$ lbs., and the sample standard deviation is $s = 1.28$ lbs. Data for this problem are in the dataset *ch6_birth_weight*.

BOX 6.4 DESCRIPTION OF *ch6_birth_weight* DATASET

The National Health and Nutrition Examination Survey (NHANES) conducted by the Centers for Disease Control and Prevention (CDC) asks, "How much did you/he/she weigh at birth?" Responses were recorded in pounds and ounces. We converted ounces to fractions of a pound to create the variable *birth_weight* (birthweight in pounds). Gender was ascertained from all participants as either "Male" or "Female." The sample in the dataset (*ch6_birth_weight*) is limited to those reporting male gender.

A What is the point estimate for μ_{male}, the mean birthweight in pounds among male babies?

B By hand, calculate a 95% confidence interval for the true mean birthweight for male babies.

C Interpret the 95% confidence interval for the true mean birthweight for males.

D Using SAS or Stata, calculate the 95% confidence interval for the true mean birthweight for males. Does the confidence interval match the hand calculation?

References

1. Webb Hooper M, Antoni MH, Okuyemi K, Dietz NA, Resnicow K. Randomized controlled trial of group-based culturally specific cognitive behavioral therapy among African American smokers. *Nicotine Tob Res*. 2016. doi:10.1093/ntr/ntw181.
2. Heatherton TF, Kozlowski LT, Frecker RC, Fagerstrom KO. The Fagerstrom Test for Nicotine Dependence: A Revision of the Fagerstrom Tolerance Questionnaire. *Br J Addict*. 1991;86:1119–1127. doi:doi:10.1111/j.1360-0443.1991.tb01879.x.
3. National Health and Nutrition Examination Survey. Hyattsville, MD: Centers for Disease Control and Prevention, National Center for Health Statistics. https://wwwn.cdc.gov/Nchs/Nhanes/Search/nhanes13_14.aspx. Published 2014. Accessed February 23, 2017.

4. Kaphingst KA, Blanchard M, Milam L, Pokharel M, Elrick A, Goodman MS. Relationships between health literacy and genomics-related knowledge, self-efficacy, perceived importance, and communication in a medically underserved population. *J Health Commun*. 2016;21 Suppl 1:58–68. doi:10.1080/10810730.2016.1144661.
5. U.S. Environmental Protection Agency. *National Air Toxics Assessment*. https://egis-hud.opendata.arcgis.com/datasets/c7e2c62560bd4a999f0e0b2f4cee2494_0. Published 2005. Accessed May 16, 2017.
6. Centers for Disease Control and Prevention. *Youth Risk Behavior Survey Questionnaire*. www.cdc.gov/yrbs. Published 2013. Accessed April 11, 2017.
7. Centers for Disease Control and Prevention. *Behavioral Risk Factor Surveillance System*. http://www.cdc.gov/brfss/annual_data/annual_data.htm. Published 2014. Accessed April 3, 2017.

7 One-sample hypothesis testing

This chapter will focus on one-sample hypothesis tests and will include the following topics:

- Basics of hypothesis testing
- Confidence intervals and hypothesis tests
- One-sample tests for the mean using software
- Inference for proportions
- One-sample test for proportions using software
- Determining power and calculating sample size

Terms

- critical value
- one-sided test
- *p*-value
- power
- rejection region
- two-sided test
- type I error
- type II error

Introduction

In the last chapter, we discussed methods of point and interval estimation for parameters of various distributions. Often, researchers have preconceived ideas about what these parameters might be and wish to test whether the data conform to these ideas. Hypothesis testing provides an objective framework for making decisions using probabilistic methods. People can form different opinions by looking at data, but hypothesis tests provide a uniform decision-making criterion that is consistent. With hypothesis tests, the research question is formulated in a framework by specifying a null hypothesis, H_0, and an alternative hypothesis.

In this workbook, we will consistently use H_1 to refer to the alternative hypothesis, but be aware that it can also be written as H_A. In a hypothesis test, we wish to compare the relative probabilities of obtaining the sample data under each of these hypothesis cases. In other words, hypothesis tests allow us to formally evaluate whether the data are consistent with the null hypothesis. In a one-sample problem, hypotheses are specified about a single distribution. In a two-sample problem, two different distributions are compared.

Basics of hypothesis testing

Hypothesis Testing: The process by which we draw some conclusion about a population parameter using information contained in a sample of observations.

- Hypothesis tests are always done under the assumption that the null hypothesis is true.
- They ask the question, "Is it likely that I would have observed my test statistic if the null hypothesis were true?" If it is likely, then we *do not reject* the null hypothesis. If it is unlikely, then we have evidence to *reject* the null hypothesis.

When we conduct a hypothesis test, we perform the following steps:

1. State the hypotheses (both the null and alternative).
2. Specify the significance level (α).
3. Draw a sample of size n.
4. Compute the test statistic.
5. Determine the p-value, compare the p-value to the significance level, and decide whether to reject or fail to reject H_0.
6. State conclusions regarding the subject matter.

We will go into each of these steps in more detail.

Step 1: State the hypothesis

- Identify the null hypothesis. This is a claim that the population parameter is equal to some quantity. For example, if we are interested in testing a mean, we can express the null hypothesis in symbols as H_0: $\mu = \mu_0$. The null hypothesis is usually what we want to disprove. It is what we don't believe, which leads to a proof by contradiction.
- Formulate the alternative hypothesis (H_1), a statement that contradicts H_0. This is usually what we do believe, or what we want to believe.

We need to set up the two hypotheses (null and alternative) to cover *all possibilities* for μ. This leads to a choice of three possible sets of null and alternative hypotheses, depending on the question we want to answer, as shown in Table 7.1.

Hypothesis tests can be either one-sided (two possible sets of null and alternative hypotheses) or two-sided (one possible set of null and alternative hypotheses).

Table 7.1 Null and alternative hypotheses for means

Confidence interval	*Null*	*Alternative*
Two-sided	H_0: $\mu = \mu_0$	H_1: $\mu \neq \mu_0$
One-sided	H_0: $\mu \geq \mu_0$	H_1: $\mu < \mu_0$
One-sided	H_0: $\mu \leq \mu_0$	H_1: $\mu > \mu_0$

Note: There are three sets of null and alternative hypotheses for tests for the mean. In a two-sided test, the alternative hypothesis is that the mean is not equal to the null mean. If the test is one-sided, the mean under the alternative is either less than or greater than the null mean.

One-Sided Test: A test in which the values of the parameters being studied under the alternative hypothesis are allowed to be on one side of the value of the parameter under the null hypothesis, or in one direction. When we look at the values being studied in a one-sided test, we consider whether the values are greater than or less than the values of the parameter under the null hypothesis, but we don't consider both cases.

- If the null hypothesis is $\mu \geq \mu_0$ and our alternative hypothesis is $\mu < \mu_0$, here we are performing a one-sided test. In our alternative hypothesis, we are examining only whether μ is less than μ_0 but not whether μ is greater than μ_0.
- If the null hypothesis is $\mu \leq \mu_0$ and our alternative hypothesis is $\mu > \mu_0$, here we are performing a one-sided test. In our alternative hypothesis, we are examining only whether μ is greater than μ_0 but not whether μ is less than μ_0.

Two-Sided Test: A test in which the values of the parameter being studied are sought in two directions (or on two sides), where the values can be greater than or less than the value of the parameter under the null hypothesis. This is the case in a scenario where the null hypothesis is $\mu = \mu_0$ and the alternative hypothesis is $\mu \neq \mu_0$. In the alternative hypothesis, values of μ can be greater or less than μ_0. In other words, in a two-sided test, we are examining both $\mu < \mu_0$ and $\mu > \mu_0$ for the alternative hypothesis.

There are various reasons for choosing a two-sided versus a one-sided test. In practice, two-sided tests are much more common. Unless the question implies that a one-sided test is more appropriate, a two-sided test should always be used.

- Two-sided tests are also more conservative; the *p*-value for a two-sided test is generally twice that of a one-sided test, making it harder to reach the significance level.

Regardless of the chosen option, always state *a priori* which type of test will be used. Once the null and alternative hypotheses are specified, we take a sample and evaluate whether the sample is more consistent with the null or with the alternative hypothesis. In other words, is the difference between the estimate of a population parameter and hypothesized value too large to be attributed to chance alone? Specifically, is the probability of obtaining the observed estimate or one that is even more extreme under the null hypothesis sufficiently small?

In actual practice, it is impossible, using the hypothesis-testing method, to prove that the null hypothesis is true. Because of this, *we do not accept the null; rather, we fail to reject it*. This difference in wording may seem trivial, but it is important to keep this in mind when interpreting the outcome of the test.

Step 2: Specify the significance level

The significance level of the test is also chosen *a priori*. By convention, the significance level is set to 0.05, or 5%. However, a smaller or larger alpha may be desirable. Other significance levels that we may see are 0.10 (10%) or 0.01 (1%). If multiple tests are involved, the level of significance for each test may be reduced to account for multiple testing (to be discussed later in Chapter 11). It is important to note that, when considering your conclusions, a distinction must be made between clinical (or scientific) and statistical significance because the two terms do not necessarily coincide. Results can be statistically significant but clinically unimportant. When sample sizes are large, small differences that are not clinically meaningful can be statistically significant. However, statistically nonsignificant results can be an indicator for more research or the need to test hypotheses with a larger sample size.

Step 3: Draw sample of size n

The sample is drawn from the general population about which we want to make an inference. In practice, the size of the sample may be determined by a variety of constraints, from practical to financial.

Step 4: Compute the test statistic

In order to get a p-value and to determine the outcome of the test, we must compute the test statistic. The formula for the test statistic will vary, depending on the test being used. So far, we have only discussed Z- and t-test statistics, but there are others that are applicable in different situations.

In Table 7.2, we see that when we are performing a one-sample test of the mean, we have a choice between using a normal test (Z-test) or a t-test. We use Z when σ is known and t when we have estimated σ with the sample standard deviation (s).

Let's assume that we have a scenario in which we know the population standard deviation; a normal test is appropriate. The test statistic Z follows a standard normal distribution, and we want to evaluate it under H_0. That is, how extreme is our statistic, assuming that the null hypothesis is true?

We know that if the null is true, 95% of the time, Z should be between -1.96 and 1.96. Therefore, if $Z > 1.96$ or $Z < -1.96$, we assume that the null hypothesis cannot be true (since such could happen only with a 5% chance). Thus, we would reject H_0 because Z has fallen in the rejection region.

Rejection Region: The range of test statistic values for which H_0 is rejected.

Finally, the critical value method of hypothesis testing is the general approach in which we compute a test statistic and determine the outcome of the test by comparing the test statistic to a critical value determined by the significance level of the test.

Table 7.2 One-sample test for the mean

Component	*Known variance*	*Unknown variance*
Test	Z-test	t-test
Test statistic	$Z = \frac{\bar{x} - \mu_0}{\frac{\sigma}{\sqrt{n}}}$	$t = \frac{\bar{x} - \mu_0}{\frac{s}{\sqrt{n}}}$
Distribution of test statistic under H_0	Standard normal	t-distribution with $n - 1$ df
Confidence interval (two-sided)	$\left(\bar{x} \pm Z_{1-\alpha/2}\frac{\sigma}{\sqrt{n}}\right)$	$\left(\bar{x} \pm t_{n-1,1-\alpha/2}\frac{s}{\sqrt{n}}\right)$

Note: There are two cases of the one-sample test for the mean: known variance and unknown variance. When the variance is known, we use a Z-test. If the variance is unknown, we use a one-sample t-test.

Abbreviation: df, degrees of freedom.

Table 7.3 Critical Z values at the 5% level of significance

Null and alternative	*Rejection criteria*
H_0: $\mu = \mu_0$ H_1: $\mu \neq \mu_0$	Reject if $\lvert z \rvert > 1.96$
H_0: $\mu \geq \mu_0$ H_1: $\mu < \mu_0$	Reject if $z < -1.645$
H_0: $\mu \leq \mu_0$ H_1: $\mu > \mu_0$	Reject if $z > 1.645$

Note: The Z-value for the rejection region depends on the choice of null and alternative hypotheses and the significance level. When $\alpha = 0.05$, the outcome of the test depends on the relationship of the test statistic to $z = 1.96$ (two-sided) or $z = 1.645$ (one-sided).

Critical Value: The value of a test statistic such that if the outcome is greater than or less than that value, the null hypothesis will be rejected. The critical value will change, depending on the significance level chosen for the test. Critical values for Z when α = 0.05 are given in Table 7.3.

Step 5: Compare p-value to α and determine to reject or fail to reject the null hypothesis

p-*Value:* The probability of obtaining the observed estimate, or one that is even more extreme, under the null hypothesis.

- The *p*-value answers the question, "What is the probability of getting as large, or a larger, discrepancy?" We compute *p*-values to assess the strength of the evidence.
- Once the *p*-value is determined, it is evaluated relative to the *a priori* selected level of significance of α (e.g., 0.05).
- If the *p*-value is less than α, then we reject the null hypothesis.
- However, if the *p*-value is greater than α, we fail to reject the null hypothesis.

Types of errors

Four outcomes of the hypothesis test are possible (Table 7.4).

- Two of the possible outcomes result in errors (type I and type II).
- If we fail to reject the null hypothesis and the null hypothesis is true or if we reject the null hypothesis when the alternative hypothesis is true, then there is not an error.

Type I Error (rejection error or α error): A false positive, the error that occurs when H_0 is rejected although H_0 is true. It is symbolized by $\alpha \equiv P$ (reject $H_0 \mid H_0$ is true). The type I error is usually set by the investigator to be 0.05 or 0.01, depending on the significance level of the test.

Type II Error: A false negative, which occurs when we fail to reject H_0 when H_0 is false. It is symbolized by β, where $\beta \equiv P$ (do not reject $H_0 \mid H_0$ is false). β is associated with a particular value in the alternative hypothesis.

Table 7.4 Four possible outcomes of a hypothesis test

	Truth	
Decision	*Null*	*Alternative*
Fail to reject	Fail to reject the null and the null is true	Fail to reject the null and the alternative is true (Type II error, β)
Reject	Reject the null and the null is true (Type I error, α)	Reject the null and the alternative is true

Note: There are four possible outcomes of a hypothesis test, two of which are erroneous. We can commit a type I or type II error if the decision from the test does not align with the truth. It is often hard or impossible to know whether an error has been committed.

Asymmetry of errors

Conventionally, a type I error is set smaller than a type II error. Because of this, we can feel confident about rejecting H_0 but not about accepting H_0. For example, if α is set at 0.05, then the probability of incorrectly rejecting H_0 is only 0.05 whereas the probability of incorrectly accepting H_0 is four times as much, 0.2.

We generally want a statistical test that makes α and β as small as possible, but this is a difficult goal because as α decreases, β increases, and vice versa. Our general strategy is to fix α at some specific level and to use the test that minimizes β or equivalently maximizes power. (See the Determining Power and Calculating Sample Size later in the chapter.)

Step 6: State conclusions regarding subject matter

The last step in conducting a hypothesis test is to state conclusions about the results. This should be done in the context of the hypothesis being tested and the available data.

Confidence intervals and hypothesis tests

A relationship exists between hypothesis testing and confidence intervals. Hypothesis testing uses the observed data to determine whether the sample statistic (e.g., the sample mean) could have happened by chance alone under the assumption that the hypothesized value is the truth. However, confidence intervals are intervals that contain values for the fixed population parameter (e.g., μ) that are plausible based on the data. Through their width, confidence intervals convey the amount of available information used to estimate a population parameter (e.g., mean) from a sample. Despite the differences, we should draw the same conclusion from a confidence interval as we would from a hypothesis test. In addition to examining the p-value, another way to determine the outcome of the hypothesis test is by using the confidence interval. Suppose that we have a problem in which we are interested in the population mean. If the null value μ_0 is in the confidence interval, we will not reject H_0 if we perform a hypothesis test. Thus, we do not reject the null hypothesis for any value of μ_0 that is contained in the confidence interval. In contrast, we would reject the null hypothesis for any value of μ_0 that is outside of the confidence interval.

One-sample tests for the mean using software

One-sample tests for the mean using SAS

We can use SAS to perform a one-sample test for the mean in addition to or instead of doing it by hand. To do so, we use PROC TTEST and the following syntax. (The mean under the null hypothesis should be specified in the "H0 =" option unless we want the default of 0.)

```
PROC TTEST DATA = dataset_name H0 = nullmean;
      VAR continuous_var;
RUN;
```

- For example, if we want to perform a one-sample *t*-test where $\mu_0 = 7.5$, we type the following:

```
PROC TTEST DATA = dataset_name H0 = 7.5;
      VAR continuous_var;
RUN;
```

- The output gives the following tables as well as a histogram and a Q–Q plot.

The TTEST Procedure
Variable: continuous_var

N	Mean	Std Dev	Std Err	Minimum	Maximum
100	6.0982	0.9777	0.0978	3.7416	8.6702

Mean	95% CL	Mean	Std Dev	95% CL	Std Dev
6.0982	5.9042	6.2922	0.9777	0.8584	1.1357

DF	t Value	Pr > |t|
99	−14.34	<.0001

- The test statistic ("t Value"), degrees of freedom ("DF"), and the *p*-value for the test ("P > |t|") are provided in the third output box.
- Two-sided tests are the default, so if we are interested in a one-sided test, we must specify SIDES = U (alternative mean is greater than null) or SIDES = L (alternative mean is lower than null) on the PROC TTEST line.
- We can also change the alpha level if we do not want the default of 0.05.

- The following code will run a one-sided test for the mean at the 0.01 level of significance where the null hypothesis is that the mean is less than or equal to 7.5:

```
PROC TTEST DATA = dataset_name H0 = 7.5 SIDES = U ALPHA = 0.01;
      VAR continuous_var;
RUN;
```

The TTEST Procedure
Variable: continuous_var

N	Mean	Std Dev	Std Err	Minimum	Maximum
100	6.0982	0.9777	0.0978	3.7416	8.6702

Mean	95% CL	Mean	Std Dev	95% CL	Std Dev
6.0982	5.8670	Infty	0.9777	0.8251	1.1928

DF	t Value	Pr > |t|
99	−14.34	1.0000

- The output for a one-sided test looks almost identical in structure to that from a two-sided test, but the confidence interval will also be one-sided and will give only a lower or upper bound.

One-sample tests for the mean using Stata

Stata can be used in two ways to conduct one-sample tests for the mean: manual input of the parameters or with a dataset loaded into the program.

- The first option is to use the calculator function and manually input the sample mean, population mean, sample standard deviation or population standard deviation (depending on whether we want a t-test or Z-test), and the alpha level.
- To do so, use the *ztesti* command for a Z-test and use the *ttesti* command for a t-test.
- Stata outputs both the one-sided and two-sided p-values by default, so there is no need to specify a one-sided or two-sided test in the code.
- The default alpha level is 0.05, so the level option can be left out unless a different alpha level is desired.

```
ztesti n mean sigma null mean, level(95)
ttesti n mean std nullmean, level(95)
```

- For example, if we want to perform a one-sample t-test using a sample of 100 observations where $\alpha = 0.05$, $\bar{x} = 6.1$, $\mu_0 = 7.5$, and $s = 0.98$, we type the following:

```
ttesti 100 6.10 0.98 7.5, level(95)
```

The following is the output:

```
One-sample t test
------------------------------------------------------------------------------
     |   Obs    Mean     Std. Err.    Std. Dev.    [95% Conf. Interval]
-----+------------------------------------------------------------------------
   x |   100     6.1        .098          .98       5.905547   6.294453
------------------------------------------------------------------------------
    mean = mean(x)                                         t = -14.2857
Ho: mean = 7.5                          degrees of freedom =        99

   Ha: mean < 7.5            Ha: mean != 7.5            Ha: mean > 7.5
Pr(T < t) = 0.0000      Pr(|T| > |t|) = 0.0000      Pr(T > t) = 1.0000
```

- The output shows test statistic ("t =") and the degrees of freedom on the right side.
- The *p*-values for two-sided and one-sided tests are provided. "P(T < t)" and "P(T > t)" give the one-sided *p*-values, and "P(|T| > |t|)" gives the two-sided *p*-value.
- The confidence interval is shown on the right side of the output above the test statistic.

The second option is to use a dataset loaded into Stata. In this case, we use the *ztest* or *ttest* command instead of *ztesti* or *ttesti*. This allows Stata to determine the sample mean, sample size, and sample standard deviation (only for *t*-test) directly from a continuous variable in a dataset without the need to manually input the values.

- The continuous variable in our dataset is specified after the *ztest* or *ttest* command.
- Two equal signs separate the name of the continuous variable from the value of the null mean.
- For a *Z*-test, the population standard deviation is also required in the *sd* option.

```
ztest continuous_var == nullmean, sd(pop_std) level(95)
ttest continuous_var == nullmean, level(95)
```

- To run the same one-sample test that we ran previously using the *ttesti* function, we use the following code:

```
ttest continuous_var == 7.5, level(95)
```

The output is below:

```
One-sample t test
------------------------------------------------------------------------------
Variable | Obs      Mean   Std. Err.   Std. Dev. [95% Conf. Interval]
---------+--------------------------------------------------------------------
contin~r | 100  6.098193   .0977677    .9776772     5.9042    6.292185
------------------------------------------------------------------------------
```

```
  mean = mean(continuous_var)                                t = -14.3381
Ho: mean = 7.5                              degrees of freedom =         99

   Ha: mean < 7.5              Ha: mean != 7.5             Ha: mean > 7.5
Pr(T < t) = 0.0000        Pr(|T| > |t|) = 0.0000       Pr(T > t) = 1.0000
```

- The output from the *ttest* function is essentially identical to that from the *ttesti* function described previously.
- Output from the *ztest* command is very similar to that from the *ttest* command.

```
One-sample z test
------------------------------------------------------------------------------
Variable | Obs        Mean    Std. Err.   Std. Dev.  [99% Conf. Interval]
---------+--------------------------------------------------------------------
contin~r | 100   6.098193          .15         1.5   5.711818    6.484567
------------------------------------------------------------------------------
    mean = mean(continuous_var)                                 z =  -9.3454
Ho: mean = 7.5

   Ha: mean < 7.5             Ha: mean != 7.5               Ha: mean > 7.5
Pr(Z < z) = 0.0000       Pr(|Z| > |z|) = 0.0000        Pr(Z > z) = 1.0000
```

- The test statistic is shown on the right after "z = ."
- The lines "P(Z < z)" and "P(Z > z)" give the one-sided p-values, and "P(|Z| > |z|)" gives the two-sided p-value.

To illustrate the process of a one-sample test of the mean, we will look at an example.

EXAMPLE PROBLEM 7.1

We want to investigate the question, "What is the mean blood calcium level for women with hypertension?" We know that blood calcium levels of U.S. residents are normally distributed with $\mu = 9.47$ mg/dL and $\sigma = 0.37$ mg/dL.[1] We have a sample of 487 women who have hypertension and whose average blood calcium level is $\bar{x}$. Our null hypothesis is that the mean calcium level for women with hypertension is the same as that of the general U.S. population. The alternative is that the mean calcium level of women with hypertension is not the same as that of the general U.S. population. In symbols, we can write H_0: $\mu = 9.47$ mg/dL and H_1: $\mu \neq 9.47$ mg/dL. We will assume the standard significance level of $\alpha = 0.05$.

A We will look at three scenarios to see how the test outcomes change depending on the sample data. What do we conclude if the following is true:

1. $\bar{x} = 9.48$ mg/dL?
2. $\bar{x} = 9.52$ mg/dL?
3. $\bar{x} = 9.41$ mg/dL?

BOX 7.1 DESCRIPTION OF EXAMPLE PROBLEM 7.1 DATA

The National Health and Nutrition Examination Survey (NHANES) collects laboratory measurements on the participants. The blood calcium level is reported in mg/dL. The survey also asks, "Have you ever been told by a doctor or other health professional that you had hypertension, also called high blood pressure?" Subjects can respond "Yes," "No," or "Don't know," or they can refuse to answer the question. Sex of each participant was recorded as either "Male" or "Female." The sample used for the data is limited to those who answered "Yes" to the hypertension question and "Female" to the sex question.

1 Our next step is to compute the test statistic. Since we know the population standard deviation, we will use a Z-statistic (as opposed to a t-statistic). We substitute in our sample mean ($\bar{x} = 9.48$ mg/dL), the hypothesized population mean ($\mu_0 = 9.47$ mg/dL), the population standard deviation ($\sigma = 0.37$ mg/dL), and the sample size ($n = 487$).

$$H_0: \mu = 9.47$$

$$H_1: \mu \neq 9.47$$

$$\alpha = 0.05$$

$$Z = \frac{\bar{x} - \mu_0}{\frac{\sigma}{\sqrt{n}}} = \frac{9.48 - 9.47}{\frac{0.37}{\sqrt{487}}} = 0.60$$

Once we have the value of the test statistic, we can use it to find the corresponding p-value. The p-value is the probability that Z is greater than 0.60 or less than −0.60. Since the normal distribution is symmetric, the probability that Z is greater than 0.60 is the same as the probability that Z is less than −0.60. Expressed in symbols, this is $P(Z > 0.60 \text{ or } Z < -0.60) = 2 \times P(Z > 0.60)$. From here, we turn to the normal distribution table to find the probability that Z is greater than 0.60.

$$P(Z > 0.60) = 0.2743$$

$$2 \times P(Z > 0.60) = 2 \times 0.2743 = 0.5485$$

$$p\text{-value} = 0.5485$$

Once we have the p-value, we compare it to the significance level to determine whether to reject H_0. Because p is greater than α, $0.5485 > 0.05$, we fail to reject the null hypothesis. We conclude that there is no evidence to suggest that the mean blood calcium level for women with hypertension is different from that of the general U.S. population.

2 Now, let the sample mean be 9.52 mg/dL. We will follow the same hypothesis-testing steps as in the scenario in Example Problem 7.1—Part (A).1 by first stating the null and alternative hypotheses and specifying alpha, then computing the test statistic given the new value of $\bar{x}$.

$$H_0: \mu = 9.47$$

$$H_1: \mu \neq 9.47$$

$$\alpha = 0.05$$

$$Z = \frac{\bar{x} - \mu_0}{\frac{\sigma}{\sqrt{n}}} = \frac{9.52 - 9.47}{\frac{0.37}{\sqrt{487}}} = 2.98$$

Next, we find the p-value. The p-value is $P(Z > 2.98 \text{ or } Z < -2.98) = 2 \times P(Z > 2.98)$. Using the normal distribution table, we need to look up the probability that Z is greater than 2.98.

$$P(Z > 2.98) = 0.0014$$

$$2 \times P(Z > 2.98) = 2 \times 0.0014 = 0.0029$$

$$p\text{-value} = 0.0029$$

In this scenario, $p < \alpha$ since 0.0029 is less than 0.05. Therefore, we reject the null hypothesis. We conclude that the mean blood calcium level for women with hypertension is different from that of the general U.S. population. Since Z is positive, the mean blood calcium level for women with hypertension is higher than that of U.S. residents in general.

3 Next, we will determine the test statistic in the case where $\bar{x} = 9.41$ mg/dL.

$$H_0: \mu = 9.47$$

$$H_1: \mu \neq 9.47$$

$$\alpha = 0.05$$

$$Z = \frac{\bar{x} - \mu_0}{\frac{\sigma}{\sqrt{n}}} = \frac{9.41 - 9.47}{\frac{0.37}{\sqrt{487}}} = -3.58$$

Next, we will determine the p-value. The p-value is $P(Z > 3.58$ or $Z < -3.58) = 2 \times P(Z > 3.58)$. Using the normal distribution table, we find the following:

$$P(Z > 3.58) = 0.0002$$

$$2 \times P(Z > 3.58) = 2 \times 0.0002 = 0.0004$$

$$p\text{-value} = 0.0004$$

In this scenario, $p < \alpha$ since 0.0004 is less than 0.05. Therefore, we reject the null hypothesis. We conclude that the mean blood calcium level for women with hypertension is different from that of the general U.S. population. Since Z is negative in this case, the mean blood calcium level for women with hypertension is lower than that of the general U.S. population.

B Now, we will use the confidence interval approach. We can compute a 95% confidence interval in each of the three scenarios in Example Problem 7.1—Part (A) and use the confidence intervals to determine whether to reject the null hypothesis.

$$P\left(\bar{x} - Z_{1-\frac{\alpha}{2}} \frac{\sigma}{\sqrt{n}}, \bar{x} + Z_{1-\alpha/2} \frac{\sigma}{\sqrt{n}}\right) = 0.95$$

$$\bar{x} \pm Z_{1-\alpha/2} \frac{\sigma}{\sqrt{n}} \rightarrow \bar{x} \pm 1.96 \frac{0.37}{\sqrt{487}} = \bar{x} \pm 0.03 = (\bar{x} - 0.03, \bar{x} + 0.03)$$

Scenario	*95% CI*
$\bar{x} = 9.48$ mg/dL	(9.45, 9.51 mg/dL)
$\bar{x} = 9.52$ mg/dL	(9.49, 9.55 mg/dL)
$\bar{x} = 9.41$ mg/dL	(9.38, 9.44 mg/dL)

What does it mean if the 95% confidence interval based on our sample does not include the assumed value for the population parameter (i.e., μ)? It could mean that we are in the 5% region of possibilities. Alternatively, it could mean that the assumed value of μ is not correct (i.e., the null hypothesis is not correct). Which is more plausible? It is more plausible that the null hypothesis is not correct. So, if the confidence interval does not include 9.47 mg/dL, we will reject the null hypothesis in favor of the alternative hypothesis. If the confidence interval contains 9.47 mg/dL, we fail to reject the null hypothesis.

Scenario	*95% CI*	*Outcome*
$\bar{x} = 9.48$ mg/dL	(9.45, 9.51 mg/dL)	Fail to reject
$\bar{x} = 9.52$ mg/dL	(9.49, 9.55 mg/dL)	Reject
$\bar{x} = 9.41$ mg/dL	(9.38, 9.44 mg/dL)	Reject

When we calculate confidence intervals, we should not forget to interpret the confidence interval in words and to state the conclusion in terms of the subject matter.

If $\bar{x} = 9.48$ mg/dL:

We are 95% confident that the interval (9.45, 9.51 mg/dL) covers the true mean blood calcium level for women with hypertension. Since this interval contains μ_0, we conclude that there is no evidence to suggest that the mean blood calcium level for women with hypertension is different from that of the general U.S. population.

If $\bar{x} = 9.52$ mg/dL:

We are 95% confident that the interval (9.49, 9.55 mg/dL) covers the true mean blood calcium level for women with hypertension. Since this interval does not contain μ_0, we conclude that the mean blood calcium level for women with hypertension is different from that of the general U.S. population. There is evidence to suggest that the mean blood calcium level for women with hypertension is greater than that of U.S. residents as a whole (because the entire interval is higher than μ_0).

If $\bar{x} = 9.41$ mg/dL:

We are 95% confident that the interval (9.38, 9.44 mg/dL) covers the true mean blood calcium level for women with hypertension. Since this interval does not contain μ_0, we conclude that the mean blood calcium level for women with hypertension is different from that of the general U.S. population. There is evidence to suggest that the mean blood calcium level for women with hypertension is less than that of the general U.S. population (because the entire interval is lower than μ_0).

EXAMPLE PROBLEM 7.2

Medical residents at a university-affiliated hospital are required to take a cultural competency self-assessment survey. For the population of hospital residents, the distribution of survey scores is approximately normal with unknown mean μ and unknown standard deviation σ. A sample of 30 residents from this hospital have a mean score $\bar{x} = 85.0$ and a standard deviation $s = 4.7$.

A Construct a 95% confidence interval for the population mean μ.

Since σ is unknown, we will use a t-distribution with $n - 1 = 30 - 1 = 29$ degrees of freedom.

$$95\%\ \text{CI} = \left(\bar{x} \pm t_{n-1,1-\alpha/2} \frac{s}{\sqrt{n}} \right) = \left(\bar{x} \pm t_{29,1-0.05/2} \frac{s}{\sqrt{n}} \right)$$

$$= \left(85.0 \pm 2.045 \frac{4.7}{\sqrt{30}} \right) = (85.0 \pm 1.8) = (83.2, 86.8)$$

We are 95% confident that the true mean cultural competency self-assessment survey score for hospital residents lies within the interval (83.2, 86.8).

B At the 0.05 level of significance, test whether the mean cultural competency self-assessment survey score for hospital residents is equal to 88.0, the mean cultural competency self-assessment survey score for hospital employees. What is the p-value of the test?

First, we will list what we know:

$\bar{x} = 85.0$

$\alpha = 0.05$

$\mu_0 = 88.0$

We would like to perform a two-sided test where H_0: $\mu = 88.0$ and H_1: $\mu \neq 88.0$.

$$t = \frac{\bar{x} - \mu_0}{\frac{s}{\sqrt{n}}} = \frac{85.0 - 88.0}{\frac{4.7}{\sqrt{30}}} = \frac{-3}{0.9} = -3.5$$

We can use the t table to find the corresponding p-value. Our test statistic follows a t-distribution with 29 degrees of freedom. From the table, we can determine that $2 \times 0.0005 < p < 2 \times 0.005$, which is equivalent to $0.001 < p < 0.01$.

C What do we conclude?

Since $p < \alpha = 0.05$, we reject H_0 and conclude that the mean cultural competency self-assessment score for hospital residents is not equal to 88.0, the mean cultural competency self-assessment score for hospital employees. In fact, there is evidence to suggest that the mean cultural competency self-assessment survey score for hospital residents is lower than that of the general population of employees (since t is negative).

D On the basis of the 95% confidence interval, would you have expected to reject or not reject the null hypothesis? Why?

The null value 88.0 does not lie inside the 95% confidence interval for μ (83.2, 86.8), so we would have expected that the null hypothesis would be rejected.

PRACTICE PROBLEM 7.1

We are concerned that there is an association between diet and total cholesterol levels and would like to investigate the possible association using hypothesis testing. We measured the total cholesterol level, in mg/dL, in a group of people who reported eating at fast food or pizza places in the last year. In a sample of 286, the mean total cholesterol level was $\bar{x} = 188.30$ mg/dL with a standard deviation s = 40.46 mg/dL.[1] In the general population, the total cholesterol levels are normally distributed with mean 183.37 mg/dL. Data for this problem are in the dataset *ch7_cholesterol_diet*.

BOX 7.2 DESCRIPTION OF *ch_cholesterol_diet* DATASET

The National Health and Nutrition Examination Survey (NHANES) collects the total cholesterol level of participants in mg/dL. The survey also asks, "In the past 12 months, did you buy food from fast food or pizza places?" The participant can respond "Yes," "No," or "Don't know," or can refuse to answer the question. The sample in the dataset *ch7_diet_cholesterol* is limited to those who reported buying food from fast food or pizza places in the past 12 months.

A By hand, test the hypothesis that people who report eating at fast food restaurants or pizza places in the last year have mean cholesterol levels different from the general population. Let $\alpha = 0.05$.

B Compute a 95% confidence interval for the true mean cholesterol level among people who have eaten at fast food or pizza places in the last year.

C Compare the results from the hypothesis test with the information available from the confidence interval.

D Write the code to run the appropriate hypothesis test in a statistical package. Check the answers to Practice Problem 7.1—Parts (A)–(C) using the output.

Inference for proportions

In the previous section, we conducted one-sample hypothesis tests for the mean. In this section, we will discuss the one-sample hypothesis test for a proportion. In Chapter 4, we introduced the binomial distribution where X is a random variable that counts the number of successes in n independent trials where each trial has probability p of success. The normal approximation to the binomial distribution holds when the sample size is sufficiently large, meaning that both np and $n(1-p)$ are greater than or equal to 5.

Using the normal approximation to the binomial, we can say that X follows an approximately normal distribution with mean np and standard deviation $\sqrt{np(1-p)}$. Thus, $Z = \frac{X - np}{\sqrt{np(1-p)}}$ follows a standard normal distribution with a mean of 0 and a standard deviation of 1.

The one-sample hypothesis test for a proportion is used for the estimation of p, the true unknown population proportion or probability of outcome. We estimate p by $\hat{p}$, which is calculated from a random sample drawn from the population. To calculate $\hat{p}$, we divide the observed number of successes by the number of trials performed. In symbols, this is represented by $\hat{p} = \frac{x}{n}$. As a result of the CLT, the sampling distribution of

$\hat{p}$ is approximately normal with mean p and standard deviation $\sigma = \sqrt{\frac{p(1-p)}{n}}$. Thus, $Z = \frac{\hat{p} - p}{\sqrt{p(1-p)/n}}$ follows a standard normal distribution.

Hypothesis testing for proportions

A one-sample test for a proportion can be one sided or two sided. The two-sided test is the most common, where we are testing the null hypothesis H_0: $p = p_0$ versus the alternative hypothesis H_1: $p \neq p_0$. After specifying the null and alternative hypotheses, we compute the test statistic. The test statistic depends on the value of $\hat{p}$, p_0, and n, and follows a standard normal distribution. The test statistic for proportions follows a standard normal distribution (instead of a t-distribution) since only one parameter (p) needs to be estimated from the data. Note that the estimates of standard deviation used in hypothesis testing are different from those used to construct confidence intervals. The components of the hypothesis test for proportions are shown in Table 7.5.

There are two methods for computing p-values for the one-sample test for proportions: The normal theory method and the exact method. Both methods have two cases, the choice of which depends on the relationship between $\hat{p}$ and p_0. Either $\hat{p} \leq p_0$ or $\hat{p} \geq p_0$, and the formula for the p-value is specific to each case. The equations for calculating p-values for two-sided, one-sample proportion tests are shown in Table 7.6.

First, decide whether the normal theory method or the exact method is appropriate. Then, select the equation that corresponds to the correct relationship between $\hat{p}$ and p_0. Use the normal theory method when $np > 5$ and $n(1-p) > 5$. Note that (ϕ) refers to the CDF of the standard normal distribution.

Table 7.5 One-sample test for a proportion

Component	*Formula*
Hypotheses	$H_0: p = p_0$ vs. $H_1: p \neq p_0$ $H_0: p \geq p_0$ vs. $H_1: p < p_0$ $H_0: p \leq p_0$ vs. $H_1: p > p_0$
Test statistic	$Z = \frac{\hat{p} - p_0}{\sqrt{\frac{p_0(1-p_0)}{n}}}$
Distribution of test statistic under H_0	Standard normal
Confidence interval (two-sided)	$\left(\hat{p} \pm Z_{1-\alpha/2}\sqrt{\frac{\hat{p}(1-\hat{p})}{n}}\right)$
Confidence interval (one-sided)	$\left(\hat{p} \pm Z_{1-\alpha}\sqrt{\frac{\hat{p}(1-\hat{p})}{n}}\right)$

Note: The components of the one-sample test for proportion are shown. There are three sets of null and alternative hypotheses for the test. The Z value in the confidence interval depends on whether the test is one-sided or two-sided.

Table 7.6 Obtaining p-values for two-sided, one-sample proportion tests

Method	*Relationship between $\hat{p}$ and p_0*	*Two-sided p-value*
Normal	$\hat{p} \leq p_0$	$p = 2 \times \phi(Z)$
	$\hat{p} \geq p_0$	$p = 2 \times [1 - \phi(Z)]$
Exact	$\hat{p} \leq p_0$	$p = 2 \times P(X \leq x) = \min\left[2\sum_{k=0}^{x}\binom{n}{k}p_0^k(1-p_0)^{n-k}, 1\right]$
	$\hat{p} \geq p_0$	$p = 2 \times P(X \geq x) = \min\left[2\sum_{k=x}^{n}\binom{n}{k}p_0^k(1-p_0)^{n-k}, 1\right]$

Note: The two methods for a one-sample test for proportions are the normal approximation method and the exact method. The formula for the p-value depends on the choice of method and the value of $\hat{p}$ relative to p_0.

One-sample tests for a proportion using SAS

We can use PROC FREQ to run a hypothesis test for a proportion. Unfortunately, there is no way to do this in SAS unless we have a dataset with a binary variable indicating the event. Some other software packages will run a test without an actual dataset as long as all of the necessary parameters are specified.

Enter the value of p_0 under the null hypothesis in the P = option and the variable name after the TABLES statement. The following code will run a one-sample test for proportions using the normal theory method.

```
PROC FREQ DATA = dataset_name;
      TABLES binary_variable / BINOMIAL(P = 0.032);
RUN;
```

If the exact method is desired, include the EXACT BINOMIAL option. The default level of significance is 0.05, but it can be specified using the ALPHA option for a different level of significance.

SAS calculates the proportion $\hat{p}$ using the lowest level of the variable by default. Thus, if we have a binary variable with levels 0 and 1, the proportion will be the proportion with *binary_variable = 0*. In order to get $\hat{p}$ to be the proportion with the event (proportion where *binary_variable = 1*), we need to add another BINOMIAL statement with a LEVEL option.

```
PROC FREQ DATA = dataset_name;
      TABLES binary_variable / BINOMIAL(P = 0.032)
            BINOMIAL (LEVEL = "1") ALPHA = 0.01;
      EXACT BINOMIAL;
RUN;
```

One-sample tests for a proportion using Stata

Unlike SAS, Stata can run a one-sample test for proportion using a binary input variable or using a series of manual inputs. If we have a dataset with a binary variable, we use the *prtest* command. We must specify the binary variable and the proportion under the null hypothesis after two equal signs.

```
prtest binary_var == nullprop, level(95)
```

If we do not have a dataset with the binary variable and instead want to manually input the parameters for the test, we use the *prtesti* command. We specify the sample size (n), sample proportion $\hat{p}$ (*prop*), and proportion under the null hypothesis p_0 (*nullprop*).

```
prtesti n prop nullprop, level(95)
```

The default alpha level for both versions is 0.05, so the level option can be omitted unless a different alpha is desired. For example, we would use the following code if we had a sample of 100 subjects (20% of whom had the event) and if it was known that 25% in the general population had the event. We also want to set $\alpha = 0.01$.

```
prtesti 100 0.20 0.25, level(99)
```

The output is below:

```
One-sample test of proportion                  x: Number of obs =        100
------------------------------------------------------------------------------
  Variable |     Mean   Std. Err.                     [99% Conf. Interval]
-------------+----------------------------------------------------------------
         x |       .2         .04                     .0969668     .3030332
------------------------------------------------------------------------------
    p = proportion(x)                                           z = -1.1547
Ho: p = 0.25

   Ha: p < 0.25              Ha: p != 0.25                Ha: p > 0.25
Pr(Z < z) = 0.1241       Pr(|Z| > |z|) = 0.2482      Pr(Z > z) = 0.8759
```

The output shows the test statistic z = on the right side. Both the one-sided ("P(Z < z)" or "P(Z > z)") and two-sided ("P(|Z| > |z|)") p-values are given by default. The confidence interval for the proportion is displayed above the test statistic on the right side of the output.

EXAMPLE PROBLEM 7.3

Suppose that we would like to examine the relationship between smoking status and education level. In particular, we wish to estimate the proportion of adults (p) who did not graduate from high school and who are current smokers. To estimate the proportions, we selected a random sample of 500 adults who did not graduate from high school. Of the adults sampled, 130 were current smokers.[2]

BOX 7.3 DESCRIPTION OF EXAMPLE PROBLEM OF 7.3 DATA

The Behavioral Risk Factor Surveillance System (BRFSS) asks each participant, "Have you smoked at least 100 cigarettes in your entire life?" Those who answer "Yes" are asked the follow-up question, "Do you now smoke cigarettes every day, some days, or not at all?" The response options are "Every day," "Some days," "Not at all," "Don't know/Not sure," or "Refused." Subjects who report smoking at least 100 cigarettes in their lifetime and who say that they currently smoke every day or some days are classified as current smokers. Education level is ascertained from the question, "What is the highest grade or year of school you completed?" Those who report "Never attended school or only kindergarten," "Grades 1 through 8 (Elementary)," or "Grades 9 through 11 (Some high school)" are classified as not having graduated from high school. The sample is limited to those who did not graduate from high school.

A Find a point estimate for the true proportion p.

$$\hat{p} = \frac{x}{n} = \frac{130}{500} = 0.26$$

B Construct a 99% confidence interval for $\hat{p}$ after first checking that the normal approximation is appropriate.

For the normal approximation to be valid, we must check that np and $n(1 - p)$ are both at least 5.

$np = 500 \times 0.26 = 130 > 5$ and $n(1 - p) = 500(1 - 0.26) = 370 > 5$. Therefore, the normal approximation is appropriate.

The 99% confidence interval is

$$\left(\hat{p} \pm Z_{1-\alpha/2}\sqrt{\frac{\hat{p}(1-\hat{p})}{n}}\right) = \left(0.26 \pm 2.58\sqrt{\frac{0.26(1-0.26)}{500}}\right) = (0.26 \pm 0.05) = (0.21, 0.31).$$

C Interpret the confidence interval.

We are 99% confident that the interval (0.21, 0.31) captures the true proportion of current smokers among adults who did not graduate from high school.

We do not know the true value of p for this population, but we do know that 16% of adults are current smokers. We would like to know whether the proportion of adults who did not graduate from high school and who smoke is the same as the proportion of adults who smoke in the general population. Since we are concerned with deviations that could occur in either direction, conduct a two-sided test at the 0.01 level of significance. Use a normal approximation.

D What are your null and alternative hypotheses?

$H_0: p = 0.16$

$H_1: p \neq 0.16$

E What is the value of your test statistic?

$$Z = \frac{\hat{p} - p_0}{\sqrt{\frac{p_0(1-p_0)}{n}}} = \frac{0.26 - 0.16}{\sqrt{\frac{0.16(1-0.16)}{500}}} = \frac{0.10}{0.016} = 6.10$$

F Draw a conclusion using the critical value method.

The critical Z value is 2.58 when $\alpha = 0.01$.
Since $z = 6.10 > 2.58$, we reject the null hypothesis.

G What is the distribution of your test statistic and the *p*-value of the test?

The test statistic follows a standard normal distribution. To calculate the *p*-value of the test, we use the code in Table 7.7.

$$p\text{-value} = 2 \times P(Z > 6.10) = 2 \times (5.30 \times 10^{-10}) = 1.06 \times 10^{-9}$$

H Do you reject or fail to reject the null hypothesis?

Because the *p*-value $< \alpha = 0.01$, we reject the null hypothesis.

I What do you conclude?

Table 7.7 *p*-value calculation for Example Problem 7.3

Using SAS	*Using Stata*
SAS Code	Stata Code

```
DATA g;
 p-value = 2*(1 - PROBNORM(6.10));
RUN;

PROC PRINT DATA = g;
RUN;
```

```
di 2*(1 - (normprob(6.10)))
```

SAS Output

Obs	*p*-value
1	1.0607E-9

Stata Output

```
1.061e-09
```

Note: The table shows the code and output used to find the *p*-value for Example Problem 7.3 Part (G).

We have statistically significant evidence that the proportion of current smokers among adults who did not graduate from high school is not equal to the proportion of current smokers in the general population. There is evidence to suggest that the proportion of smokers among adults who did not graduate from high school is higher than the proportion of smokers in the general adult population (the test statistic is positive).

J Does the confidence interval contain p_0? Would you expect it to?

The confidence interval does not contain the null value $p_0 = 0.16$, and we would not expect it to since we reject the null hypothesis.

PRACTICE PROBLEM 7.2

Suppose that we are interested in investigating the prevalence of regular secondhand smoke exposure in the United States and its association with race. In particular, we wish to estimate the proportion of African American children between ages 3 and 11 who are regularly exposed to secondhand smoke. To do this, a random sample of 600 African Americans aged 3 to 11 years was chosen, and of the 600 children, 420 were regularly exposed to secondhand smoke.

A Find a point estimate for the true proportion p.

B Construct a 95% confidence interval for p after first checking that the normal approximation is appropriate.

C Interpret the confidence interval.

Although we do not know the true value of p for this population, we know that in the United States, 40% of children between ages 3 and 11 are regularly exposed to secondhand smoke according to the CDC.[3] We would like to know whether the proportion of African American children regularly exposed to secondhand smoke is the same as that of the general population. Conduct a two-sided test at the 0.05 level of significance using the normal approximation.

D What are the null and alternative hypotheses?

E What is the value of the test statistic?

F Draw a conclusion using the critical value method.

G What is the distribution of the test statistic?

H What is the p-value of the test?

I Do we reject or fail to reject the null hypothesis? What do we conclude?

J Does the confidence interval contain p_0? Would we expect it to?

Determining power and calculating sample size

We previously introduced the two types of errors that can arise from an incorrect conclusion of a hypothesis test. A type I error, called α, occurs when we reject H_0 although H_0 is true. The type I error rate is usually set by the investigator. A type II error, denoted as β, occurs when we fail to reject H_0 although H_0 is false. The complement of the type II error is power.

Power: The probability of rejecting the null hypothesis when it is false. Mathematically, power $= P$ (reject $H_0 \mid H_0$ is false) $= 1 - \beta$.

- In practice, we would like the power to be as high as possible; power levels are typically set at 80% or 90%.
- The power of a test tells us how likely it is that a statistically significant difference will be detected based on a finite sample size (n) if the alternative hypothesis is true. For example, in the case of a test for the mean, power indicates how likely it is that we will detect a statistically significant difference based on the sample size if the true mean differs from the mean under the null hypothesis.
- Power is often used to plan a study before any data have been obtained. It is important to make sure that the study is not underpowered, meaning that a null finding is due to having too few observations.
- If the power is too low, there is little chance of finding a significant difference even if real differences exist between the true mean and the null mean.
- Inadequate sample size is usually the cause of low power. However, obtaining a larger sample is not the only aspect that contributes to increased power.

Power depends on four factors: The distance between real μ and the hypothesized μ_0, the sample size, the standard deviation, and the type I error rate. The power of a test increases as the following occur:

1 $|\mu_0 - \mu_1|$ increases
2 n increases
3 σ decreases
4 α increases

Calculating power

When we calculate power, we assume the standard deviation is known without having any data to estimate it. Like a hypothesis test, power calculation requires that specified steps be performed.

Power is the area under the curve of a normal distribution with the mean equal to the specified alternative that falls into the rejection region. The formulas for calculating power are in Table 7.8. Figure 7.1 illustrates the case if $\mu_1 > \mu_0$. In this situation, the area under the alternative curve to the night of the cut-off is the power, or $1 - \beta$, shown at the bottom of the figure. Figure 7.2 shows the opposite situation, where $\mu_1 < \mu_0$. We can see from the bottom of the figure that the area under the alternative curve to the right of the cut-off is β; the area to the left of the cut-off is power

Table 7.8 Power formulas for one-sample tests

Situation	*Type*	*Power*
Mean	One-sided	$\phi\left(-Z_{1-\alpha} + \frac{\lvert\mu_0 - \mu_1\rvert\sqrt{n}}{\sigma}\right)$
	Two-sided	$\phi\left(-Z_{1-\alpha/2} + \frac{\lvert\mu_0 - \mu_1\rvert\sqrt{n}}{\sigma}\right)$
Proportion	One-sided	$\phi\left[\sqrt{\frac{p_0(1-p_0)}{p_1(1-p_1)}}\left(-Z_{1-\alpha} + \frac{\lvert p_0 - p_1\rvert\sqrt{n}}{\sqrt{p_0(1-p_0)}}\right)\right]$
	Two-sided	$\phi\left[\sqrt{\frac{p_0(1-p_0)}{p_1(1-p_1)}}\left(-Z_{1-\alpha/2} + \frac{\lvert p_0 - p_1\rvert\sqrt{n}}{\sqrt{p_0(1-p_0)}}\right)\right]$

Note: The power of a one-sample test for a mean depends on alpha, the null and alternative means, the sample size, and the standard deviation. For a one-sample test for a proportion, the power depends on the alpha, the null and alternative proportions, and the sample size. Before computing power for a proportion, check $np_0(1 - p_0) \geq 5$.

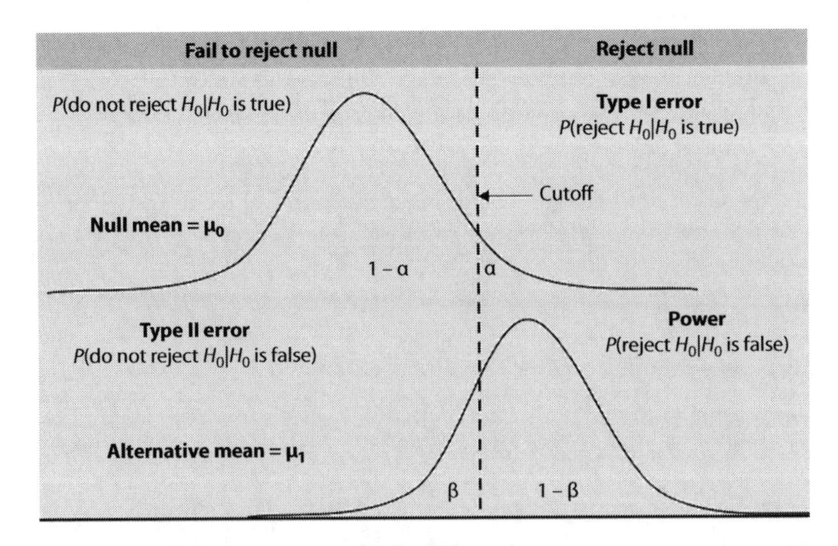

Figure 7.1 **Power diagram for case where $\mu_1 > \mu_0$.** The figure illustrates the four possible outcomes of the hypothesis test using normal curves. When $\mu_1 > \mu_0$, the power of a test is the area under the curve to the right of the test statistic under the alternative mean.

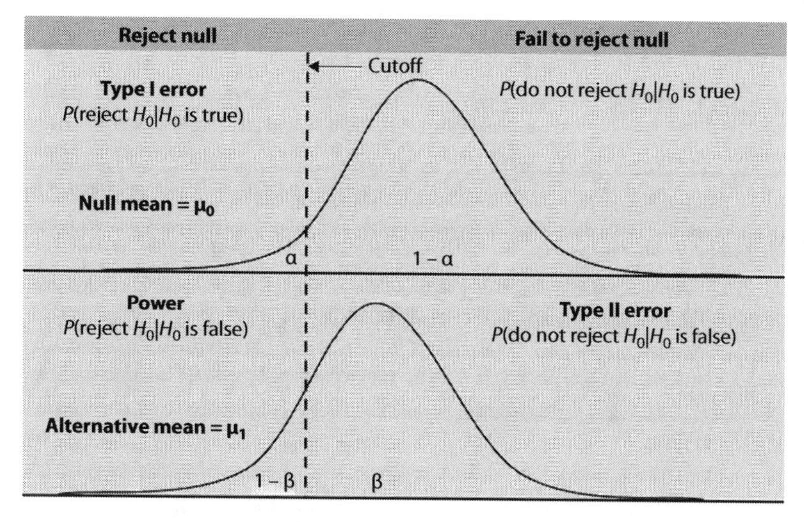

Figure 7.2 **Power diagram for case where $\mu_1 < \mu_0$.** The figure illustrates the four possible outcomes of the hypothesis test using normal curves. When $\mu_1 < \mu_0$, the power of a test is the area under the curve to the left of the test statistic under the alternative mean.

The 10 steps to finding the power of a test are below:

1. State the null and alternative hypothesis.
2. Determine whether the test will be one sided or two sided.
3. Specify the significance level (α).
4. Write down the information you are given in the problem.
   a. n—sample size
   b. μ_0—mean under the null hypothesis
   c. μ_1—mean under the alternative hypothesis
   d. σ—standard deviation
5. Find the corresponding Z value for the significance level of your test.
6. Determine the cutoff value equivalent to the Z value in Step 5 under the *null* hypothesis.
7. Use the cutoff from Step 6 to find the Z-statistic under the *alternative* hypothesis.
8. Specify β.
   a. If $\mu_1 > \mu_0$, the area under the curve to the left of the test statistic is β.
   b. If $\mu_1 < \mu_0$, the area under the curve to the right of the test statistic is β.
9. Calculate power = $1 - \beta$.
10. Interpret the power in words.

EXAMPLE PROBLEM 7.4

Participants are enrolled in a health coaching program for eight weeks to try to improve physical health and overall wellness. At the end of the trial period, the participants take a personal health improvement survey. The mean health improvement survey score for all participants in the program is 74.4 with a standard deviation of 10.3. We have reason to think that one of the health coaches (Coach A) who participated in an additional training program will have subjects who have higher health improvement survey scores than the overall program average. We know that Coach A trains 30 subjects, but, among a sample of five of those subjects, the average health improvement survey score is 80.1. We want to test the hypothesis that subjects who work with Coach A have higher health improvement survey scores compared with the rest of the program participants. We are also interested to know what the power of the test is at the 0.05 level of significance.

A **What is the null hypothesis? What is the alternative hypothesis?**

The null hypothesis is that the average health improvement survey score among Coach A's trainees is less than or equal to the overall program average. We want to test this against the alternative hypothesis that the mean health improvement survey score among Coach A's trainees is greater than the overall program average.

B **Would you conduct a one-sided or two-sided test?**

In this situation, a one-sided test is appropriate.

C **What would be the power of the test? Interpret the power in words.**

To find the power of the test, we use the following steps for finding the power of a test. We have a case where $\mu_1 > \mu_0$.

10 steps to finding the power of a one-sample, one-sided test

1 Write down the null and alternative hypotheses.

$H_0: \mu \leq 74.4$

$H_1: \mu > 74.4$

2 Is your test one sided or two sided?
Here, a one-sided test is appropriate based on the hypotheses.

3 Specify alpha.

$\alpha = 0.05$

4 List other parameters that you are given in the problem.

$n = 5, \mu_0 = 74.4, \mu_1 = 80.1, \sigma = 10.3$

5 Find the corresponding Z value for the significance level of your test.

$z = 1.645$

6 Determine the cutoff value equivalent to the Z value in Example Problem 7.4—Part (C) Step 5 under the *null* hypothesis. In other words, for what values of $\bar{x}$ would you reject the null hypothesis?

$$Z=\frac{\bar{x}-\mu_0}{\frac{\sigma}{\sqrt{n}}}\rightarrow 1.645=\frac{\bar{x}-74.4}{\frac{10.3}{\sqrt{5}}}\rightarrow \bar{x}=\frac{1.645\times 10.3}{\sqrt{5}}+74.4\rightarrow \bar{x}=81.98$$

is the cutoff.

We would reject the null hypothesis if the mean among Coach A's trainees is greater than 81.98.

7 Use this same cutoff to find the Z statistic under the *alternative* hypothesis.

$$Z=\frac{\bar{x}-\mu_1}{\frac{\sigma}{\sqrt{n}}}=\frac{81.98-80.1}{\frac{10.3}{\sqrt{5}}}=\frac{1.88}{4.6}=0.41$$

8 The area under the curve to the right of the test statistic is $1-\beta$, since $\mu_1 > \mu_0$. Specify β.

Figure 7.3 shows the power diagram when $Z = 0.41$ and $\mu_1 > \mu_0$.

$$\beta=\phi(0.41)=0.659$$

9 Power is $1-\beta$. Specify the power.

Power = 1 – 0.659 = 0.341

10 Interpret the power in words.

The power is 34.1% to detect a mean health improvement survey score greater than 74.4 under the alternative of 80.1 with a sample size of 5.

D How could you increase the power?

Increase $\mu_1 - \mu_0$ (difference between null and alternative mean).
Increase n (sample size).
Decrease s (standard deviation).
Increase α (significance level of the test).

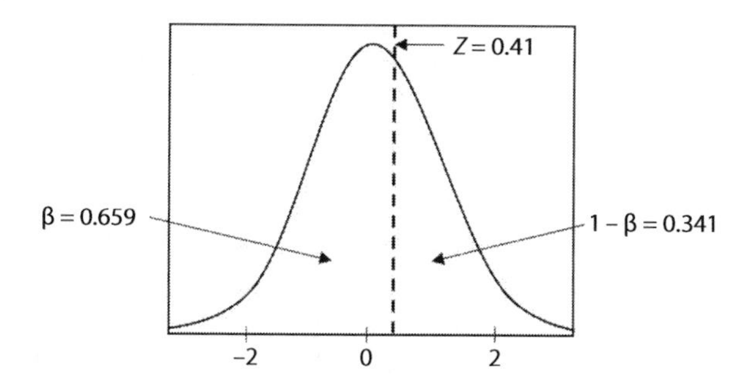

Figure 7.3 **Power diagram for Problem 7.6—Part (C).** The Z value under the alternative hypothesis is $Z = 0.41$. In this case $\mu_1 > \mu_0$, so the area under the curve to the right of 0.41 is equal to the power, or $1-\beta$. β is the area that lies to the left of 0.41.

Calculating sample size

We frequently need some idea of an appropriate sample size before a study begins. With sample size calculations, we want to know what sample size is needed to be able to detect a significant difference with probability $1 - \beta$, given a set level of significance α and a true alternative mean expected to be μ_1. That is, we want to solve for n given α, β, σ, μ_0, and μ_1.

It is also necessary to know whether the test will be one sided or two sided, as the sample size for a two-sided test is always larger than the sample size for a one-sided test. When performing a sample size calculation, it is important to always round up to the nearest whole number. Just as with power calculations, many factors affect the sample size. The sample size increases as the following occur:

1. σ increases
2. α decreases
3. power $= 1 - \beta$ increases
4. $|\mu_1 - \mu_0|$ decreases

The formulas for sample size are shown in Table 7.9.

Table 7.9 Sample size formulas for one-sample tests

Situation	*Type*	*Sample size*
Mean	One-sided	$n = \left[\frac{[Z_{1-\alpha} + Z_{1-\beta}]\sigma}{(\mu_1 - \mu_0)} \right]^2$
	Two-sided	$n = \left[\frac{[Z_{1-\alpha/2} + Z_{1-\beta}]\sigma}{(\mu_1 - \mu_0)} \right]^2$
	Two-sided confidence limit based	$n = 4Z^2_{1-\alpha/2} \frac{s^2}{L^2}$
Proportion	One-sided	$n = \frac{p_0(1-p_0)\left(Z_{1-\alpha} + Z_{1-\beta}\sqrt{\frac{p_1(1-p_1)}{p_0(1-p_0)}} \right)^2}{(p_1 - p_0)^2}$
	Two-sided	$n = \frac{p_0(1-p_0)\left(Z_{1-\alpha/2} + Z_{1-\beta}\sqrt{\frac{p_1(1-p_1)}{p_0(1-p_0)}} \right)^2}{(p_1 - p_0)^2}$

Note: The sample size for a one-sample test for a mean depends on alpha, power, the null and alternative means, and the standard deviation. An alternative method allows us to find the sample size from the sample standard deviation, width of the confidence interval, and alpha level. For a one-sample test for a proportion, the sample size depends on alpha, power, and the null and alternative proportions.

EXAMPLE PROBLEM 7.5

Let's continue with the situation introduced in Example Problem 7.4, the health-coaching intervention. We would like to find the sample size needed to detect a significant difference in health improvement survey scores at various levels of power.

A **How many health improvement survey scores do we need from participants who had Coach A in order to have 90% power for the hypothesis test?**

We have a one-sided test at the $\alpha = 0.05$ level of significance with 90% power, so we will use $Z_{1-\alpha} = 1.645$ and $Z_{1-\beta} = 1.28$. Once again, $\mu_0 = 74.4$, $\mu_1 = 80.1$, and $\sigma = 10.3$.

$$n = \left[\frac{[Z_{1-\alpha} + Z_{1-\beta}]\sigma}{(\mu_1 - \mu_0)}\right]^2 = \left[\frac{[1.645 + 1.28]10.3}{(80.1 - 74.4)}\right]^2 = 27.9$$

We should always round the sample size up, so we need health improvement survey scores from 28 participants who trained with Coach A.

B **Suppose that we are willing to have 80% power. What value does this change?**

Changing to 80% power means that β changes from 0.10 to 0.20.

C **How will the sample size change?**

For $\beta = 0.20$, $Z_{1-\beta} = 0.84$.

$$n = \left[\frac{[Z_{1-\alpha} + Z_{1-\beta}]\sigma}{(\mu_1 - \mu_0)}\right]^2 = \left[\frac{[1.645 + 0.84]10.3}{(80.1 - 74.4)}\right]^2 = 20.2$$

Thus, in order to have 80% power, we will need health improvement survey scores from 21 participants who trained with Coach A.

Approximate sample size based on confidence interval width

It is also possible to estimate the required sample size, given how wide we would like the confidence interval to be. Suppose that we wish to estimate the mean of a normal distribution with sample variance s^2 and require the two-sided $100\%(1 - \alpha)$ confidence interval for μ to be no wider than a set number of units (L).

The number of subjects needed is approximately $n = 4Z^2_{1-\alpha/2}\frac{s^2}{L^2}$.

Power and sample size for one-sample tests for the mean using SAS

We can calculate power and sample size for a one-sample test for the mean using PROC POWER in SAS. The SIDES = U option specifies that it is a one-sided test (U [upper] indicates that the alternative mean is higher than the null; L [lower] indicates that the alternative is lower than the null). For a two-sided test, omit the SIDES option.

Enter the null mean value, sample mean, standard deviation, desired power, alpha (not necessary as default is 0.05), and sample size. PROC POWER can calculate either the sample size or the power, depending on which value is set to missing. For example, the following will calculate the total number of subjects needed for a one-sided, one-sample test for the mean at 90% power:

```
PROC POWER;
  ONESAMPLEMEANS TEST = T
  SIDES = U
  NULLMEAN = 11.79
  MEAN = 12.29
  STDDEV = 0.85
  POWER = 0.90
  ALPHA = 0.05
  NTOTAL = . ;
RUN;
```

The POWER Procedure
One-Sample *t* Test for Mean

Fixed Scenario Elements	
Distribution	Normal
Method	Exact
Number of Sides	U
Null Mean	11.79
Alpha	0.05
Mean	12.29
Standard Deviation	0.85
Nominal Power	0.9

Computed N Total	
Actual Power	N Total
0.908	27

The "Computed N Total" box provides the sample size in the "N Total" column. If, instead, we would like to calculate the level of power that corresponds to a certain number of subjects, we can set the POWER = option to missing.

```
PROC POWER;
  ONESAMPLEMEANS TEST = T
  SIDES = U
  NULLMEAN = 11.79
  MEAN = 12.29
  STDDEV = 0.85
  POWER = .
  ALPHA = 0.05
  NTOTAL = 20;
RUN;
```

The POWER Procedure
One-Sample *t* Test for Mean

Fixed Scenario Elements	
Distribution	Normal
Method	Exact
Number of Sides	U
Null Mean	11.79
Alpha	0.05
Mean	12.29
Standard Deviation	0.85
Total Sample Size	20

Computed Power
Power
0.813

The "Computed Power" box shows the power of the test.

Power and sample size for one-sample tests for the mean using Stata

The power command with the *onemean* option will perform power or sample size calculations for a one-sample test for a mean. The mean under the null hypothesis is specified first and then the alternative mean. Enter the standard deviation in *sd( )*. The *onesided* option will produce a calculation assuming a one-sided hypothesis test. For a two-sided test, omit the *onesided* option. If we would like a sample size calculation, specify the power level in *power( )*.

```
power onemean 11.79 12.29, power(0.9) sd(0.85)
power onemean 11.79 12.29, power(0.9) sd(0.85) onesided
```

The output below is for a one-sided test:

```
Estimated sample size for a one-sample mean test
t test
Ho: m = m0  versus  Ha: m > m0

Study parameters:

        alpha =    0.0500
        power =    0.9000
        delta =    0.5882
           m0 =   11.7900
           ma =   12.2900
           sd =    0.8500

Estimated sample size:

            N =        27
```

The output shows the null and alternative hypotheses at the top and the input parameters below. The estimated sample size is shown at the bottom of the output. For power calculations, specify the sample size in *n( )*.

```
power onemean 11.79 12.29, n(20) sd(0.85)
power onemean 11.79 12.29, n(20) sd(0.85) onesided
```

The output below is for a one-sided test:

```
Estimated power for a one-sample mean test
t test
Ho: m = m0  versus  Ha: m > m0

Study parameters:

        alpha =    0.0500
            N =        20
        delta =    0.5882
           m0 =   11.7900
           ma =   12.2900
           sd =    0.8500

Estimated power:

        power =    0.8134
```

The estimated power is shown at the bottom of the output.

Power and sample size for one-sample tests for a proportion using SAS

We can also use PROC POWER to do power and sample size calculations for tests for a proportion. The ONESAMPLEFREQ option specifies that the test is a one-sample test for a proportion, and the METHOD = normal option indicates that the normal approximation will be used.

Specify the NULLPROPORTION (p_0) and the PROPORTION (p_1), also as either the level of power or the total sample size. The option set to missing will be calculated. The SIDES = option can also be added if we are interested in conducting a one-sided test. For example, the following sample codes calculate the power (when n = 500) or sample size (when power = 80%) for a two-sided, one-sample test for proportion where p_0 = 0.25 and p_1 = 0.30.

```
PROC POWER;
        ONESAMPLEFREQ TEST = z METHOD = normal
        NULLPROPORTION = 0.25
        PROPORTION = 0.30
        NTOTAL = 500
        POWER = .;
RUN;
```

The POWER Procedure
Z Test for Binomial Proportion

Fixed Scenario Elements	
Method	Normal approximation
Null Proportion	0.25
Binomial Proportion	0.3
Total Sample Size	500
Variance Estimate	Null Variance
Number of Sides	2
Alpha	0.05

Computed Power
Power
0.722

The power level is shown in the bottom box labeled "Computed Power." If we need to calculate a sample size rather than a power level, we leave the NTOTAL option blank.

```
PROC POWER;
        ONESAMPLEFREQ TEST = z METHOD = normal
        NULLPROPORTION = 0.25
        PROPORTION = 0.30
        NTOTAL = .
        POWER = 0.80;
RUN;
```

The POWER Procedure
Z Test for Binomial Proportion

Fixed Scenario Elements	
Method	Normal approximation
Null Proportion	0.25
Binomial Proportion	0.3
Nominal Power	0.8
Variance Estimate	Null Variance
Number of Sides	2
Alpha	0.05

Computed N Total	
Actual Power	N Total
0.800	610

The sample size needed is shown in the "Computed N Total" output box in the "N Total" column.

Power and sample size for one-sample tests for a proportion using Stata

To perform power or sample size calculation for a one-sample test for a proportion, we use the power command with the *oneproportion* option. Specify the null proportion and the alternative proportion after the *oneproportion* option. For a power calculation, input the sample size in *n( )*. If we want another alpha level besides 0.05, we can add an alpha option to the code. The default is a two-sided test. If a one-sided test is desired, use the *onesided* option.

```
power oneproportion 0.25 0.30, n(500) alpha(0.01) onesided
power oneproportion 0.25 0.30, n(500)
```

The output below is for a two-sided test:

```
Estimated power for a one-sample proportion test
Score z test
Ho: p = p0  versus  Ha: p != p0

Study parameters:

        alpha =    0.0500
            N =       500
        delta =    0.0500
```

```
           p0 =      0.2500
           pa =      0.3000

Estimated power:

        power =      0.7217
```

The power of the test is shown at the bottom of the output in the "power =" line. For a sample size calculation, we omit the *n( )* statement and instead specify the power level. Otherwise, the structure of the command is identical to the power calculation command. It is possible to omit the *power( )* statement if we wish to accept the default power level of 80%.

```
power oneproportion 0.25 0.30, alpha(0.01) power(0.9) onesided
power oneproportion 0.25 0.30, power(0.9)
```

The output is below is for a two-sided test:

```
Estimated sample size for a one-sample proportion test
Score z test
Ho: p = p0  versus  Ha: p != p0

Study parameters:

        alpha =      0.0500
        power =      0.9000
        delta =      0.0500
           p0 =      0.2500
           pa =      0.3000

Estimated sample size:

            N =         825
```

The necessary sample size is on the bottom line of the output.

RECAP

- Always draw a conclusion for each hypothesis test in context, and state the direction when you reject the null hypothesis. For example, "The mean cholesterol level in men with heart disease is significantly higher than that of the disease-free population."
- Be sure to follow all of the steps for a hypothesis test, including stating the null and alternative hypotheses. This is important to do even if the question does not specifically ask for H_0 and H_1.
- Always interpret the confidence interval in words.

PRACTICE PROBLEM 7.3

The Gini index is a measure of income inequality in a location, ranging from a value of 0 (total equality) to 1 (total inequality). According to the American Community Survey (ACS) 2009 to 2014 estimates,[4] the mean Gini index among counties in the United States was 0.442 with a standard deviation $\sigma = 0.036$. We are interested in determining whether the mean Gini index of counties in southern states is different from the mean Gini index in the country as a whole. A random sample of 50 counties in southern states has a mean Gini index of 0.460. Assume $\alpha = 0.05$ for all analyses.

A What are the null and alternative hypotheses that we would like to test?

B Perform the hypothesis test.

C What is the power of the test in Practice Problem 7.3—Part (A)?

D What is the minimum sample size necessary to have 80% power?

E Suppose that we take a random sample of 100 counties and the mean Gini index is 0.451. Would we reject or fail to reject the null hypothesis?

F Suppose that we take a random sample of 100 counties and the mean Gini index is 0.448. Calculate a 95% confidence interval. On the basis of this interval, would we reject or fail to reject the null hypothesis?

G What is the power of the test in Practice Problem 7.3—Part (F)?

PRACTICE PROBLEM 7.4

A national survey from 2014 reports that 39% of U.S. adults had received a flu shot or a flu vaccine sprayed in the nose in the past 12 months.[2] We want to conduct a study to test whether the proportion of men who received flu vaccinations is the same as the proportion of all adults who received flu vaccinations in the general population. We have data from a sample of 200 men, and 88 of the 200 men reported receiving a flu vaccine in the past 12 months. Assume $\alpha = 0.05$. The data are in the file *ch7_flu_shot*.

BOX 7.4 DESCRIPTION OF *ch7_flu_shot* DATASET

The Behavioral Risk Factor Surveillance System (BRFSS) asks each participant, "During the past 12 months, have you had either a flu shot or a flu vaccine that was sprayed in your nose? (A new flu shot came out in 2011 that injects vaccine into the skin with a very small needle. It is called Fluzone Intradermal vaccine. This is also considered a flu shot.)" Participants can answer "Yes," "No," or "Don't know," or they can refuse to respond. Those who respond "Yes" are given a value of *flu_shot* = *1*, and those who respond "No" are coded *flu_shot* = *0*. All respondents are categorized as male or female sex. The sample in the dataset *ch7_flu_shot* is limited to those who indicate they are of male sex and report receiving a flu vaccination in the past 12 months.

A We would like to conduct a one-sample, two-sided hypothesis test. What are the null and alternative hypotheses?

B Find a point estimate for the true proportion p of men who received the flu vaccine in the past 12 months.

C What are the value and distribution of the test statistic?

D What is the p-value of the test?

E Do we reject or fail to reject the null hypothesis? What do we conclude?

F Write the SAS or Stata code to perform the hypothesis test. Then, check that the output matches the hand calculations.

G What is the 95% confidence interval for p?

PRACTICE PROBLEM 7.5

The birthweight for the population of babies born in the United States has a mean μ = 7.32 lbs.[1] We are interested in determining whether there is an association between babies' birthweight and mothers' age at birth using a sample of birthweights from 100 babies born to mothers age 35 and older. In the sample, the sample mean birthweight is $\bar{x} = 7.23$ lbs., and the sample standard deviation is $s = 1.35$ lbs. Assume $\alpha = 0.05$ for the analyses. Data for this problem are in the dataset *ch7_birth_weight*.

> **BOX 7.5 DESCRIPTION OF *ch7_birth_weight* DATASET**
>
> The National Health and Nutrition Examination Survey (NHANES) conducted by the Centers for Disease Control and Prevention (CDC) asks caregivers of children aged 15 or younger, "How much did he/she weigh at birth?" Responses are recorded in pounds and ounces. We converted ounces to fractions of a pound to create the variable *birth_weight* (birthweight in pounds). In order to determine the age of the mother at the time of the child's birth, the respondents are asked the question "How old was {participant's name} biological mother when {she or /he} was born?" The sample in the dataset *ch7_birth_weight* is limited to those whose mothers were at least aged 35 at the time of birth.

A By hand, test the hypothesis that babies born to mothers age 35 and older have mean birthweights different from the general population.

B Compute a 95% confidence interval for the true mean birthweight among babies born to mothers age 35 and older.

C Compare the results from the hypothesis test with the information available from the confidence interval.

D Write the SAS or Stata code that will run the appropriate hypothesis test. Check the answer to Practice Problem 7.5—Parts (A) and (B) against the output.

PRACTICE PROBLEM 7.6

In the United States in 2014, 9.5% of residents aged 65 and older were living in poverty, according to the ACS.[5] We would like to determine whether the proportion of residents aged 65 and older living in poverty in our city is different from the national population. Of 400 local seniors surveyed, 28 were living in poverty. In all analyses, we will assume $\alpha = 0.05$.

A Compute the power of the test by hand.

B What sample size would be needed if we want 80% power? Compute n by hand.

C Write and run the SAS or Stata code to determine the power of the test, and check your answer to Practice Problem 7.6—Part (A) against the output.

D Check the sample size calculation in Practice Problem 7.6—Part (B) using SAS or Stata.

References

1. National Health and Nutrition Examination Survey. Hyattsville, MD: Centers for Disease Control and Prevention, National Center for Health Statistics. https://wwwn.cdc.gov/Nchs/Nhanes/Search/nhanes13_14.aspx. Published 2014. Accessed February 23, 2016.
2. Behavioral Risk Factor Surveillance System. Atlanta, GA: Centers for Disease Control and Prevention. http://www.cdc.gov/brfss/annual_data/annual_data.htm. Published 2014. Updated September 11, 2015. Accessed February 23, 2016.
3. Centers for Disease Control and Prevention. Secondhand smoke facts. http://www.cdc.gov/tobacco/data_statistics/fact_sheets/secondhand_smoke/general_facts/. Updated August 20, 2015. Accessed September 22, 2016.
4. United States Census Bureau. American Community Survey 2014: Gini index of income inequality, 2009–2014. http://www.socialexplorer.com/tables/ACS2014_5yr/R11234719?ReportId=R11234719. Accessed March 18, 2016.
5. United States Census Bureau. American Community Survey 2014: Poverty status in 2014 for population age 65 and over. http://www.socialexplorer.com/tables/ACS2014/R11234722?ReportId=R11234722. Accessed March 18, 2016.

Lab C: One-sample hypothesis testing, power, and sample size

PRACTICE PROBLEM C.1

Along with exercise, consuming a healthy diet is a key part of maintaining a healthy weight. The weights of U.S. men aged 18 or older who self-report having an excellent, very good, or good diet were measured.[1] In a sample of 216 adult men who self-report having an excellent, very good, or good diet, the mean weight is 83.74 kg with a standard deviation of 19.98 kg. The data can be found in the *labc_diet_weight* file.

> **BOX C.1 DESCRIPTION OF *labc_diet_weight* DATASET**
>
> The National Health and Nutrition Examination Survey (NHANES) asks, "In general, how healthy is your overall diet?" The response is a seven-level categorical variable with options "Excellent," "Very Good," "Good," "Fair," "Poor," "Don't know," and "Refused." Those who reported having an excellent, very good, or good diet were classified as eating a healthy diet (*good_diet* = 1). Respondents who selected "Fair" or "Poor" were given a value of *good_diet* = 0. The body weight of each respondent was also measured during the survey and was captured in the variable *weight*. The sample in the dataset *labc_diet_weight* was additionally limited to those who selected "Male" as their gender.

A Assume that the distribution of weight in the general population is normal. If the mean weight in the general population of adult males is 89.02 kg, test the hypothesis that the group of men who report excellent, very good, or good diets have weights different from those in the general population.

B What is the 95% confidence interval for the true mean weight among men who report an excellent, very good, or good diet?

C Use the confidence interval to make a conclusion about whether adult men with excellent, very good, or good diets have weights different from those of the general population of adult males.

PRACTICE PROBLEM C.2

In 2014, the age-adjusted percentage of women who had ever been diagnosed with breast cancer was 1.3%.[2] Suppose that among 10,000 black women, 90 reported having been diagnosed with breast cancer. Since we are concerned about racial variations in cancer prevalence, we wish to determine whether there is a difference between the proportion of black women who have been diagnosed with breast cancer and the proportion in the general population. The data are in the file *labc_breast_cancer*. The variable *cancer* is 1 for women who reported ever being diagnosed with breast cancer and 0 for women who did not.

A State the hypothesis to use in answering this question.

B Is a one-sided or two-sided test appropriate here?

C Perform the hypothesis test using a statistical package. What is your conclusion?

D Interpret the confidence interval for the true proportion of black women who have received a diagnosis of breast cancer.

PRACTICE PROBLEM C.3

We know that the proportion of women who have ever been diagnosed with breast cancer in the general population is 0.013 or 1.3%. We think that a meaningful difference in proportion of women who have ever been diagnosed with breast cancer is $|p_0 - p_1| = 0.02$, or two percentage points difference. For all calculations, let $\alpha = 0.05$.

A What sample size is needed to have 90% power to detect this difference, assuming that we use a two-sided test?

B If we have a set sample size of 280 subjects, how much power does the test have?

PRACTICE PROBLEM C.4

We created a series of materials with the goal of increasing health literacy in a medically underserved population, and we enrolled participants to see whether there is a change in their health literacy before and after using the materials. Ten participants took a health literacy assessment before and after receiving the materials. The mean change in health literacy score on the assessment was 3.50 points with a standard deviation of 4.12 points. We would now like to implement this health literacy intervention again.

A Let μ_d be the true mean difference in the health literacy assessment score before and after the intervention. How many participants are needed to have a 90% chance of detecting a significant difference using a one-sided test with a significance level of 5%? Assume that the true mean and standard deviation of the difference in the health literacy assessment score are the same as observed in the initial study of 10 subjects.

B Suppose that the sample size is set at 13 participants. What is the probability that we will be able to reject H_0 using a one-sided test at the 5% level if the true mean and standard deviation of the health literacy score difference are the same as in the initial study of 10 subjects?

C Suppose that we would like to do the test with 90% power but would like to perform a two-sided test as opposed to a one-sided test. How many participants would be needed? Are more or fewer needed compared to those needed for a one-sided test?

PRACTICE PROBLEM C.5

Suppose that we are interested in the distribution of the mother's age at the child's birth for low birthweight babies. Low birthweight babies are those with a weight less than 5.5 pounds at birth. Assume that the distribution of the mother's age is approximately normal with unknown mean and standard deviation. Furthermore, we know that in the general population, the mean mother's age at the child's birth is 27.52 years, and we want to know whether the mean mother's age at the child's birth for low birthweight babies is equal to that in the general population.[3] A random sample of 50 low birthweight babies has a mean mother's age at child's birth of $\bar{x} = 28.00$ years and standard deviation $s = 7.61$ years. Perform an appropriate hypothesis test at the 0.05 level of significance.

BOX C.2 DESCRIPTION OF PRACTICE PROBLEM C.5 DATA

The National Health and Nutrition Examination Survey (NHANES) asks, "How much did he/she weigh at birth?" to caregivers of respondents aged 15 and younger. Responses were recorded in pounds and ounces. Ounces were converted to fractions of a pound to create the variable *birth_weight* (birthweight in pounds). The survey also asks, "How old was the respondent's mother when he/she was born?" Answers could be a numeric value, or the response could be "Don't know" or a refusal to answer the question. The sample of low birthweight babies was limited to respondents who weighed less than 5.5 pounds at birth.

A Is a one-sided or two-sided test more appropriate?

B State the null hypothesis.

C State the alternative hypothesis.

D Calculate the test statistic by hand. What is the distribution of the test statistic?

E Calculate and interpret the p-value of your test statistic.

F Write the SAS or Stata code to test the hypothesis.

G Compare the results from the hand calculation to the following output:

SAS output:

The TTEST Procedure

Variable: mothers_age (Mother's Age at Child's Birth)

N	Mean	Std Dev	Std Err	Minimum	Maximum
50	28.0000	7.6104	1.0763	16.0000	45.0000

Mean	95% CL Mean		Std Dev	95% CL Std Dev	
28.0000	25.8371	30.1629	7.6104	6.3572	9.4836

DF	*t Value*	*Pr > |t|*
49	0.45	0.6576

Stata output:

```
One-sample t test
------------------------------------------------------------------------------
Variable |     Obs      Mean    Std. Err.   Std. Dev.    [95% Conf. Interval]
---------+--------------------------------------------------------------------
mother~e |      50        28    1.076275    7.610412     25.83714    30.16286
------------------------------------------------------------------------------
    mean = mean(mothers_age)                                   t =    0.4460
Ho: mean = 27.52                              degrees of freedom =        49

  Ha: mean < 27.52            Ha: mean != 27.52           Ha: mean > 27.52
Pr(T < t) = 0.6712       Pr(|T| > |t|) = 0.6576        Pr(T > t) = 0.3288
```

PRACTICE PROBLEM C.6

Next, we wish to look at birthweight in relation to maternal smoking status. The mean birthweight in the population of babies is known to be 7.18 pounds.[3] We want to investigate whether the mean birthweight of babies whose mothers did smoke while pregnant is lower than that of the general population of babies. In a sample of 100 babies whose mothers smoked while pregnant, the sample mean birthweight is $\bar{x} = 6.75$ pounds with a sample standard deviation of $s = 1.26$. The data are in the file *labc_smoking_bw*.

BOX C.3 DESCRIPTION OF THE *labc_smoking_bw* DATASET

The National Health and Nutrition Examination Survey (NHANES) asks, "How much did he/she weigh at birth?" to caregivers of respondents age 15 and younger. Responses were recorded in pounds and ounces. Ounces were converted to fractions of a pound to create the variable *birth_weight* (birth weight in pounds). The survey also asks, "Did the respondent's biological mother smoke at any time while she was pregnant with him/her?" The response options were "Yes," "No," "Don't know," or refusal to answer the question. The sample in the dataset *labc_smoking_bw* was limited to records where the mother was reported to be a smoker (*mother_smoked* = 1).

A Is a one-sided or two-sided test more appropriate?

B State the null hypothesis.

C State the alternative hypothesis.

D Calculate the test statistic by hand. What is the distribution of the test statistic?

E Calculate and interpret the *p*-value of your test statistic.

F Perform the hypothesis test in SAS or Stata. Do the results match?

G What is the 95% confidence interval for the true mean birthweight of babies whose mothers smoked while pregnant?

H Would your conclusion have changed if you had performed a different test from Practice Problem C.6—Part (A) (one sided or two sided)?

PRACTICE PROBLEM C.7

Suppose that we are planning a new study to determine the mean blood lead level for the population of families living below the poverty line. We know that the mean blood lead level in the general population is $\mu = 1.10$ ug/dL, and the standard deviation is $\sigma = 2.95$ ug/dL.[1] We want to design the study so that we have 80% power to detect a difference in means of 0.50 ug/dL.

BOX C.4 DESCRIPTION OF PRACTICE PROBLEM C.7 DATA

Respondents in the National Health and Nutrition Examination Survey (NHANES) reported their annual family income and the number of people in the family. These values were then used to calculate a ratio of the family income to the federal poverty guidelines. The laboratory component of the survey measured the blood lead level, in µg/dL, of participants.

A Assuming that we would like to conduct a two-sided test with $\alpha = 0.05$, what is the sample size needed to achieve the desired power?

B Suppose that we have evidence that the mean blood lead levels will be higher for those whose families are in poverty. What sample size would be needed for a one-sided test?

C What sample size would be needed to achieve 90% power for the one-sided test?

PRACTICE PROBLEM C.8

A List three ways in which the power of a test can be increased.

B Which of these are under the control of the investigator?

References

1. National Health and Nutrition Examination Survey. Hyattsville, MD: Centers for Disease Control and Prevention, National Center for Health Statistics. 2014. https://wwwn.cdc.gov/Nchs/Nhanes/Search/nhanes13_14.aspx. Accessed February 23, 2016.
2. Centers for Disease Control and Prevention. National Center for Health Statistics. National Health Interview Survey: Tables of summary health statistics, Table A-3. 2014. http://ftp.cdc.gov/pub/Health_Statistics/NCHS/NHIS/SHS/2014_SHS_Table_A-3.pdf.
3. National Health and Nutrition Examination Survey. Hyattsville, MD: Centers for Disease Control and Prevention, National Center for Health Statistics. 2012. http://wwwn.cdc.gov/nchs/nhanes/search/nhanes11_12.aspx.

8 Two-Sample Hypothesis Testing

This chapter will focus on two-sample hypothesis testing and will include the following topics:

- Dependent samples (paired tests)
- Independent samples
- Sample size and power for two-sample test of means

Terms

- cross-sectional study
- independent data
- longitudinal (follow-up) study
- paired (dependent) data

Introduction

In Chapter 7, we discussed one-sample hypothesis testing, where we generate a hypothesis about a single distribution. A two-sample hypothesis testing problem allows the comparison of the underlying parameters of two different populations, neither of whose values is assumed known. Two-sample tests are appropriate in many common study designs, including longitudinal and cross-sectional studies.

Longitudinal (Follow-Up) Study: A study in which the same group of people is followed over time.

Paired (Dependent) Samples: Term used to describe two samples where each data point of the first sample has a corresponding unique data point in the second sample. In this case, there are two measurements taken on the same sample.

Let's say that we are interested in comparing an individual's body weight before and after an exercise intervention. The subject's body weight is measured initially (Sample 1) and then again after a set number of weeks (Sample 2). In order to test whether there is a difference in weight due to the intervention, we must use a test that takes into account the dependent nature of the data. The observations (body weights) from the second sample are not independent from the observations from the first sample since they are measured in the same individual. This is a case of paired, or dependent, samples.

Cross-Sectional Study: A study in which the participants are seen at only one point in time. Cross-sectional studies are considered suggestive because other confounding factors may influence the outcome and cause an apparent difference to be found when none is actually present.

Independent Samples: Term used to describe two samples where the data points in one sample are unrelated to the data points in the second sample. In this case, there are two samples with the same measurement taken on different participants.

Let's examine a variation on the exercise intervention just described. Instead of following the same subjects over time, we enrolled one group of participants in the exercise intervention and kept one group as an inactive control. To compare whether there is a difference in mean body weight between the two groups, we will use a two-sample test for independent data. The subjects in the intervention group are not related to the subjects in the control group, and we are not examining measures within subjects over time.

When comparing means from two samples, we need to determine whether to use normal tests or t-tests just as we did in the one-sample situation. If the population variance is known, we use a normal test (Z-test). If the population variance is unknown, a t-test will be appropriate. The t-test does assume that the underlying distribution is normally distributed. Keep in mind that when the sample size is sufficiently large, the CLT holds; therefore, a normal test can be used even if the variance is unknown.

Dependent samples (paired tests)

With two-sample tests that have dependent data, we want to investigate whether the two populations have equal means.

- We will denote the difference between the means of the two populations, $\mu_1 - \mu_2$, by the Greek letter delta (δ).
- We estimate $\delta = \mu_1 - \mu_2$ with $\bar{d} = \bar{x}_1 - \bar{x}_2$.

We follow the same basic steps of hypothesis testing as we did in the one-sample case, starting with specifying the null and alternative hypotheses.

- The null hypothesis is that the difference in the population means is 0, or H_0: $\delta = 0$.
- The corresponding two-sided alternative hypothesis is that the difference in population means is not equal to zero, or H_1: $\delta \neq 0$.
- Once the hypotheses and significance level are specified, we use the sample to compute the test statistic.
- The formulas for the test statistics that are appropriate for paired data are in Table 8.1.
- Note that the tests for dependent data are essentially one-sample hypothesis tests based on the differences.
- When using paired data, n is the number of pairs.
- For the paired t-test, we must calculate $\bar{d}$ (Equation 8.1) and the sample standard deviation of the observed differences (s_d; Equation 8.2).

Table 8.1 Tests for dependent (paired) data

Component	*Known variance*	*Unknown variance*
Hypotheses	H_0: $\delta = 0$ vs. H_1: $\delta \neq 0$ H_0: $\delta \geq 0$ vs. H_1: $\delta < 0$ H_0: $\delta \leq 0$ vs. H_1: $\delta > 0$	H_0: $\delta = 0$ vs. H_1: $\delta \neq 0$ H_0: $\delta \geq 0$ vs. H_1: $\delta < 0$ H_0: $\delta \leq 0$ vs. H_1: $\delta > 0$
Hypothesis test	Paired normal test	Paired t-test
Test statistic	$Z = \frac{\bar{d} - \delta}{\sigma_d / \sqrt{n}}$	$t = \frac{\bar{d} - \delta}{s_d / \sqrt{n}}$
Distribution of test statistic	Standard normal	t-distribution with $n - 1$ df
Confidence interval (two-sided)	$\bar{d} \pm Z_{1-\frac{\alpha}{2}} \frac{\sigma_d}{\sqrt{n}}$	$\bar{d} \pm t_{n-1,1-\alpha/2} \frac{s_d}{\sqrt{n}}$

Note: There are two cases of the two-sample test with dependent data: Known variance and unknown variance. When the variance is known, we use a paired normal test. If the variance is unknown, we use a paired t-test.
Abbreviation: df, degrees of freedom.

$$\bar{d} = \bar{x}_1 - \bar{x}_2 \tag{8.1}$$

$$s_d = \frac{\sqrt{\sum_{i=1}^{n} d_i^2 - \frac{1}{n}\left(\sum_{i=1}^{n} d_i\right)^2}}{n-1} \tag{8.2}$$

Using SAS with dependent samples

Two primary ways exist to conduct a two-sample test for dependent data in SAS. These approaches give identical results. The first way is to run a one-sample t-test on the difference variable, and another is to run a t-test using a PAIRED statement. In either option, by default, SAS will run a two-sided test.

- If a one-sided test is desired, add the SIDES = U or SIDES = L option into the PROC TTEST line.
- Note that the confidence interval output will also be one sided when using the SIDES option.
- The first approach is to create a difference variable equal to the difference between the first and second observation and to, then, perform a one-sample t-test to test whether the difference is equal to 0.
- The H0 option will always be set to 0.

```
PROC TTEST DATA = dataset_name H0 = 0;
    VAR diff;
RUN;
```

The TTEST Procedure
Variable: diff

N	Mean	Std Dev	Std Err	Minimum	Maximum
50	–1.1842	2.6371	0.3729	–7.7213	4.5146

Mean	95% CL Mean		Std Dev	95% CL Std Dev	
–1.1842	–1.9337	–0.4348	2.6371	2.2028	3.2861

DF	t Value	Pr > |t|
49	–3.18	0.0026

- The output is identical in format to the output from the one-sample *t*-tests introduced in Chapter 7.
- The *p*-value is shown in the third output box under the "Pr > |t|" heading.
- The second approach is to use the PAIRED statement. Both the variable of interest from Sample 1 (*pre*) and the variable from Sample 2 (*post*) must be specified.

```
PROC TTEST DATA = dataset_name;
     PAIRED x_post*x_pre;
RUN;
```

The TTEST Procedure
Difference: x_post – x_pre

N	Mean	Std Dev	Std Err	Minimum	Maximum
50	–1.1842	2.6371	0.3729	–7.7213	4.5146

Mean	95% CL Mean		Std Dev	95% CL Std Dev	
–1.1842	–1.9337	–0.4348	2.6371	2.2028	3.2861

DF	t Value	Pr > |t|
49	–3.18	0.0026

- The output is very similar, but notice the "Difference" heading after the "The TTEST Procedure" title. This tells us the variables that are being used to calculate the difference for the paired *t*-test.
- The *p*-value is shown in the third output box under the "Pr > |t|" heading.

Using Stata with dependent samples

To perform a paired *t*-test in Stata, we create a variable for the difference between the two sets of observations and, then, perform a one-sample *t*-test where the mean difference under the null hypothesis is equal to 0. The code to run this test was described in Chapter 7, but to recap, we can either manually input the sample size, the mean of the differences, the standard deviation of the differences, and the null mean, or we can set the difference variable as the continuous variable and simply specify the null mean.

```
ttesti n mean std nullmean, level(95)
ttest diff_var == nullmean, level(95)
```

- Remember that the level option can be dropped as long as we are assuming $\alpha = 0.05$.
- Since the null mean will always be 0 for the paired test, we have the following:

```
ttest diff_var == 0
```

The output follows:

```
One-sample t test
------------------------------------------------------------------------------
Variable |  Obs       Mean    Std. Err.   Std. Dev.   [95% Conf. Interval]
---------+--------------------------------------------------------------------
  diff   |   50  -1.184235   .3729389    2.637076    -1.933684   -.4347865
------------------------------------------------------------------------------
    mean = mean(diff_var)                                     t =   -3.1754
Ho: mean = 0                                degrees of freedom =        49

    Ha: mean < 0              Ha: mean != 0                 Ha: mean > 0
Pr(T < t) = 0.0013       Pr(|T| > |t|) = 0.0026          Pr(T > t) = 0.9987
```

- The output for the *ttest* and *ttesti* commands is almost identical.
- The one-sided and two-sided p-values are shown on the last line of the output.

EXAMPLE PROBLEM 8.1

We are interested in examining health insurance coverage rates before and after the passage of the Patient Protection and Affordable Care Act. Data on prevalence of health insurance coverage for all 50 states plus Puerto Rico and the District of Columbia come from the American Community Survey.[1,2] We are interested in comparing the prevalence rates for each state in 2009 versus 2014. The dataset is called *ch8_insurance_coverage*.

Let μ_1 be the true mean prevalence of insurance coverage in 2014 and μ_2 be the true mean prevalence of insurance coverage in 2009. The observed average difference in prevalence of health insurance coverage was 3.20 percentage points with a sample standard deviation of 1.53 percentage points. Assume that we are only interested in determining whether the coverage rates have increased over time. Conduct a test at the $\alpha = 0.05$ significance level.

A What type of test will you perform?

A paired t-test is appropriate for this scenario, as the data in the two "samples" are measurements on the same states at different time points (years).

B State the null and alternative hypotheses.

Let $\delta = \mu_{2014} - \mu_{2009}$. We would like to test the null hypothesis H_0: $\delta \leq 0$ versus the alternative hypothesis H_1: $\delta > 0$ since the premise of the problem indicates a one-sided test (Have insurance rates increased over time?).

C What is the value of your test statistic?

$$t = \frac{\bar{d} - \delta}{s_d / \sqrt{n}} = \frac{3.20 - 0}{1.53 / \sqrt{52}} = \frac{3.20}{0.2122} = 15.08$$

D What is the distribution of your test statistic?

The test statistic follows a t_{n-1} distribution. Because 52 observations are in our sample, the test statistic follows a $t_{52-1} = t_{51}$ distribution.

E What is the *p*-value for your test?

The *p*-value is $P(t_{51} > 15.08) < 0.0001$.

F Do you reject or fail to reject the null hypothesis?

Because $p < 0.0001 < \alpha = 0.05$, we reject the null hypothesis.

G What conclusion can you draw from this test?

We have statistically significant evidence to conclude that the mean prevalence of health insurance coverage was higher in 2014 compared to 2009.

H What code would be used to perform the desired test in SAS or Stata?

To run the test in SAS, we use PROC TTEST with the mean under the null hypothesis set to 0. We also include the SIDES option for a one-sided test.

```
PROC TTEST DATA = ch8_insurance_coverage H0 = 0 SIDES = U;
    VAR coverage_difference;
RUN;
```

The TTEST Procedure
Variable: coverage_difference

N	Mean	Std Dev	Std Err	Minimum	Maximum
52	3.2027	1.5281	0.2119	0.3800	7.2800

Mean	95% CL Mean		Std Dev	95% CL Std Dev	
3.2027	2.8477	Infty	1.5281	1.2806	1.8951

DF	t Value	Pr > |t|
51	15.11	<.0001

From the last box in the SAS output for the TTEST procedure, we can check that the value of the test statistic is $t = 15.11$ (our hand calculation is off due to rounding) and that the p-value is < 0.0001.

In Stata, we use the *ttest* command, specifying the variable *coverage_difference* as the continuous difference variable and 0 as the mean under the null hypothesis.

```
ttest coverage_difference == 0
```

The output follows:

```
One-sample t test
------------------------------------------------------------------------------
Variable |  Obs       Mean    Std. Err.    Std. Dev.    [95% Conf. Interval]
---------+--------------------------------------------------------------------
covera~e |   52   3.202692     .2119129     1.528126     2.777259   3.628125
------------------------------------------------------------------------------
    mean = mean(coverage_difference)                          t =    15.1132
Ho: mean = 0                                     degrees of freedom =       51

    Ha: mean < 0                 Ha: mean != 0                  Ha: mean > 0
Pr(T < t) = 1.0000         Pr(|T| > |t|) = 0.0000          Pr(T > t) = 0.0000
```

The test statistic calculated by Stata is $t = 15.11$. The p-value is shown next to "Pr(T > t)" and is <0.0001.

I How could you have used the confidence interval for the true difference in means to test the null hypothesis?

We can either calculate the confidence interval by hand or use a statistical package. In SAS, the code from Example Problem 8.1—Part (H) produces a confidence interval in addition to the test for the mean. Because we are interested in whether rates have increased over time, we have a one-sided confidence interval with a lower bound.

Mean	95% CL Mean		Std Dev	95% CL Std Dev	
3.2027	2.8477	Infty	1.5281	1.2806	1.8951

The output from the Stata code in Example Problem 8.1—Part (H) gives the two-sided 95% confidence interval rather than the one-sided interval. Since the lower bound of a one-sided 95% confidence interval is equal to the lower bound of a 90% two-sided confidence interval, we set alpha to 0.10 and ran the code again to get the lower bound.

```
ttest coverage_difference == 0, level(90)
```

The output follows:

```
One-sample t test
------------------------------------------------------------------------------
Variable |  Obs       Mean    Std. Err.    Std. Dev.     [90% Conf. Interval]
---------+--------------------------------------------------------------------
covera~e |   52   3.202692    .2119129     1.528126      2.847678    3.557707
------------------------------------------------------------------------------
```

We can see from the abbreviated output that the lower bound of the 95% confidence interval is 2.85.

We are 95% confident that the true mean difference in health insurance coverage prevalence between 2009 and 2014 is more than 2.85. This interval does not contain the null value of 0; therefore, we reject H_0.

PRACTICE PROBLEM 8.1

Data on life expectancy were collected for 77 communities in Chicago, Illinois, at two time points: 2000 and 2010. We are interested in determining whether the mean life expectancy was the same in 2010 as it was in 2000. Let $\alpha = 0.01$ for this analysis. The dataset is called *ch8_life_expectancy*. The dataset includes a variable for the life expectancy at 2000 (*life_expectancy_2000*), a variable for the life expectancy at 2010 (*life_expectancy_2010*), and a variable for the difference in life expectancy between 2000 and 2010 (*change_2000_2010 = life_expectancy_2010 – life_expectancy_2000*).

A What type of test is appropriate? State the corresponding null and alternative hypotheses.

B Perform the hypothesis test using a statistical package. What is the value of the test statistic and its distribution?

C What is the *p*-value for the test? What conclusion can we draw from this?

D Check that the outcome of the test matches the conclusion drawn from the confidence interval.

Independent samples

For independent samples, it seems reasonable to base the significance test on the difference between the two sample means. If the difference is far from zero, then the null hypothesis will be rejected. There are two cases of two-sample tests for independent data: situations in which we assume the two samples have equal variances and situations in which we assume the two samples have unequal variances.

Tests assuming unequal variances are more conservative. Therefore, tests with unequal variances are usually chosen unless we are certain that the variances are equal. Before conducting a two-sample test, we could perform a test for the equality of two variances to determine which case we have, or we could just conduct a test for unequal variances (being conservative) and skip this step.

Testing for the equality of two variances

When testing for the equality of variances, we make the assumption that the two samples are independent random samples from a $N(\mu_1, \sigma_1^2)$ and a $N(\mu_2, \sigma_2^2)$ distribution. We would like to test the null hypothesis that the two variances are equal, $H_0: \sigma_1^2 = \sigma_2^2$. The alternative hypothesis is that the two variances are not equal, $H_1: \sigma_1^2 \neq \sigma_2^2$.

The best test is based on the ratio of the sample variances $\left(\frac{s_1^2}{s_2^2}\right)$. Thus, the null is rejected when the variance ratio is either too large or too small. The distribution of the variance ratio $\left(\frac{s_1^2}{s_2^2}\right)$ follows an F distribution under the null hypothesis (Table 8.2).

Like the t distribution, there is no unique F distribution; instead, there is a family of F distributions. The F distributions are indexed by two parameters termed the *numerator degrees of freedom* and the *denominator degrees of freedom*. Let n_1 be the sample size of the first sample and n_2 the sample size of the second sample. The variance ratio follows an F distribution with $n_1 - 1$ (numerator df) and $n_2 - 1$ (denominator df), which is written as an F_{n_1-1,n_2-1} distribution.

Since we are conducting a two-sided test, it does not make a difference which sample is selected as the numerator or the denominator. However, variance ratios greater than 1 are usually more convenient, so the sample with the larger variance is generally chosen to be Sample 1. To find values of the F distribution, we can use either the F table (Table A.6) or statistical software.

The F table is a matrix with the numerator df (df_1) in the first row and the denominator df (df_2) in the first column. The various percentiles (p) are shown in the second column. Note that the F table gives only the area in the upper tail of the distribution, but the symmetric properties of the F distribution make it possible to derive the area in the lower tail of any F distribution from the corresponding upper tail value. The lower p^{th} percentile of an F distribution is the same as the inverse of the upper p^{th} percentile of an F distribution with the degrees of freedom reversed. In symbols:

$$F_{d_1,d_2,p} = \frac{1}{F_{d_2,d_1,1-p}} \tag{8.3}$$

Table 8.2 Test for the equality of two variances

Component	*Formula*
Hypotheses	$H_0: \sigma_1^2 = \sigma_2^2$ vs. $H_1: \sigma_1^2 \neq \sigma_2^2$
Test statistic	$F = \frac{s_1^2}{s_2^2}$
Distribution of test statistic	F distribution with $n_1 - 1$, $n_2 - 1$ df

Note: We conduct the test for the equality of two variances before the two-sample test of means with independent data. If the conclusion is to reject the null hypothesis, we assume unequal variances.

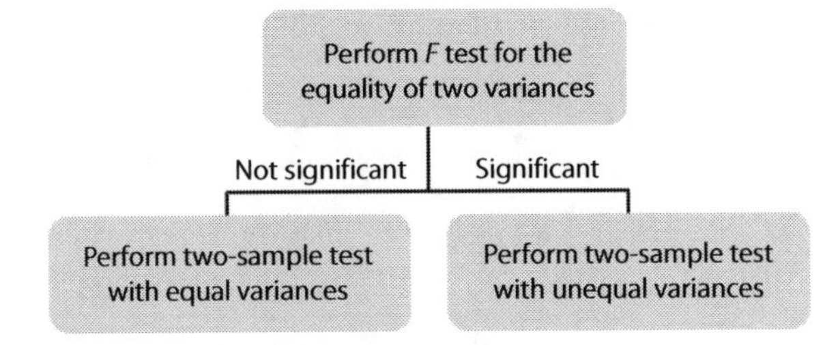

Figure 8.1 **Steps for choosing a hypothesis test for two independent, normally distributed samples.** Because the two-sample test of means with independent data depends on whether the variances are equal, we typically first conduct a test for the equality of variances. If the *p*-value is significant, we perform a two-sample test with unequal variances. If the *p*-value is not significant, we perform a two-sample test with equal variances.

If the *p*-value is significant and the conclusion of the test is to reject the null hypothesis, then, subsequently, a two-sample test for independent data with unequal variances should be used. If the test for equality of variances fails to reject the null hypothesis, then a two-sample test with equal variances is appropriate. In SAS, the hypothesis test for the equality of two variances will be conducted by default as a part of the two-sample *t*-test procedure. Figure 8.1 is a flowchart of the testing process for two independent samples.

Test for equality of variances in stata

- The *sdtest* command runs the test for equality of variances.
- Specify the continuous variable and the grouping variable after *sdtest*.
- If alpha is not 0.05, we can include the level option.

```
sdtest continuous_variable, by(group_variable) level(95)
```

The output follows:

```
Variance ratio test
------------------------------------------------------------------------------
   Group |  Obs     Mean    Std. Err.   Std. Dev.   [95% Conf. Interval]
---------+--------------------------------------------------------------------
    0    |  50   16.91534     .15896     1.124017    16.59589    17.23478
    1    |  50   15.13702   .1269282     .8975182    14.88195    15.39209
---------+--------------------------------------------------------------------
combined| 100   16.02618   .1350043     1.350043    15.7583     16.29406
------------------------------------------------------------------------------
    ratio = sd(0) / sd(1)                                  f =    1.5684
Ho: ratio = 1                            degrees of freedom =    49, 49

    Ha: ratio < 1               Ha: ratio != 1                Ha: ratio > 1
Pr(F < f) = 0.9407         2*Pr(F > f) = 0.1186          Pr(F > f) = 0.0593
```

The *p*-value for the test is listed after "2*Pr(F > f)." If the *p*-value is less than α, we will assume that the variances are not equal for the two-sample *t*-test. If the *p*-value is greater than α, we assume that the variances are equal for the two-sample *t*-test.

CASE I: EQUAL VARIANCES

After the equality of variance test is performed and we have failed to reject the null hypothesis that the variances are equal, we can perform a two-sample test for independent data with equal variance. In a two-sided situation, we would like to test the null hypothesis that the mean in Group 1 is equal to the mean in Group 2, H_0: $\mu_1 = \mu_2$. Note that this equation can be rearranged and written as H_0: $\mu_1 - \mu_2 = 0$. Our alternative hypothesis is that the means in the two groups are not equal: H_1: $\mu_1 \neq \mu_2$ or H_1: $\mu_1 - \mu_2 \neq 0$. In this test, we make three key assumptions:

1 The two samples are independent of each other.
2 Both samples are normally distributed.
3 The samples have equal variance, which we have previously tested and have reason to believe is the case.

Under the equal variances assumption, we can find the distribution of the difference in the sample means. We know $\bar{X}_1 \sim N\left(\mu_1, \sigma^2/n_1\right)$ and $\bar{X}_2 \sim N\left(\mu_2, \sigma^2/n_2\right)$. Thus, $\bar{X}_1 - \bar{X}_2 \sim N\left(\mu_1 - \mu_1, \sigma^2\left[\frac{1}{n_1} + \frac{1}{n_2}\right]\right)$.

Under the null hypothesis, we know that $\mu_1 = \mu_2$; hence, $\bar{X}_1 - \bar{X}_2 \sim N\left(0, \sigma^2\left[\frac{1}{n_1} + \frac{1}{n_2}\right]\right)$.

When the variance of the population is unknown, which is most often the case, we must find the pooled variance before computing the test statistic. The pooled variance, s_p^2, is a weighted average of the two sample variances, where the weights are the number of degrees of freedom in each sample (Equation 8.4).

$$s_p^2 = \frac{(n_1 - 1)s_1^2 + (n_2 - 1)s_2^2}{n_1 + n_2 - 2} \tag{8.4}$$

If the conclusion of the test is to reject the two-sided null hypothesis, we can conclude that there is evidence of a statistically significant difference in means in the two groups. Failing to reject the null hypothesis means that there is no evidence to suggest that there is a difference in the means of the two groups.

t-Test with equal variances in SAS

In SAS, the test for independent data with equal variances is done using PROC TTEST. Sample code and output are shown below. The continuous variable of interest goes in the VAR line, and the dichotomous variable that indicates the two groups goes in the CLASS statement.

```
PROC TTEST DATA = dataset_name;
       VAR continuous_variable;
       CLASS group_variable;
RUN;
```

The TTEST Procedure
Variable: continuous_variable

group_variable	N	Mean	Std Dev	Std Err	Minimum	Maximum
0	50	16.9153	1.1240	0.1590	14.1380	20.0997
1	50	15.1370	0.8975	0.1269	13.1709	17.6702
Diff (1–2)		1.7783	1.0171	0.2034		

group_ variable	Method	Mean	95% CL Mean		Std Dev	95% CL Std Dev	
0		16.9153	16.5959	17.2348	1.1240	0.9389	1.4007
1		15.1370	14.8819	15.3921	0.8975	0.7497	1.1184
Diff (1–2)	Pooled	1.7783	1.3746	2.1820	1.0171	0.8925	1.1825
Diff (1–2)	Satterthwaite	1.7783	1.3744	2.1822			

Method	Variances	DF	t Value	Pr > |t|
Pooled	Equal	98	8.74	<.0001
Satterthwaite	Unequal	93.424	8.74	<.0001

Equality of Variances				
Method	Num DF	Den DF	F Value	Pr > F
Folded F	49	49	1.57	0.1186

The first step in interpreting the output is to look at the test for equality of variances in the last section of the output. The *p*-value should not be significant in order to continue with a two-sample test with equal variances. After this is confirmed, look at the test for the "Pooled" method in the third output box. The degrees of freedom, test statistic value, and *p*-value are given on the "Pooled" line.

t-Test with equal variances in Stata

The *ttest* and *ttesti* commands will run a *t*-test assuming equal variances. List the name of the continuous variable after the *ttest* command, and specify the grouping variable in the by statement. The level option can be used to change the α level, if desired.

```
ttest continuous_variable, by(group_variable) level(95)
```

For the *ttesti* command, specify the sample size, mean, and standard deviation in the first sample, and then the sample size, mean, and standard deviation in the second sample.

```
ttesti n1 xbar1 std1 n2 xbar2 std2, level(95)
```

The output follows:

```
Two-sample t test with equal variances
------------------------------------------------------------------------------
 Group    | Obs     Mean     Std. Err.   Std. Dev.  [95% Conf. Interval]
----------+-------------------------------------------------------------------
     0    |  50  16.91534   .15896      1.124017    16.59589     17.23478
     1    |  50  15.13702  .1269282     .8975182    14.88195     15.39209
----------+-------------------------------------------------------------------
combined  | 100  16.02618   .1350043   1.350043     15.7583      16.29406
----------+-------------------------------------------------------------------
    diff  |      1.778316   .2034184                1.374639     2.181993
------------------------------------------------------------------------------
    diff = mean(0) - mean(1)                                  t =   8.7422
Ho: diff = 0                                 degrees of freedom =       98

    Ha: diff < 0              Ha: diff != 0              Ha: diff > 0
Pr(T < t) = 1.0000     Pr(|T| > |t|) = 0.0000      Pr(T > t) = 0.0000
```

The test statistic and degrees of freedom are shown towards the lower right side. Both one-sided and two-sided p-values are given. The two-sided p-value appears in the "Pr(|T| > |t|)" line.

CASE II: UNEQUAL VARIANCES

If we have a situation with unequal variances, we need to take that into account when performing the hypothesis test. Two of the three assumptions for a two-sample test for independent data with unequal variance are the same as in the equal variance case. We assume the following:

1. The samples are independent.
2. Both samples come from data that are normally distributed (have a normal distribution).
3. The variances of the two samples are unequal.

The null and alternative hypotheses are the same as in the equal variance case. Under the null hypothesis, the exact distribution of the test statistic t is difficult to derive when the variances are assumed not to be equal. Several approximate solutions have been proposed that have the appropriate type I error.

Here, we present only the commonly used Satterthwaite approximation for calculating the degrees of freedom for the test statistic. A major advantage of the Satterthwaite approximation is its easy implementation using the ordinary t table. When the variance is unknown, the test statistic follows a t distribution with ν degrees of freedom. The degrees of freedom ν are a function of the sample standard deviations and the sample sizes.

The following formula is used to calculate ν. The degrees of freedom should be rounded down to the nearest integer.

$$\nu = \frac{\left[\left(\frac{s_1^2}{n_1}\right)+\left(\frac{s_2^2}{n_2}\right)\right]^2}{\left[\frac{\left(\frac{s_1^2}{n_1}\right)^2}{(n_1-1)}+\frac{\left(\frac{s_2^2}{n_2}\right)^2}{(n_2-1)}\right]} \tag{8.5}$$

The conclusion of the test under the unequal variance assumption is the same as the conclusion under the equal variance assumption. Table 8.3 provides a summary for conducting hypothesis test under the equal variance assumption and Table 8.4 for conducting hypothesis test under the unequal variance assumption.

t-Test with unequal variances in SAS

The same SAS code that is used to run a two-sample test for independent data with equal variance is also used for the test assuming unequal variance.

The TTEST Procedure
Variable: continuous_variable

group_variable	N	Mean	Std Dev	Std Err	Minimum	Maximum
0	50	22.9153	1.1240	0.1590	20.1380	26.0997
1	50	25.5481	3.5901	0.5077	17.6834	35.6808
Diff (1–2)		–2.6327	2.6601	0.5320		

group_variable	Method	Mean	95% CL Mean		Std Dev	95% CL Std Dev	
0		22.9153	22.5959	23.2348	1.1240	0.9389	1.4007
1		25.5481	24.5278	26.5684	3.5901	2.9989	4.4737
Diff (1–2)	Pooled	–2.6327	–3.6885	–1.5770	2.6601	2.3341	3.0927
Diff (1–2)	Satterthwaite	–2.6327	–3.6975	–1.5680			

Method	Variances	DF	t Value	Pr > |t|
Pooled	Equal	98	–4.95	<.0001
Satterthwaite	Unequal	58.515	–4.95	<.0001

Equality of Variances				
Method	Num DF	Den DF	F Value	Pr > F
Folded F	49	49	10.20	<.0001

Table 8.3 Tests for independent data with equal variances

Component	*Known variance*	*Unknown variance*
Hypotheses	$H_0: \mu_1 = \mu_2$ vs. $H_1: \mu_1 \neq \mu_2$ $H_0: \mu_1 \leq \mu_2$ vs. $H_1: \mu_1 > \mu_2$ $H_0: \mu_1 \geq \mu_2$ vs. $H_1: \mu_1 < \mu_2$	$H_0: \mu_1 = \mu_2$ vs. $H_1: \mu_1 \neq \mu_2$ $H_0: \mu_1 \leq \mu_2$ vs. $H_1: \mu_1 > \mu_2$ $H_0: \mu_1 \geq \mu_2$ vs. $H_1: \mu_1 < \mu_2$
Test	Two-sample normal test with equal variances	Two-sample t-test with equal variances
Test statistic	$Z = \frac{(\bar{x}_1 - \bar{x}_2) - (\mu_1 - \mu_2)}{\sqrt{\sigma^2\left[\left(\frac{1}{n_1}\right)+\left(\frac{1}{n_2}\right)\right]}}$	$t = \frac{(\bar{x}_1 - \bar{x}_2) - (\mu_1 - \mu_2)}{\sqrt{s_p^2\left[\left(\frac{1}{n_1}\right)+\left(\frac{1}{n_2}\right)\right]}}$
Distribution of test statistic	Standard normal	t-distribution with $n_1 + n_2 - 2$ df
Confidence interval (two-sided)	$(\bar{X}_1 - \bar{X}_2) \pm Z_{1-\alpha/2}\sqrt{\sigma^2\left(\frac{1}{n_1}\right)+\left(\frac{1}{n_2}\right)}$	$(\bar{x}_1 - \bar{x}_2) \pm t_{n_1+n_2-2,1-\alpha/2}\sqrt{s_p^2\left[\left(\frac{1}{n_1}\right)+\left(\frac{1}{n_2}\right)\right]}$

Note: There are two cases of the two-sample test of means assuming equal variances: Known variance and unknown variance. When the variance is known, we use a two-sample normal test with equal variances. If the variance is unknown, we use a two-sample t-test with equal variances.

Table 8.4 Tests for independent data with unequal variances

Component	*Known variance*	*Unknown variance*
Hypotheses	$H_0: \mu_1 = \mu_2$ vs. $H_1: \mu_1 \neq \mu_2$ $H_0: \mu_1 \leq \mu_2$ vs. $H_1: \mu_1 > \mu_2$ $H_0: \mu_1 \geq \mu_2$ vs. $H_1: \mu_1 < \mu_2$	$H_0: \mu_1 = \mu_2$ vs. $H_1: \mu_1 \neq \mu_2$ $H_0: \mu_1 \leq \mu_2$ vs. $H_1: \mu_1 > \mu_2$ $H_0: \mu_1 \geq \mu_2$ vs. $H_1: \mu_1 < \mu_2$
Test	Two-sample normal test with unequal variances	Two-sample t-test with unequal variances
Test statistic	$Z = \frac{(\bar{x}_1 - \bar{x}_2) - (\mu_1 - \mu_2)}{\sqrt{\left(\frac{\sigma^2}{n_1}\right)+\left(\frac{\sigma^2}{n_2}\right)}}$	$t = \frac{(\bar{x}_1 - \bar{x}_2) - (\mu_1 - \mu_2)}{\sqrt{\left(\frac{s_1^2}{n_1}\right)+\left(\frac{s_2^2}{n_2}\right)}}$
Distribution of test statistic	Standard normal	t-distribution with ν df
Confidence interval (two-sided)	$(\bar{X}_1 - \bar{X}_2) \pm Z_{1-\alpha/2}\sqrt{\frac{\sigma_1^2}{n_1}+\frac{\sigma_2^2}{n_2}}$	$(\bar{x}_1 - \bar{x}_2) \pm t_{\nu,1-\alpha/2}\sqrt{\left(\frac{s_1^2}{n_1}\right)+\left(\frac{s_2^2}{n_2}\right)}$

Note: There are two cases of the two-sample test of means assuming unequal variances: known variance and unknown variance. When the variance is known, we use a two-sample normal test with unequal variances. If the variance is unknown, we use a two-sample t-test with unequal variances.

In the output, there should be a significant *p*-value in the "Equality of Variances" box. For the *t*-test, the appropriate output appears on the "Satterthwaite" line in the third section. This line shows the degrees of freedom, the test statistic value, and the *p*-value for the two-sample *t*-test assuming unequal variances.

t-Test with unequal variances in Stata

The two-sample test with unequal variances uses the same code as the *t*-test with equal variances with the addition of the unequal option.

```
ttesti n1 xbar1 std1 n2 xbar2 std2, unequal level(95)
ttest continuous_variable, by(group_variable) unequal level(95)
```

The output follows:

```
Two-sample t test with unequal variances
------------------------------------------------------------------------------
 Group    |   Obs       Mean      Std. Err.     Std. Dev.    [95% Conf. Interval]
---------+--------------------------------------------------------------------
    0     |    50    22.91534       .15896      1.124017     22.59589    23.23478
    1     |    50    25.54808     .5077129      3.590073     24.52779    26.56837
---------+--------------------------------------------------------------------
combined |   100    24.23171     .2958865      2.958865      23.6446    24.81881
---------+--------------------------------------------------------------------
    diff |          -2.632743    .5320157                   -3.697489   -1.567997
------------------------------------------------------------------------------
    diff = mean(0) - mean(1)                                     t =  -4.9486
Ho: diff = 0                       Satterthwaite's degrees of freedom =  58.5151

    Ha: diff < 0                 Ha: diff != 0                 Ha: diff > 0
 Pr(T < t) = 0.0000         Pr(|T| > |t|) = 0.0000          Pr(T > t) = 1.0000
```

The test statistic *t* and corresponding degrees of freedom (Satterthwaite's degrees of freedom) are in the lower right. The bottom line of the output shows the *p*-value for both the one-sided and two-sided tests.

EXAMPLE PROBLEM 8.2

We are interested in the association between body mass index (BMI) and smoking. Suppose that we wish to determine whether the mean BMI among adults who have smoked at least 100 cigarettes in their lifetime is equal to the mean BMI among adults who have not smoked at least 100 cigarettes. For brevity, we will call the former group "ever smokers" and the latter group "nonsmokers." In each group, the distribution of BMI is approximately normal, but we cannot assume that the variances are equal. We obtained a random sample of 139 ever smokers and 128 nonsmokers.[3] The ever smokers had mean BMI $\bar{x}_1 = 26.88\ \text{kg/m}^2$ with standard deviation $s_1 = 4.80\ \text{kg/m}^2$; the nonsmokers had mean BMI $\bar{x}_2 = 27.36\ \text{kg/m}^2$ with standard deviation $s_2 = 6.67\ \text{kg/m}^2$. Assuming $\alpha = 0.05$, use a statistical software package to conduct the appropriate hypothesis test. The dataset name is *ch8_bmi_smoking*.

BOX 8.1 DESCRIPTION OF THE *cb8_bmi_smoking* DATASET

The Behavioral Risk Factor Surveillance System (BRFSS) asks each respondent, "Have you smoked at least 100 cigarettes in your entire life?" The response categories are "Yes," "No," or "Don't know/Not sure," or the respondent can refuse to answer the question. Those who reported smoking at least 100 cigarettes are considered ever smokers (*smoke100* = *1*). Those who answered "No" are coded as *smoke100* = *0*. Respondents were also asked to report their weight and height, which was used to calculate their body mass index (BMI). Those who had a recorded BMI and who answered "Yes" or "No" to having smoked 100 cigarettes in their lifetime were eligible for the sample in the dataset *cb8_bmi_smoking*.

A What type of test will you perform?

A two-sample *t*-test for independent data is appropriate.

B State your null and alternative hypotheses.

H_0: $\mu_1 = \mu_2$

H_1: $\mu_1 \neq \mu_2$

C Does the assumption of equal variances appear reasonable?

The variance in the ever smoker group is $4.80^2 = 23.04$.
In the sample of nonsmokers, the variance is $6.67^2 = 44.49$.
Because these two variances are fairly different from each other, we suspect that the assumption of equal variances is not reasonable.

D Write the appropriate SAS or Stata code, and test for the equality of variances.

In SAS, the test for equality of variances comes as part of the output from PROC TTEST. The continuous variable is *bmi*, and the grouping variable is *smoke100*.

```
PROC TTEST DATA = bmi_smoking;
VAR bmi;
CLASS smoke100;
RUN;
```

Equality of Variances				
Method	Num DF	Den DF	F Value	Pr > F
Folded F	213	152	1.93	<.0001

The "Equality of Variances" output table shows the results of the test for equality of variances. Because $p < 0.0001 < \alpha = 0.05$, we reject the null hypothesis that the variances are equal and conduct a two-sample *t*-test with unequal variances.

The *sdtest* command runs the test in Stata. The grouping variable *smoke100* goes in the by option.

```
sdtest bmi, by(smoke100)
```

The output follows:

```
Variance ratio test
------------------------------------------------------------------------------
   Group |     Obs        Mean    Std. Err.   Std. Dev.   [95% Conf. Interval]
---------+--------------------------------------------------------------------
       0 |     214    27.36333    .4558699    6.668802    26.46474    28.26193
       1 |     153     26.8775    .3878745    4.797743    26.11118    27.64382
---------+--------------------------------------------------------------------
combined |     367    27.16079    .3110098    5.958091     26.5492    27.77238
------------------------------------------------------------------------------
    ratio = sd(0) / sd(1)                                         f =   1.9321
Ho: ratio = 1                                  degrees of freedom =  213, 152

    Ha: ratio < 1               Ha: ratio != 1                 Ha: ratio > 1
  Pr(F < f) = 1.0000         2*Pr(F > f) = 0.0000           Pr(F > f) = 0.0000
```

The p-value calculated by Stata is <0.0001. Because $p < \alpha = 0.05$, we reject the null hypothesis that the variances are equal and conduct a two-sample t-test with unequal variances.

E From the output, what are the value and distribution of the test statistic for the two-sample t-test?

The TTEST Procedure
Variable: bmi (Body Mass Index [BMI])

SMOKE100	N	Mean	Std Dev	Std Err	Minimum	Maximum
0	214	27.3633	6.6688	0.4559	15.6955	54.8576
1	153	26.8775	4.7977	0.3879	12.1616	42.5879
Diff (1–2)		0.4858	5.9614	0.6311		

SMOKE100	Method	Mean	95% CL Mean		Std Dev	95% CL Std Dev	
0		27.3633	26.4647	28.2619	6.6688	6.0912	7.3684
1		26.8775	26.1112	27.6438	4.7977	4.3137	5.4051
Diff (1–2)	Pooled	0.4858	–0.7553	1.7270	5.9614	5.5586	6.4277
Diff (1–2)	Satterthwaite	0.4858	–0.6912	1.6629			

Method	Variances	DF	t Value	Pr > |t|
Pooled	Equal	365	0.77	0.4419
Satterthwaite	Unequal	364.98	0.81	0.4175

```
Two-sample t test with unequal variances
------------------------------------------------------------------------------
   Group |     Obs        Mean    Std. Err.   Std. Dev.   [95% Conf. Interval]
---------+--------------------------------------------------------------------
       0 |     214    27.36333    .4558699    6.668802    26.46474    28.26193
       1 |     153     26.8775    .3878745    4.797743    26.11118    27.64382
---------+--------------------------------------------------------------------
combined |     367    27.16079    .3110098    5.958091     26.5492    27.77238
---------+--------------------------------------------------------------------
    diff |            .4858297    .5985516               -.6912131    1.662872
------------------------------------------------------------------------------
    diff = mean(0) - mean(1)                                      t =   0.8117
Ho: diff = 0                     Satterthwaite's degrees of freedom =  364.982

    Ha: diff < 0                 Ha: diff != 0                 Ha: diff > 0
 Pr(T < t) = 0.7912         Pr(|T| > |t|) = 0.4175          Pr(T > t) = 0.2088
```

In Example Problem 8.3—Part (D), we determined that the two-sample test with unequal variances is appropriate. In SAS, the results on the line labeled "Satterthwaite" are for the unequal variance test using the Satterthwaite approximation. The value of the test statistic is $t = 0.81$. The test statistic follows a t distribution with 364.98 degrees of freedom. We see similar results in the Stata output.

F **What is the p-value for your test?**

The p-value is 0.4175.

G **Do you reject or fail to reject the null hypothesis? What conclusion can you draw from this study?**

Since $p > \alpha = 0.05$, we fail to reject the null hypothesis. We do not have evidence to suggest that the mean BMI among persons who have smoked at least 100 cigarettes in their lifetime is different from that of the mean BMI among persons who have never smoked at least 100 cigarettes.

H **How could you have used the confidence interval for the true difference in means to test the null hypothesis?**

The confidence interval for the true difference in means is (–0.69, 1.66). This is found in the SAS output in the line beginning "Diff(1 – 2) Satterthwaite" under the heading "95% CL Mean" or in the Stata output in the "diff" line under "95% Conf. Interval." This confidence interval contains the null value, 0; therefore, we fail to reject H_0.

I **Would your results have changed if you had incorrectly assumed *equal* variances?**

The SAS output in Example Problem 8.2—Part (E) shows that if we had incorrectly assumed equal variances, the p-value would have been 0.4419.

To find the p-value in Stata, we can run the same code for the *ttest* command again but leave out the unequal option.

```
ttest bmi, by(smoke100)
```

The abbreviated output is shown:

```
     Ha: diff < 0             Ha: diff != 0             Ha: diff > 0
 Pr(T < t) = 0.7790    Pr(|T| > |t|) = 0.4419     Pr(T > t) = 0.2210
```

We see that Stata gives 0.4419 as the p-value, assuming equal variances.

Thus, the test assuming equal variances leads to the same conclusion as the unequal variances test. However, this is not always the case. There are situations in which the variance assumption will lead to contradictory hypothesis test outcomes, so it is important to check the test for equality of variances before assuming equal variances.

Modern convention says that there is no need to conduct a variance ratio test. Always assume unequal variances, as this is the more conservative test.

PRACTICE PROBLEM 8.2

We have a sample of 266 adults with diabetes who are from an outpatient clinic.[4] Among the calculated variables from the data collected was the Medication Regimen Complexity Index (MRCI), a scale used to quantify the complexity of a patient's medication-taking routine. We are interested in exploring whether the mean MRCI is different in adults with diabetes who have had at least one visit to the ED in the past year versus adults with diabetes who have had no ED visits. Of the 266 subjects, 105 did not visit the ED, and 161 subjects did have at least one visit to an ED in the past year. Let $\alpha = 0.05$. The dataset is called *ch8_mrci_ed_visits*.

A What type of test is appropriate in this situation?

B State the null and alternative hypotheses.

C Test for the equality of variances. Can we assume equal variances in this situation?

D Perform the hypothesis test. What is the value of the test statistic and its distribution?

E What is the p-value for the test?

F Do you reject or fail to reject the null hypothesis? State the results in terms of the subject matter.

G What is the confidence interval for the difference in means?

H Check to make sure that the conclusion from the confidence interval matches that from the hypothesis test.

Table 8.5 Sample size for two-sample test of means

Type	*Situation*	*Formula*
One-sided	Equal groups	$n = \frac{(\sigma_1^2 + \sigma_2^2)(Z_{1-\alpha} + Z_{1-\beta})^2}{\Delta^2}$
	Unequal groups	$n_1 = \frac{\left(\sigma_1^2 + \sigma_2^2/k\right)(Z_{1-\alpha} + Z_{1-\beta})^2}{\Delta^2}$ $n_2 = \frac{(k\sigma_1^2 + \sigma_2^2)(Z_{1-\alpha} + Z_{1-\beta})^2}{\Delta^2}$
Two-sided	Equal groups	$n = \frac{(\sigma_1^2 + \sigma_2^2)\left(Z_{1-\alpha/2} + Z_{1-\beta}\right)}{\Delta^2}$
	Unequal groups	$n_1 = \frac{\left(\sigma_1^2 + \sigma_2^2/k\right)\left(Z_{1-\alpha/2} + Z_{1-\beta}\right)^2}{\Delta^2}$ $n_2 = \frac{(k\sigma_1^2 + \sigma_2^2)\left(Z_{1-\alpha/2} + Z_{1-\beta}\right)^2}{\Delta^2}$

Note: The sample size for the two-sample test of means with a balanced design depends on the variance of each group, the significance level, power, and the difference between the group means. If we would like unequal groups, then we also take into account the allocation ratio.

Sample size and power for two-sample test of means

Chapter 7 introduced the notion of sample size and power for a one-sample test. Here, we expand the concept to two-sample tests. Let Δ be the absolute value of the true difference in means between the two groups, $|\mu_1 - \mu_2|$. Displayed in Table 8.5 is the sample size needed for comparing the means of two normally distributed samples using one-sided or two-sided tests with significance level α and power $1 - \beta$. In other words, the appropriate sample size in each group to have a probability of $1 - \beta$ of finding a significant difference when one exists, based on a test with significance level α, if the absolute value of the true difference in means between the two groups is $\Delta = |\mu_1 - \mu_2|$.

In many instances, we anticipate an imbalance between the groups, and we predict in advance that the number of people in one group will be k times the number of people in the other group for some number $k \neq 1$. In other words, $k = \frac{n_2}{n_1}$ is the projected ratio of the two sample sizes. In this scenario, there is a different formula for the sample size of each group, which yields a smaller sample, n_1, and a larger sample, n_2.

In many situations, a predetermined sample size is available for study. In this case, we need to determine how much power the study will have for detecting specific alternatives. Power for comparing the means of two normally distributed samples with

Table 8.6 Power for two-sample test of means

Type	*Formula*
One-sided	$\phi\left(-Z_{1-\alpha}+\dfrac{\Delta}{\sqrt{\dfrac{\sigma_1^2}{n_1}+\dfrac{\sigma_2^2}{n_2}}}\right)$
Two-sided	$\phi\left(-Z_{1-\alpha/2}+\dfrac{\Delta}{\sqrt{\dfrac{\sigma_1^2}{n_1}+\dfrac{\sigma_2^2}{n_2}}}\right)$

Note: Power for a two-sample test of means depends on the significance level, the variance of each group, the difference between the group means, and the sample size of each group.

significance level α is shown in Table 8.6. The variances σ_1^2 and σ_2^2 are assumed known along with the specified alternative, $\Delta = |\mu_1 - \mu_2|$.

Because the calculations can get very complicated, we usually use statistical software to calculate sample size and power.

Using SAS for sample size and power for two-sample test of means

Many options can be specified in the SAS code, depending on the design (balanced or unbalanced), level of power, equal or unequal variance assumption, and so forth. By default, the level of significance is set at 0.05, so the ALPHA option is optional unless a different level of significance is desired. The TEST = diff_satt option specifies that we will have a *t*-test with unequal variances that uses the Satterthwaite approximation.

The GROUPMEANS option specifies the means of the two groups, and the GROUPSTDDEVS indicates the standard deviations of the two groups. For a balanced design with unequal variances, sample code may look like the following.

```
PROC POWER;
        TWOSAMPLEMEANS TEST = diff_satt
        GROUPMEANS = 10 | 20
        GROUPSTDDEVS = 5 | 8
        POWER = 0.90
        ALPHA = 0.05
        NPERGROUP = .;
RUN;
```

The POWER Procedure
Two-Sample *t* Test for Mean Difference
with Unequal Variances

Fixed Scenario Elements	
Distribution	Normal
Method	Exact
Nominal Alpha	0.05
Group 1 Mean	10
Group 2 Mean	20
Group 1 Standard Deviation	5
Group 2 Standard Deviation	8
Nominal Power	0.9
Number of Sides	2
Null Difference	0

Computed N per Group		
Actual Alpha	Actual Power	N per Group
0.0496	0.909	11

The "N per Group" column shows the number of subjects needed in each group. From the total sample size, we can calculate the sample size for each of the unbalanced groups. For an unbalanced design with unequal variances, the NPERGROUP option can be replaced by NTOTAL, and the GROUPWEIGHTS option is needed to specify the ratio of subjects. If we would like to input the difference between the group means rather than the means of the two groups, we can use the MEANDIFF option instead of the GROUPMEANS option.

```
PROC POWER;
       TWOSAMPLEMEANS TEST = diff_satt
       MEANDIFF = 10
       GROUPSTDDEVS = 5 | 8
       GROUPWEIGHTS = (1 3)
       POWER = 0.90
       NTOTAL = .;
RUN;
```

The POWER Procedure
Two-Sample *t* Test for Mean Difference
with Unequal Variances

Fixed Scenario Elements	
Distribution	Normal
Method	Exact
Mean Difference	10
Group 1 Standard Deviation	5
Group 2 Standard Deviation	8
Group 1 Weight	1
Group 2 Weight	3
Nominal Power	0.9
Number of Sides	2
Null Difference	0
Nominal Alpha	0.05

Computed N per Group		
Actual Alpha	Actual Power	N Total
0.0501	0.911	24

The total sample size is given under the "N Total" column. Just as in the one-sample hypothesis test described in Chapter 7, if we are interested in finding the power instead of the sample size, we can switch the option that is omitted.

```
PROC POWER;
      TWOSAMPLEMEANS TEST = diff_satt
      GROUPMEANS = 10 | 20
      GROUPSTDDEVS = 5 | 8
      POWER = .
      NTOTAL = 15;
RUN;
```

The POWER Procedure
Two-Sample *t* Test for Mean Difference
with Unequal Variances

Fixed Scenario Elements	
Distribution	Normal
Method	Exact
Group 1 Mean	10
Group 2 Mean	20
Group 1 Standard Deviation	5
Group 2 Standard Deviation	8
Nominal Total Sample Size	15
Actual Total Sample Size	14
Null Difference	0
Nominal Alpha	0.05
Group 1 Weight	1
Group 2 Weight	1
Nominal Alpha	0.05

Computed Power	
Actual Alpha	Power
0.0487	0.708

The "Computed Power" box shows the power level of the test.

Using Stata for sample size and power for two-sample test of means

The *power* command with the *twomeans* option runs power and sample size calculations. To determine the necessary sample size, we must specify the means of the two groups after the *twomeans* option, followed by the standard deviations of the groups. The default alpha level is 0.05, and the default power level is 0.80.

```
power twomeans 10 20, sd1(5) sd2(8) alpha(0.05) power(0.9)
```

The output follows:

```
Estimated sample sizes for a two-sample means test
Satterthwaite's t test assuming unequal variances
```

```
Ho: m2 = m1   versus   Ha: m2 != m1
Study parameters:

        alpha =     0.0500
        power =     0.9000
        delta =    10.0000
           m1 =    10.0000
           m2 =    20.0000
          sd1 =     5.0000
          sd2 =     8.0000

Estimated sample sizes:

            N =         22
  N per group =         11
```

We can also specify the difference between the means rather than both means, but unlike SAS, we must also specify the mean in Group 1 after the *twomeans* statement.

```
power twomeans 10, diff(10) sd1(5) sd2(8) alpha(0.05) power(0.9)
```

- If the groups are unbalanced, the *nratio* option is added to specify the ratio $k = \frac{n_2}{n_1}$.

```
power twomeans 10 20, sd1(5) sd2(8) alpha(0.05) power(0.9) nratio(3)
```

The output follows:

```
Estimated sample sizes for a two-sample means test
Satterthwaite's t test assuming unequal variances
Ho: m2 = m1   versus   Ha: m2 != m1

Study parameters:

        alpha =     0.0500
        power =     0.9000
        delta =    10.0000
           m1 =    10.0000
           m2 =    20.0000
          sd1 =     5.0000
          sd2 =     8.0000
        N2/N1 =     3.0000

Estimated sample sizes:

            N =         24
           N1 =          6
           N2 =         18
```

The total sample size and the size of each of the groups appear at the bottom of the output. To compute power rather than sample size, we substitute the *n* option for the *power* option.

```
power twomeans 10 20, sd1(5) sd2(8) alpha(0.05) n(15)
```

The output follows:

```
Estimated power for a two-sample means test
Satterthwaite's t test assuming unequal variances
Ho: m2 = m1  versus  Ha: m2 != m1

Study parameters:

        alpha =    0.0500
            N =        15
        delta =   10.0000
           m1 =   10.0000
           m2 =   20.0000
          sd1 =    5.0000
          sd2 =    8.0000

Actual sample sizes:

            N =        14
  N per group =         7

Estimated power:

        power =    0.7159
```

The power of the test is shown on the bottom line of the output.

EXAMPLE PROBLEM 8.3

Suppose that we are planning a new study to determine the difference between mean fasting glucose levels (mg/dL) among U.S. adults older than 18 years old who eat a healthy diet and those who eat a poor diet. We know that the standard deviation of fasting glucose level in the general population of U.S. adults who eat a healthy diet is σ_1 = 28.58 mg/dL.[5] The mean for those eating a healthy diet is 102.83 mg/dL. Among U.S. adults eating a poor diet, we know that the standard deviation of fasting glucose level is σ_2 = 22.28 mg/dL. We want to design the study so that it will have 80% power to detect a difference in means of 5.00 mg/dL.

BOX 8.2 DESCRIPTION OF EXAMPLE PROBLEM 8.3 DATA

The laboratory component of the National Health and Nutrition Examination Survey (NHANES) collects respondents' fasting glucose levels in mg/dL. Respondents are also asked, "In general, how healthy is your overall diet?" The response is a seven-level categorical variable, ranging from "Excellent" to "Poor" with options for "Don't know" and "Refused." Those who reported having an excellent, very good, or good diet were classified as eating a healthy diet. Respondents who selected "Fair" or "Poor" were categorized as having a poor diet. Additionally, the age of each respondent was recorded during the survey.

A Assuming that we do a two-sided test at the 0.05 level of significance, what is the sample size needed to achieve the desired power? We would like to have balanced groups. Calculate the sample size by hand, and use a statistical package.

First, we should list the information that we know. Then, we will use the equation for a two-sided test with equal groups.

$\alpha = 0.05$ $\quad Z_{1-\beta} = 0.84$

$Z_{1-\alpha/2} = 1.96$ $\quad \sigma_1 = 28.58$ mg/dL

$\beta = 0.20$ $\quad \sigma_2 = 22.28$ mg/dL

$\Delta = |\mu_1 - \mu_2| = 5.00$ mg/dL

$$n = \frac{(\sigma_1^2 + \sigma_2^2)(Z_{1-\alpha/2} + Z_{1-\beta})}{\Delta^2} = \frac{(28.58^2 + 22.28^2)(1.96 + 0.84)^2}{5.00^2}$$

$$= \frac{10295.60}{25.00} = 411.82$$

To achieve 80% power, 412 subjects in each group are needed.

Using SAS, we can check our calculation. Because both groups will be equal, we can use the NPERGROUP option to get the sample size in each group.

```
PROC POWER;
     TWOSAMPLEMEANS TEST = diff_satt
     MEANDIFF = 5.00
     GROUPSTDDEVS = 28.58 | 22.28
     POWER = 0.80
     ALPHA = 0.05
     NPERGROUP = .;
RUN;
```

The POWER Procedure
Two-Sample *t* Test for Mean Difference
with Unequal Variances

Fixed Scenario Elements	
Distribution	Normal
Method	Exact
Nominal Alpha	0.05
Mean Difference	5
Group 1 Standard Deviation	28.58
Group 2 Standard Deviation	22.28
Nominal Power	0.8
Number of Sides	2
Null Difference	0

Computed N per Group		
Actual Alpha	Actual Power	N per Group
0.0501	0.801	414

The output shows that 414 subjects are needed in each group in order to achieve 80% power. A slight difference between the hand calculations and the output from the statistical packages is due to the use of the *Z* distribution in the hand calculations.

In Stata, we use the *power* command with the *twomeans* option. Since alpha is 0.05 and power is 0.80, we can drop the alpha and *power* options from the code. We specify the mean in the first group, the difference that we want to detect, and the standard deviation in each group.

```
power twomeans 102.83, diff(5) sd1(28.58) sd2(22.28)
```

The output follows:

```
Estimated sample sizes for a two-sample means test
Satterthwaite's t test assuming unequal variances
Ho: m2 = m1  versus  Ha: m2 != m1

Study parameters:

        alpha =    0.0500
        power =    0.8000
        delta =    5.0000
           m1 =  102.8300
```

```
             m2 =   107.8300
           diff =     5.0000
            sd1 =    28.5800
            sd2 =    22.2800

Estimated sample sizes:

              N =        828
    N per group =        414
```

The output gives a value of 414 subjects per group, for a total sample size of 828 subjects.

B Let's take a variation on the scenario. Assume that, instead of a balanced design, we know that there will be an unbalanced design in which there will be only one subject with a healthy diet for every two subjects with a poor diet. What sample size is needed in each of the groups in this case, assuming all of the other parameters are the same?

Once again, we first write out what we know.

$\alpha = 0.05$ $\qquad \Delta = |\mu_1 - \mu_2| = 5.00 \text{ mg/dL}$

$Z_{1-\alpha/2} = 1.96$ $\qquad \beta = 0.20$

$\sigma_1 = 28.58 \text{ mg/dL}$ $\qquad Z_{1-\beta} = 0.84$

$\sigma_2 = 22.28 \text{ mg/dL}$ $\qquad k = 2/1 = 2$

For Group 1, those with healthy diets:

$$n_1 = \frac{\left(\sigma_1^2 + \sigma_2^2/k\right)\left(Z_{1-\alpha/2} + Z_{1-\beta}\right)^2}{\Delta^2} = \frac{\left(28.58^2 + 22.28^2/2\right)(1.96 + 0.84)^2}{5.00^2}$$

$$= \frac{8349.72}{25.00} = 333.99$$

After rounding up, 334 adults with healthy diets will be needed.
For Group 2, those with poor diets:

$$n_2 = \frac{\left(k\sigma_1^2 + \sigma_2^2\right)\left(Z_{1-\alpha/2} + Z_{1-\beta}\right)^2}{\Delta^2} = \frac{(2 * 28.58^2 + 22.28^2)(1.96 + 0.84)^2}{5.00^2}$$

$$= \frac{16699.44}{25.00} = 667.98$$

After rounding up, 668 adults with poor diets are needed to achieve 80% power.

We can check this calculation using the following SAS code. The unbalanced design means that we should use the GROUPWEIGHTS option to specify the subject ratio of the two groups and the NTOTAL option to find the total sample size.

```
PROC POWER;
     TWOSAMPLEMEANS TEST = diff_satt
     MEANDIFF = 5.00
     GROUPSTDDEVS = 28.58 | 22.28
     GROUPWEIGHTS = (1 2)
     POWER = 0.80
     ALPHA = 0.05
     NTOTAL = .;
RUN;
```

The POWER Procedure
Two-Sample *t* Test for Mean Difference with Unequal Variances

Fixed Scenario Elements	
Distribution	Normal
Method	Exact
Nominal Alpha	0.05
Mean Difference	5
Group 1 Standard Deviation	28.58
Group 2 Standard Deviation	22.28
Group 1 Weight	1
Group 2 Weight	2
Nominal Power	0.8
Number of Sides	2
Null Difference	0

Computed N Total		
Actual Alpha	Actual Power	N Total
0.05	0.801	1008

SAS calculates that 1008 total subjects are required to have 80% power. Given our ratio of one healthy diet to two poor diets, we need 336 adults with healthy diets and 672 adults with poor diets.

In Stata, we add in the *nratio* option to specify that the design is unbalanced with twice as many adults with poor diets.

```
power twomeans 102.83, diff(5) sd1(28.58) sd2(22.28) nratio(2)
```

The output follows:

```
Estimated sample sizes for a two-sample means test
Satterthwaite's t test assuming unequal variances
Ho: m2 = m1  versus  Ha: m2 != m1

Study parameters:

        alpha =    0.0500
        power =    0.8000
        delta =    5.0000
           m1 =  102.8300
           m2 =  107.8300
         diff =    5.0000
          sd1 =   28.5800
          sd2 =   22.2800
        N2/N1 =    2.0000

Estimated sample sizes:

            N =      1008
           N1 =       336
           N2 =       672
```

The output shows that to have 80% power we need 336 adults who eat a healthy diet and 672 who do not, for a total sample size of 1008 total subjects.

The calculation done in statistical software requires more participants since they are based on the *t*-test (unknown variance) while hand calculations use z-statistic (known variance). In practice we always use statistical software for power and sample size calculations.

BOX 8.3 DESCRIPTION OF PRACTICE PROBLEM 8.3 DATA

The National Health and Nutrition Examination Survey (NHANES) asks each respondent aged 20 and older, "What is the highest grade or level of school you have completed or the highest degree you have received?" The response is a seven-level categorical variable, ranging from "Less than 9th Grade" to "College Graduate or Above" with options for "Don't know" and "Refused." The survey also asks, "During the past 30 days, how much money {did your family/did you} spend at supermarkets or grocery stores? Please include purchases made with food stamps." Numerical values are specified for the answers. Also, participants can report that they do not know or can refuse to answer the question.

PRACTICE PROBLEM 8.3

We are planning a study to investigate the association between food consumption behaviors and education levels. Monthly spending at grocery stores or supermarkets will be measured and compared between adults with no college degree and college graduates. Among U.S. adults aged 20 years and older with no college degree, the mean amount spent at grocery stores or supermarkets is $453.88/month with a standard deviation of σ_1 = $324.80/month.[5] For U.S. adults aged 20 years and older who have a college degree, the standard deviation is $\sigma_2 = 310.20$.

A There is a predetermined sample size of 200 U.S. adults in each education group, for a total of 400 subjects. What level of power would we need to have to detect a difference in grocery spending of $100/month? Set the level of significance at 0.05.

B Assume now that we want to have 80% power to detect a difference in grocery spending of $100/month. Keep $\alpha = 0.05$. How many subjects are needed in each group in order to achieve the desired level of power?

References

1. United States Census Bureau. American Community Survey: Health insurance, 2009. http://www.socialexplorer.com/tables/ACS2009/R11239760?ReportId=R11239760. Accessed March 9, 2016.
2. United States Census Bureau. American Community Survey: Health insurance, 2014. http://www.socialexplorer.com/tables/ACS2014/R11239768?ReportId=R11239768. Accessed March 9, 2016.
3. Behavioral Risk Factor Surveillance System. 2014 BRFSS Survey Data and Documentation. Atlanta, GA: Centers for Disease Control and Prevention. http://www.cdc.gov/brfss/annual_data/annual_2014.html. September 11, 2015. Accessed February 23, 2016.
4. Fan JH, Lyons S, Goodman MS, Blanchard MS, Kaphingst KA. Relationship between health literacy and unintentional and intentional medication nonadherence in medically underserved patients with type 2 diabetes. *Diabetes Educ.* 2016;42(2):199–208. doi:10.1177/0145721715624969.
5. National Health and Nutrition Examination Survey. Hyattsville, MD: Centers for Disease Control and Prevention, National Center for Health Statistics. https://wwwn.cdc.gov/Nchs/Nhanes/Search/nhanes13_14.aspx. Published 2014. Accessed February 23, 2016.

9 Nonparametric hypothesis testing

This chapter will focus on nonparametric statistical methods and will include the following topics:

- Types of data
- Parametric vs. nonparametric tests
- Nonparametric tests for paired data
- Nonparametric tests for independent data

Terms

- cardinal data
- interval scale
- nominal scale
- nonparametric statistical methods
- ordinal data
- parametric statistical methods
- ratio scale

Introduction

Thus far, we have assumed that data come from some underlying distribution, such as the normal or binomial distribution, whose general form is known. The methods of estimation and hypothesis tests introduced up to this point have been based on these assumptions. These procedures are called *parametric statistical methods* because the parametric form of the distribution is assumed to be known.

Parametric Statistical Methods: Methods that assume the data come from a probability distribution.

If these assumptions about the shape of the distribution are not made, or if the CLT seems inapplicable because of small sample size, we must use nonparametric statistical methods. Nonparametric methods make fewer assumptions about the distribution shape.

Nonparametric Statistical Methods: Methods that do not assume that data follow a particular probability distribution.

Types of data

Another assumption is that it is meaningful to measure the distance between possible data values. This assumption is particularly characteristic of cardinal data.

Cardinal Data: Numeric data where it is meaningful to measure the distance between possible data values.

There are two types of cardinal data:

- Interval scale data
- Ratio scale data

Interval Scale: For cardinal data, if the 0 point is arbitrary, then the data are on an interval scale. For example, degrees in Fahrenheit are on an interval scale.

Ratio Scale: If the 0 point is meaningful, then the cardinal data are on a ratio scale. Money is one common example of data measured on a ratio scale.

For data on a ratio scale, it is meaningful to measure ratios between specific data values, but such measurement is not meaningful on an interval scale. However, it is appropriate to use means and standard deviations for cardinal data of either scale type.

Ordinal Data: Data that can be ordered but that do not have specific numeric values.

Therefore, common arithmetic cannot be performed with ordinal data as it would be with a cardinal data. For example, means and standard deviations are not meaningful for ordinal data. Specifically, methods of estimation and hypothesis testing based on normal distributions cannot be used. For ordinal data, we can measure the relative ordering of different categories of a variable.

Nominal Scale: A scale used for different data values that can be classified into categories without the categories having specific ordering. For instance, race and gender are commonly used nominal variables, as there is no inherent order to the levels.

Parametric vs. nonparametric tests

Parametric tests can be used only if the underlying distributions of the data are known or can be assumed to be normally distributed based on the CLT. In nonparametric tests, there are fewer assumptions about the underlying distribution. At most, in nonparametric tests, the populations must have the same shape. Nonparametric tests are less sensitive to measurement error because they rely only on signs and ranks, rather than the specific values of the variables. They can also be used for ordinal as well as continuous data, and they generally compare medians rather than means. In addition, the basic steps for hypothesis testing that we introduced in Chapter 7 still hold when conducting a nonparametric test.

It is also important to note disadvantages of nonparametric methods. If parametric assumptions are valid (i.e., the data really are normally distributed), then nonparametric tests are less powerful. This means that they need larger sample sizes to reject a false null hypothesis. For example, the Wilcoxon rank-sum test has 95% the power of a *t*-test (its parametric counterpart) if data are approximately normal. Nonparametric tests have less specific hypotheses and do not use all of the information provided by the data. Additionally, ties in ranks lead to overestimates of σ and require a correction term (beyond the scope of this book).

Table 9.1 Nonparametric tests for paired data

Component	*Sign test*	*Wilcoxon signed-rank test*
Hypotheses	H_0: median difference = 0 vs. H_1: median difference ≠ 0	H_0: median difference = 0 vs. H_1: median difference ≠ 0
Summary of observed data	D: # positive differences	T: smaller of the sums of the positive or negative ranks
Mean	$\mu_D = \frac{n}{2}$	$\mu_T = \frac{n(n+1)}{4}$
Standard deviation	$\sigma_D = \sqrt{\frac{n}{4}}$	$\sigma_T = \sqrt{\frac{n(n+1)(2n+1)}{24}}$
Test statistic	$Z_+ = \frac{D - \mu_D}{\sigma_D}$	$Z_T = \frac{T - \mu_T}{\sigma_T}$
Distribution of test statistic (large n)	Standard normal	Standard normal
Valid if	$np(1-p) \geq 5$ $\frac{n}{4} \geq 5$ where n is the number of nonzero differences	$n > 6$ where n is the number of nonzero differences

Note: The sign test and the Wilcoxon signed-rank test are two nonparametric tests for paired data.

Nonparametric tests for paired data

Nonparametric tests extend our work on the comparison of two samples in the case where there are two groups to be compared but the assumption of normality is questionable. The two main nonparametric tests for continuous paired data are the sign test and the Wilcoxon signed-rank test. Both test the null hypothesis that the median difference is equal to 0. Table 9.1 outlines the two tests.

Sign test

The sign test uses the plus (+) or minus (–) sign for the differences only and does not consider the magnitude of the differences. It should be noted that the test is not used often. The null and alternative hypotheses for the test can be seen as a special case of the one-sample binomial test where H_0: $p = \frac{1}{2}$ and H_1: $p \neq \frac{1}{2}$. Under H_0, $p = \frac{1}{2}$, $E(C) = np = \frac{n}{2}$, $Var(C) = npq = \frac{n}{4}$, thus $C \sim N\left(\frac{n}{2}, \frac{n}{4}\right)$.

To carry out the sign test, perform the following four steps:

1 Calculate the difference for each pair of observations.
2 Assign a sign to each pair.
  a If the difference is greater than 0, the pair is assigned a plus sign.
  b If the difference is less than 0, the pair is assigned a minus sign.

c Differences of exactly 0 provide no information and are, thus, excluded from the analysis. Note that if differences are excluded, the sample size must be adjusted accordingly.

3 Count the number of plus signs in the sample. This total is denoted by D.

4 When the number of nonzero differences divided by 4 is less than 5 $\left(\frac{n}{4}<5\right)$, the exact method is appropriate. In this case, use binomial distribution to calculate p-value for D. If n is large such that $\frac{n}{4}\geq 5$, then the normal approximation to the binomial distribution holds. In this case, use the test statistic $Z_+ = \frac{D-\mu_D}{\sigma_D}$ and find the corresponding p-value.

Wilcoxon signed-rank test

The Wilcoxon signed-rank test is the nonparametric analogue to the paired t-test. This test incorporates the magnitude of the differences via ranks and is more powerful than the sign test. Thus, it is preferable to use the Wilcoxon signed-rank test when given a choice between the two. The test is nonparametric because it is based on the ranks of the observations rather than the actual values of the observations.

To conduct the Wilcoxon signed-rank test, perform the following steps:

1 Calculate the difference for each pair of observations.
2 Ignoring the signs of the differences, rank the pairs in terms of their absolute values from smallest to largest.
  a A difference of 0 is not ranked and is eliminated from the analysis. If this occurs, the sample size must be reduced by 1 for each pair eliminated.
  b If two observations have the same absolute value, then they are assigned an average rank. For example, if we have 4 difference values of 4.5, 4.8, 4.8, and 5.0, then 4.5 is ranked 1, 4.8 is ranked 2.5 (the average of ranks 2 and 3), 4.8 is ranked 2.5 (the average of ranks 2 and 3), and 5.0 is ranked 4.
3 Assign each rank a minus or plus sign, depending on the sign of the difference.
4 Compute the sum of the positive ranks.
5 Compute the sum of the negative ranks.
  a The smaller of the quantities from Steps 4 and 5 is denoted T.
6 Depending on the sample size, use the table of critical values (Appendix Table A.7) to calculate a p-value or compute the test statistic.
  a For a small n, use the Wilcoxon signed-rank table in the Appendix (Table A.7) to calculate the p-value of T. This method should be used if the number of nonzero differences is 6 or less. To use the table, find the column corresponding to n, the number of nonzero differences, and the row corresponding to the value of T. The entries in the table give the one-sided p-value for the given sample size and T. For a two-sided hypothesis test, multiply the value found in the table by 2 to get the p-value.
  b If n is sufficiently large (i.e., the number of nonzero differences is more than 6), use the test statistic $Z_T = \frac{T-\mu_T}{\sigma_T}$ and obtain the corresponding p-value for the test using the standard normal table (Appendix Table A.3).

c Sometimes, a $-\frac{1}{2}$ term is added when computing the test statistic, which serves as a continuity correction to better approximate the binomial distribution (a discrete distribution) by the normal distribution (a continuous distribution).

Performing nonparametric tests for paired data in SAS

We can use PROC UNIVARIATE to perform the sign test and the Wilcoxon signed-rank test in SAS. It is necessary to first create a variable that is the difference for each pair of observations.

```
PROC UNIVARIATE DATA = dataset_name;
      VAR difference_variable;
RUN;
```

The UNIVARIATE Procedure
Variable: difference_variable

Moments			
N	16	Sum Weights	16
Mean	6.875	Sum Observations	110
Std Deviation	7.02258262	Variance	49.3166667
Skewness	–0.6376653	Kurtosis	–0.512439
Uncorrected SS	1496	Corrected SS	739.75
Coeff Variation	102.146656	Std Error Mean	1.75564566

Basic Statistical Measures			
Location		Variability	
Mean	6.875000	Std Deviation	7.02258
Median	8.500000	Variance	49.31667
Mode	.	Range	23.00000
		Interquartile Range	10.00000

Tests for Location: Mu0=0				
Test	Statistic		*p*-Value	
Student's t	t	3.915938	Pr > |t|	0.0014
Sign	M	5	Pr >= |M|	0.0213
Signed Rank	S	55	Pr >= |S|	0.0027

A table with quantiles and extreme observations will also be produced. By default, SAS will provide three tests for location in the output in the box with the heading "Tests for Location: Mu0=0."

The second test listed is the sign test, and the third test is the Wilcoxon signed-rank test. The two-sided p-value for the sign test is in the "Pr >= |M|" line, and the two-sided p-value for the Wilcoxon signed-rank test is in the "Pr >= |S|" line. We should note that for the sign test, SAS gives a test statistic M, where

$$M = \frac{\#\text{ of } + \text{ differences} - \#\text{ of } - \text{ differences}}{2}$$

SAS calculates the p-value from the binomial distribution (exact test), so the output may differ from the p-value when the normal approximation is used. For the Wilcoxon signed-rank test, SAS gives a test statistic S equal to $T - \mu_T$ and will compute the exact p-value when $n \le 20$. When there are more than 20 nonzero differences, SAS uses the t-distribution to estimate the p-value. Because of this, the p-value that SAS gives for the Wilcoxon signed-rank test may be somewhat different from the one computed by hand using the method described in this chapter.

Performing nonparametric tests for paired data in Stata

To perform the sign test, we use the *signtest* command and specify the names of the two variables that we would like to compare.

```
signtest post_variable = pre_variable
```

The output follows:

```
Sign test

        sign |    observed    expected
-------------+------------------------
    positive |          13           8
    negative |           3           8
        zero |           0           0
-------------+------------------------
         all |          16          16

One-sided tests:
  Ho: median of post_var~e - pre_variable = 0 vs.
  Ha: median of post_var~e - pre_variable > 0
      Pr(#positive >= 13) =
         Binomial(n = 16, x >= 13, p = 0.5) =  0.0106

  Ho: median of post_var~e - pre_variable = 0 vs.
  Ha: median of post_var~e - pre_variable < 0
      Pr(#negative >= 3) =
         Binomial(n = 16, x >= 3, p = 0.5) =  0.9979
```

```
Two-sided test:
  Ho: median of post_var~e - pre_variable = 0 vs.
  Ha: median of post_var~e - pre_variable != 0
      Pr(#positive >= 13 or #negative >= 13) =
         min(1, 2*Binomial(n = 16, x >= 13, p = 0.5)) =  0.0213
```

The output gives information for both one-sided and two-sided tests. The *p*-value for the sign test is given on the last line of the output. Stata calculates the *p*-value from the binomial distribution (exact test), so the output may differ from the *p*-value when the normal approximation is used. The Wilcoxon signed-rank test is performed with the *signrank* command. The two variables whose medians are being compared are placed on either side of the equals sign.

```
signrank post_variable = pre_variable
```

The output follows:

```
Wilcoxon signed-rank test

        sign |      obs   sum ranks    expected
-------------+---------------------------------
    positive |       13         123          68
    negative |        3          13          68
        zero |        0           0           0
-------------+---------------------------------
         all |       16         136         136

unadjusted variance      374.00
adjustment for ties        0.00
adjustment for zeros       0.00
                     ----------
adjusted variance        374.00

Ho: post_variable = pre_variable
             z =   2.844
    Prob > |z| =   0.0045
```

The number of positive and negative differences are shown in the column labeled "obs," and the sums of the ranks are in the "sum ranks" column. The smaller of the sums of the ranks is T. The value of μ_T appears in the "expected" column on the line corresponding to the smaller sum of ranks. The variance σ_T^2 appears on the "adjusted variance" line. The test statistic, Z_T, is shown on the second to the last line. The last line of the output shows the two-sided *p*-value.

EXAMPLE PROBLEM 9.1

Suppose that we are interested in examining mental health resources in Europe and the change in the number of resources over time. We have data from the World Health

Organization on the number of psychiatrists working in the mental health sector per 100,000 population, and we wish to look at data from 2011 and 2014 from 15 countries.[1] Table 9.2 gives the country name, value for 2011, and value for 2014. The corresponding dataset is *ch9_europe_mental_health*.

A Are the data dependent or independent? Why?

We have dependent data because each country is measured at two time points. Therefore, each observation from 2011 is paired with a corresponding observation from 2014 for that country.

B Using the sign test, evaluate the null hypothesis that the median difference in the number of psychiatrists working in the mental health sector per 100,000 population is 0 for the two time points.

H_0: median difference = 0
H_1: median difference ≠ 0

First, we must calculate the difference between the value at 2011 and the value at 2014. So that increases in mental health resources over time are positive values, the difference will be the value in 2014 minus the value in 2011. Once we calculate the difference, we assign each observation either a positive or negative sign, depending on the difference (Table 9.3).

Table 9.2 Data for Example Problem 9.1

	Psychiatrists working in the mental health sector (No./100,000 pop.)	
Country	*2011*	*2014*
Belarus	8.77	7.66
Denmark	14.12	9.57
Finland	28.06	18.37
France	22.35	14.12
Greece	12.88	14.09
Italy	7.81	10.85
Latvia	10.85	12.05
Monaco	36.47	40.98
Norway	30.77	29.69
Poland	5.13	5.07
Portugal	6.14	4.49
Romania	6.45	5.98
San Marino	15.85	15.8
Serbia	9.61	7.35
Slovenia	7.06	10.21

Note: The table shows the number of psychiatrists per 100 000 population working in the mental health sector in 2011 and in 2014. A sample of 16 countries is displayed.
Abbreviation: pop., population.

Table 9.3 Sign test for Example Problem 9.1

	Psychiatrists working in the mental health sector (No./100,000 pop.)			
Country	*2011*	*2014*	*Difference*	*Sign*
Belarus	8.77	7.66	–1.11	–
Denmark	14.12	9.57	–4.55	–
Finland	28.06	18.37	–9.69	–
France	22.35	14.12	–8.23	–
Greece	12.88	14.09	1.21	+
Italy	7.81	10.85	3.04	+
Latvia	10.85	12.05	1.2	+
Monaco	36.47	40.98	4.51	+
Norway	30.77	29.69	–1.08	–
Poland	5.13	5.07	–0.06	–
Portugal	6.14	4.49	–1.65	–
Romania	6.45	5.98	–0.47	–
San Marino	15.85	15.8	–0.05	–
Serbia	9.61	7.35	–2.26	–
Slovenia	7.06	10.21	3.15	+

Note: The difference column is equal to the value in 2014 minus the value in 2011. The sign column indicates whether the difference is positive or negative.
Abbreviation: pop., population.

There are no differences of exactly 0 in our dataset. Next, we count the number of plus signs; D is 5. We should check to see whether our sample size allows use of the normal approximation to the binomial. There are 15 nonzero differences, so $\frac{15}{4} = 3.75 < 5$. Thus, we must use the exact method.

We found that $\hat{p}_+ = \frac{5}{15}$, and under the null hypothesis $p_0 = \frac{1}{2}$.

If $\hat{p}_+ < p_0$, then p-value = $2 \times P[X \leq x]$ where $X \sim \text{Bin}\left(n = 15, p_0 = \frac{1}{2}\right)$.

$$
\begin{aligned}
p\text{-value} &= 2 \times P[X \leq x] = 2 \times P[X \leq 5] \\
&= 2 \times [P(X=0) + P(X=1) + P(X=2) + P(X=3) + P(X=4) + P(X=5)] \\
&= 2 \times [0.00003 + 0.00046 + 0.00320 + 0.01389 + 0.04166 + 0.09164] \\
&= 2 \times 0.15088 = 0.30176
\end{aligned}
$$

Since p-value = $0.30176 > \alpha = 0.05$, we fail to reject the null hypothesis. We have no evidence of a statistically significant change in the number of psychiatrists per 100,000 population working in the mental health sector in European countries between 2011 and 2014.

C Evaluate the same hypothesis using the Wilcoxon signed-rank test.

First, we need to calculate the difference between the 2011 and 2014 values and rank the differences lowest to highest in terms of absolute value. We then assign each rank a plus or minus sign, depending on the sign of the difference (Table 9.4).

The sum of the positive ranks is 7 + 10 + 6 + 12 + 11 = 46.

The sum of the negative ranks is 5 + 13 + 15 +14 + 4 + 2 + 8 + 3 + 1 + 9 = 74.

Thus, T is the sum of the positive ranks since 46 < 74.

We have 15 nonzero differences, so the normal approximation is valid for the Wilcoxon signed-rank test ($n > 6$). Next, we must compute the mean and standard deviation of T.

$$\mu_T = \frac{n(n+1)}{4} = \frac{15(15+1)}{4} = 60$$

$$\sigma_T = \sqrt{\frac{n(n+1)(2n+1)}{24}} = \sqrt{\frac{15(15+1)(2\times 15+1)}{24}} = \sqrt{310} = 17.61$$

Table 9.4 Wilcoxon signed-rank test for Example Problem 9.1

	Psychiatrists working in the mental health sector (No./100,000 pop.)					
Country	*2011*	*2014*	*Difference*	*|Difference|*	*Rank*	*Sign*
Belarus	8.77	7.66	−1.11	1.11	5	−
Denmark	14.12	9.57	−4.55	4.55	13	−
Finland	28.06	18.37	−9.69	9.69	15	−
France	22.35	14.12	−8.23	8.23	14	−
Greece	12.88	14.09	1.21	1.21	7	+
Italy	7.81	10.85	3.04	3.04	10	+
Latvia	10.85	12.05	1.20	1.20	6	+
Monaco	36.47	40.98	4.51	4.51	12	+
Norway	30.77	29.69	−1.08	1.08	4	−
Poland	5.13	5.07	−0.06	0.06	2	−
Portugal	6.14	4.49	−1.65	1.65	8	−
Romania	6.45	5.98	−0.47	0.47	3	−
San Marino	15.85	15.8	−0.05	0.05	1	−
Serbia	9.61	7.35	−2.26	2.26	9	−
Slovenia	7.06	10.21	3.15	3.15	11	+

Note: The difference column is equal to the value in 2014 minus the value in 2011. The absolute value of the difference is also shown. The absolute values of the differences are then ranked, with "1" signifying the smallest absolute difference. The sign of the difference indicates whether it is positive or negative.

Abbreviation: pop., population.

The test statistic follows a standard normal distribution and has a value of the following:

$$Z_T = \frac{T - \mu_T}{\sigma_T} = \frac{46 - 60}{17.61} = -0.80$$

The p-value is $P(Z \leq -0.80 \text{ or } Z \geq 0.80) = 2 \times P(Z \geq 0.80) = 2 \times 0.21 = 0.42$.

Since p-value $= 0.42 > \alpha = 0.05$, we fail to reject the null hypothesis. We have no evidence that the median difference in number of psychiatrists working in the mental health sector per 100,000 population between 2011 and 2014 in Europe is not equal to 0.

D Do we reach the same conclusion in each case? Which test is preferable?

Yes, both the sign test and the Wilcoxon signed-rank test led to the same conclusion. In both cases, we failed to reject the null hypothesis. The Wilcoxon signed-rank test considers both the magnitude and the direction of the differences, so it is preferable to the sign test.

E Run both the sign test and Wilcoxon signed-rank test in SAS or Stata.

To run the tests in SAS, we must first make a variable that is the difference between the number of psychiatrists per 100,000 population in 2011 and in 2014.

```
DATA europe_mental_health;
  SET europe_mental_health;
  difference = psychiatrists_2014 - psychiatrists_2011;
RUN;

PROC UNIVARIATE DATA = europe_mental_health LOCCOUNT;
          VAR difference;
RUN;
```

Tests for Location: Mu0=0				
Test		Statistic	*p*-Value	
Student's t	t	-1.04942	Pr > |t|	0.3118
Sign	M	-2.5	Pr >= |M|	0.3018
Signed Rank	S	-14	Pr >= |S|	0.4543

The "Tests for Location" box gives the results from the tests. The sign test has a p-value of 0.3018, which is identical to the p-value that we calculated by hand in Example Problem 9.1—Part (A). The p-value for the signed-rank test is 0.4543, which is similar to the value calculated by hand.

In Stata, we use the *signtest* command to run the sign test. The two variables being compared are *psychiatrists_2011* and *psychiatrists_2014*.

```
signtest psychiatrists_2014 = psychiatrists_2011
```

The output follows:

```
Sign test

        sign |    observed    expected
-------------+------------------------
    positive |           5         7.5
    negative |          10         7.5
        zero |           0           0
-------------+------------------------
         all |          15          15

One-sided tests:
  Ho: median of psych~2014 - psychiatrists_2011 = 0 vs.
  Ha: median of psych~2014 - psychiatrists_2011 > 0
      Pr(#positive >= 5) =
         Binomial(n = 15, x >= 5, p = 0.5) =  0.9408

  Ho: median of psych~2014 - psychiatrists_2011 = 0 vs.
  Ha: median of psych~2014 - psychiatrists_2011 < 0
      Pr(#negative >= 10) =
         Binomial(n = 15, x >= 10, p = 0.5) =  0.1509

Two-sided test:
  Ho: median of psych~2014 - psychiatrists_2011 = 0 vs.
  Ha: median of psych~2014 - psychiatrists_2011 != 0
      Pr(#positive >= 10 or #negative >= 10) =
         min(1, 2*Binomial(n = 15, x >= 10, p = 0.5)) =  0.3018
```

The p-value is shown in the last line of the output. The sign test has a p-value of 0.3018, which is identical to the p-value that we calculated by hand in Example Problem 9.1—Part (A).

To run the Wilcoxon signed-rank test, we use the *signrank* command.

```
signrank psychiatrists_2014 = psychiatrists_2011
```

The output follows:

```
Wilcoxon signed-rank test

        sign |      obs   sum ranks    expected
-------------+---------------------------------
    positive |        5          46          60
    negative |       10          74          60
        zero |        0           0           0
-------------+---------------------------------
         all |       15         120         120
```

```
unadjusted variance          310.00
adjustment for ties            0.00
adjustment for zeros           0.00
                         ----------
adjusted variance            310.00
Ho: psychiatrists_2014 = psychiatrists_2011
             z =  -0.795
    Prob > |z| =   0.4265
```

We see that $T = 46$ (first row under "sum ranks") and $\mu_T = 60$ (first row under "expected"). The variance $\sigma_T^2 = 310$, which is the square of the standard deviation of $\sigma_T = 17.61$ calculated by hand. The test statistic for the Wilcoxon signed-rank test is $z = -0.795$. The p-value for the test is 0.4265, which is similar to the value calculated by hand.

PRACTICE PROBLEM 9.1

As part of an intervention to train community members about research methods and public health, tests were administered before and after each training session.[2] We are interested in determining whether there was a significant change in knowledge about the subject from before the instruction to afterward. The pretest and posttest scores for a session on clinical trials and biobanks are shown in Table 9.5. The data are also in the dataset *ch9_clinical_trials_session*. We do not wish to assume that the data are normally distributed. All tests should be two sided with $\alpha = 0.05$.

A We want to conduct a Wilcoxon signed-rank test to evaluate our research question. What are the null and alternative hypotheses?

Table 9.5 Data for Practice Problem 9.1

ID	*Pretest score*	*Posttest score*	*Difference*	*|Difference|*	*Rank*	*Sign*
1	60	70				
2	70	100				
3	90	90				
4	90	90				
5	90	90				
6	80	80				
7	90	90				
8	50	70				
9	30	70				
10	50	90				
11	50	60				
12	60	90				
13	90	80				
14	50	70				
15	60	100				
16	50	50				

Note: Sixteen community members enrolled in a research training program have a pretest score and posttest score. We want to examine whether the session caused a change in scores.

B Calculate the difference between the pretest and posttest scores for each subject, and rank the differences from smallest to largest in terms of absolute value. Assign signs to each subject.

C Compute the sum of both the positive and negative ranks. What is T?

D Compute the test statistic, Z_T.

E What is the p-value of the test?

F What do you conclude?

G Compare the results of the Wilcoxon signed-rank test to the outcome of the sign test using a statistical package. Do we come to the same conclusion?

H If we had made the assumptions necessary for a parametric test, what test would we have used instead?

Nonparametric tests for independent data

We can use nonparametric tests when we have independent data as well. The Wilcoxon rank-sum test is commonly used in scenarios where we have two samples but do not want to make the assumptions about their distributions that are necessary to conduct a two-sample t-test.

Wilcoxon rank-sum test

The Wilcoxon rank-sum test, also called the Mann–Whitney test, is the nonparametric equivalent to the two-sample t-test. The test assumes that the distributions of the two populations have the same shape, but it does not make assumptions about what specific distribution the samples follow. The null hypothesis for the Wilcoxon rank-sum test is that the medians of the two samples are equal. The alternative hypothesis is that the medians are not equal.

The Wilcoxon rank-sum test can be conducted with the following steps:

1 Combine the two samples into one large group, and order the observations from smallest to largest.
2 Assign a rank to each observation.
   a The smallest value is ranked "1," and the largest value is ranked "n," where n is the total number of observations from both groups combined.
   b If there are tied observations, assign an average rank to all measurements with the same value.

Table 9.6 Nonparametric tests for independent data

Component	*Wilcoxon rank-sum test*
Hypotheses	H_0: median$_1$ = median$_2$ vs. H_1: median$_1$ ≠ median$_2$
Summary of observed data	W: smaller of the sums of the ranks in the two samples
Mean	$\mu_W = \frac{n_S(n_S + n_L + 1)}{2}$ where n_S = sample size in the smaller of the two samples and n_L = sample size in the larger of the two samples
Standard deviation	$\sigma_W = \sqrt{\frac{n_S n_L (n_S + n_L + 1)}{12}}$
Test statistic	$Z_W = \frac{W - \mu_W}{\sigma_W}$
Distribution of test statistic (large n)	Standard normal
Valid if	$\text{Min}(n_1, n_2) \geq 10$ Underlying distribution is continuous

Note: The Wilcoxon rank-sum test is a nonparametric test for independent data. The test compares the medians of two populations.

3 Calculate the sum of the ranks corresponding to the original samples. Denote the smaller of the two sums by W.
4 Use the test statistic given in Table 9.6 or use Table A.8 in the Appendix to determine the p-value.
   a If both samples have at least 10 data points, then we calculate the test statistic Z_W, which follows a standard normal distribution. Then, the two-sided p-value is $2 \times P(Z > |Z_W|)$. The one-sided p-value is $P(Z > |Z_W|)$.
   b However, if either sample size is less than 10, the normal approximation is not valid. Thus, if n is small, use the W distribution table to calculate a p-value for W. Find the values that corresponds to W, n_1, and n_2. The entries in Table A.8 in the Appendix give the one-sided p-value for the given sample sizes and W. For a two-sided hypothesis test, multiply the value found in Table A.8 in the Appendix by 2 to get the p-value.

Performing nonparametric tests for independent data in SAS

The Wilcoxon rank-sum test is performed in SAS using PROC NPAR1WAY. The WILCOXON option requests the Wilcoxon rank-sum test, and use of the continuity correction can be specified in the CORRECT = option. For small samples, the line requesting the exact test can be added.

```
PROC NPAR1WAY DATA = dataset_name WILCOXON CORRECT = NO;
      CLASS binary_var;
      VAR continuous_var;
      **EXACT WILCOXON;
RUN;
```

The NPAR1WAY Procedure

Wilcoxon Scores (Rank Sums) for Variable continuous_var Classified by Variable binary_var					
binary_var	N	Sum of Scores	Expected Under H0	Std Dev Under H0	Mean score
1	47	2280.50	2185.50	128.017957	48.521277
2	45	1997.50	2092.50	128.017957	44.388889
Average scores were used for ties.					

Wilcoxon Two-Sample Test	
Statistic	1997.5000
Normal Approximation	
Z	–0.7421
One-Sided Pr < Z	0.2290
Two-Sided Pr > |Z|	0.4580
t Approximation	
One-Sided Pr < Z	0.2300
Two-Sided Pr > |Z|	0.4599

Kruskal–Wallis Test	
Chi-Square	0.5507
DF	1
Pr > Chi-Square	0.4580

The first two boxes of output are most relevant for the Wilcoxon rank-sum test. The sums of the ranks in each group are shown under "Sums of Scores" in the first output box, and W is the smaller of the two values. W can also be found in the "Statistic" line in the second output table.

The "Expected under H0" column of the first table shows the value of μ_W in the row corresponding to the group with the smaller sum of ranks. The value of σ_W appears in the "Std Dev under H0" column in the row corresponding to the group with the smaller sum of ranks. The two-sided p-value for the test, using the normal approximation, can be found in the line "Two-Sided Pr > |Z|" under the "Normal Approximation" heading in the second table.

Performing nonparametric tests for independent data in Stata

We perform the Wilcoxon rank-sum test in Stata using the *ranksum* command. The continuous variable is specified after the *ranksum* statement and then the binary variable indicating the two groups is listed in a by option.

```
ranksum continuous_var, by(binary_var)
```

The output follows:

```
Two-sample Wilcoxon rank-sum (Mann-Whitney) test
  binary_var |      obs    rank sum    expected
-------------+---------------------------------
           1 |       47      2280.5      2185.5
           2 |       45      1997.5      2092.5
-------------+---------------------------------
    combined |       92        4278        4278
unadjusted variance     16391.25
adjustment for ties        -2.65
                        ----------
adjusted variance       16388.60
Ho: contin~r(binary~r==1) = contin~r(binary~r==2)
             z =   0.742
    Prob > |z| =   0.4580
```

The sum of the ranks are shown in the "rank sum" column of the output table, and the smaller of the two sums is W. The "expected" column of the output table shows the value of μ_W in the row corresponding to the group with the smaller sum of ranks. The value of σ_W^2 appears in the "adjusted variance" line. The output gives the test statistic Z_w on the second to last line. Note that the value of the test statistic in the output is the absolute value of the test statistic calculated by hand or in SAS. This is due to the way Stata presents the test statistic, but it will not affect the *p*-value. The two-sided *p*-value of the test is on the last line.

EXAMPLE PROBLEM 9.2

From a nationally representative sample of U.S. residents, we obtained information on self-reported asthma and the ratio of family income to the poverty level for a subset of the respondents.[3] We are interested in looking at socioeconomic status (SES) among those with asthma and those without asthma. We are not willing to assume that these distributions are necessarily normal. In the dataset, there are 427 respondents without self-reported asthma and 73 respondents with self-reported asthma. Use a two-sided test conducted at the $\alpha = 0.05$ level of significance to test the hypothesis that the median family income-to-poverty level among those with and without asthma is equivalent. The dataset is called *ch9_income_asthma*.

BOX 9.1 DESCRIPTION OF *ch9_income_asthma* DATASET

The National Health and Nutrition Examination Survey System (NHANES) asks, "Has a doctor or health professional ever told you that you have asthma?" Possible responses are "Yes," "No," or "Don't know," or participants could refuse to answer the question. Those who report having been told they had asthma by a doctor or health professional are coded as *asthma = 1*. Those who answer "No" are coded *asthma = 0*. Respondents also report their annual family income and the number of people in the family. These values are, then, used to calculate the ratio of the family income to the federal poverty guidelines. This variable is called *income_poverty_ratio*. All respondents in the sample *ch9_income_asthma* had nonmissing information on the income-to-poverty ratio and answered either "Yes" or "No" to the asthma question.

A Are the data independent or dependent? What parametric and nonparametric tests are available for this type of data?

In this case, we have independent data. The appropriate parametric test for this situation would be a two-sample *t*-test, and the nonparametric equivalent is the Wilcoxon rank-sum test.

B Which type of statistical test is most appropriate for this type of data and why?

The nonparametric test, the Wilcoxon rank-sum test, should be used because the problem states that we should not assume normality.

C What are the null and alternative hypotheses?

We want to test the null hypothesis that the median family income-to-poverty level ratio among those with self-reported asthma is equal to the median family income-to-poverty level ratio among those without self-reported asthma.

H_0: $median_{asthma} = median_{no\ asthma}$

H_1: $median_{asthma} \neq median_{no\ asthma}$

D Run the test in SAS or Stata. What is the value of *W*?

In SAS, we use PROC NPAR1WAY to run the Wilcoxon rank-sum test. The binary variable indicating the two groups is called *asthma*, and the continuous variable is *income_poverty_ratio*.

```
PROC NPAR1WAY DATA = ch9_income_asthma WILCOXON CORRECT = NO;
              CLASS asthma;
              VAR income_poverty_ratio;
RUN;
```

THE NPAR1WAY PROCEDURE

Wilcoxon Scores (Rank Sums) for Variable income_poverty_ratio Classified by Variable Asthma

Asthma	N	Sum of Scores	Expected under H0	Std Dev under H0	Mean Score
0	427	110267.50	106963.50	1138.76057	258.237705
1	73	14982.50	18286.50	1138.76057	205.239726

Average scores were used for ties.

Wilcoxon Two-Sample Test	
Statistic	14982.5000
Normal Approximation	
Z	-2.9014
One-Sided Pr < Z	0.0019
Two-Sided Pr > |Z|	0.0037
t Approximation	
One-Sided Pr < Z	0.0019
Two-Sided Pr > |Z|	0.0039

In Stata, we use the *ranksum* command and specify the variable *income_poverty_ratio* as the continuous variable and *asthma* as the binary variable.

```
ranksum income_poverty_ratio, by(asthma)
```

The output follows:

```
Two-sample Wilcoxon rank-sum (Mann-Whitney) test

      asthma |      obs    rank sum    expected
-------------+---------------------------------
           0 |      427    110267.5    106963.5
           1 |       73     14982.5     18286.5
-------------+---------------------------------
    combined |      500      125250      125250

unadjusted variance  1301389.25
adjustment for ties    -4613.62
                     ----------
adjusted variance    1296775.63

Ho: income~o(asthma==0) = income~o(asthma==1)
             z =   2.901
    Prob > |z| =   0.0037
```

W is the smaller of the sums of the ranks of the two samples. Thus, W = 14982.50 which is the sums of the ranks in the *asthma* group since 14982.5 < 110,267.50.

E **What are μ_W and σ_W?**

The value of μ_W can be found in the SAS output in the "Expected under H0" column or in the Stata output in the "expected" column. We can see that μ_W = 18286.5. The standard deviation is shown in the SAS output "Std Dev Under H0." In Stata, we take the square root of the variance provided in the "adjusted variance" line. Thus, σ_W = 1138.76.

F **What is the p-value of the test?**

The p-value for the test is 0.0037.

G **What conclusion can we make?**

Because the p-value is 0.0037, which is less than α = 0.05, we reject the null hypothesis. We conclude that the median family income-to-poverty level ratio for those with asthma is not equal to the median family income-to-poverty level ratio for those without asthma. We have reason to believe that the median family income-to-poverty level ratio is higher among persons without asthma (sum of ranks = 110267.5 for no asthma vs. 14982.5 for asthma in this sample).

PRACTICE PROBLEM 9.2

A sample of 32 adults were asked whether they participate in vigorous physical activity (VPA).[3] Of the 32 respondents, 11 said that they do engage in VPA, and the remaining

21 reported no VPA. All of the subjects had their 60-second pulse rate measured. The measurements are recorded in Table 9.7.

BOX 9.2 DESCRIPTION OF PRACTICE PROBLEM 9.2 DATA

The National Health and Nutrition Examination Survey System (NHANES) asks, "Do you do any vigorous-intensity sports, fitness, or recreational activities that cause large increases in breathing or heart rate like running or basketball for at least 10 minutes continuously?" Possible responses are "Yes," "No," or "Don't know," or participants can refuse to answer the question. Those who report engaging in a vigorous physical activity (VPA) are coded as *vpa* = *"yes,"* and those who say that they do not participate in VPA are coded as *vpa* = *"no."* The examination component of the survey measures the 60-second pulse rates of the respondents, and this information is contained in the variable *pulse_rate*. The data given in the problem come from a random sample of 32 adults whose pulse rates were measured and who answered "Yes" or "No" to the VPA question.

Table 9.7 Data for Practice Problem 9.2

60-Second pulse rate				
Vigorous physical activity[a] *(n = 11)*		*No. vigorous physical activity*[b] *(n = 21)*		
54	70	58	74	80
58	76	60	76	82
64	82	64	76	82
64	90	66	76	84
66		66	76	84
68		72	76	84
68		72	78	100

Note: Eleven subjects reported engaging in vigorous physical activity, and their 60-second pulse rates are shown in the left columns. The right columns shows the pulse measurements for 21 individuals who reported that they do not get vigorous physical activity.

[a] Each number represents the pulse rate of a person who reported vigorous physical activity.

[b] Each number represents the pulse rate of a person who reported no vigorous physical activity.

A Conduct a Wilcoxon rank-sum test to test the null hypothesis that the median 60-second pulse rate of the population of individuals who engage in VPA is equal to the median 60-second pulse rate of individuals who get no VPA. What are the null and alternative hypotheses?

B In Table 9.8, we combine all of the observations and rank them from smallest to largest. There are many tied pulse rate values, so those observations are given average ranks.

Calculate the sum of the ranks corresponding to the original samples. What is W?

C Show that the normal approximation valid in this cases?

D Calculate μ_W, σ_W, and the test statistic Z_W.

E What is the p-value?

F What do we conclude?

G Check the answers against the following SAS or Stata output.
SAS:

```
PROC NPAR1WAY DATA = ch9_vpa_pulse WILCOXON CORRECT = NO;
             CLASS vpa;
             VAR pulse_rate;
RUN;
```

The NPAR1WAY Procedure

Wilcoxon Scores (Rank Sums) for Variable pulse_rate Classified by Variable vpa

vpa	N	Sum of Scores	Expected Under H0	Std Dev Under H0	Mean Score
0	21	392.0	346.50	25.086092	18.666667
1	11	136.0	181.50	25.086092	12.363636

Average scores were used for ties.

Table 9.8 Wilcoxon rank-sum test for Practice Problem 9.2

VPA	*60-Second pulse rate*	*Rank*
yes	54	1
yes	58	2.5
no	58	2.5
no	60	4
yes	64	6
yes	64	6
no	64	6
no	66	9
no	66	9
yes	66	9
yes	68	11.5
yes	68	11.5
yes	70	13
no	72	14.5
no	72	14.5
no	74	16
no	76	19.5
no	76	19.5
no	76	19.5
no	76	19.5
no	76	19.5
yes	76	19.5
no	78	23
no	80	24
no	82	26
no	82	26
yes	82	26
no	84	28.5
no	84	28.5
yes	90	30
no	94	31
no	100	32

Note: The 32 subjects are listed from lowest pulse rate to highest. Then, a rank is assigned to each line. If multiple subjects have the same pulse rate, they receive the average rank.

Abbreviation: VPA, vigorous physical activity.

Wilcoxon Two-Sample Test	
Statistic	136.0000
Normal Approximation	
Z	–1.8138
One-Sided Pr < Z	0.0349
Two-Sided Pr > |Z|	0.0697
t Approximation	
One-Sided Pr < Z	0.0397
Two-Sided Pr > |Z|	0.0794

Stata:

```
ranksum pulse_rate, by(vpa)
```

The output follows:

```
Two-sample Wilcoxon rank-sum (Mann-Whitney) test

         vpa |      obs    rank sum    expected
-------------+---------------------------------
          no |       21         392       346.5
         yes |       11         136       181.5
-------------+---------------------------------
    combined |       32         528         528
unadjusted variance      635.25
adjustment for ties       -5.94
                     ----------
adjusted variance        629.31

Ho: pulse_~e(vpa==no) = pulse_~e(vpa==yes)
             z =   1.814
    Prob > |z| =   0.0697
```

PRACTICE PROBLEM 9.3

The modified retail food environment index (mRFEI) is a measure of healthy food options in an area.[4] The mRFEI is calculated as the percentage of healthy food retailers out of the total number of food retailers in a census tract. We have census tracts from two parts of the same city, and we are interested in investigating whether there is a significant difference in the median mRFEI between the two samples. There are 7 census tracts in the north part of the city and 10 census tracts in the south part. The data are in the dataset *ch9_mrfei*.

A What type of nonparametric test is appropriate for this scenario?

B What are the null and alternative hypotheses?

C Perform the test. Because of the small sample size, use the tables rather than the normal approximation to determine the *p*-value.

D What do you conclude from the test?

E Perform the test in SAS or Stata, and compare your output to the calculations in Practice Problem 9.3—Part (C).

F If you were to use a two-sample *t*-test instead of the nonparametric alternative, would the conclusion be different? Use a statistical package to perform a two-sample *t*-test for comparison.

PRACTICE PROBLEM 9.4

The Social Security Administration (SSA) releases claim information for SSA disability benefits by state and fiscal year.[5] The data include the filing rate of eligible adults, which is the number of claims received by the state during that fiscal year per 100 eligible adults (i.e., those who are aged 18 to 64 years and not already receiving benefits). We are interested in the change in the filing rate for eligible adults over time, specifically between 2010 and 2015. The dataset includes data from all 50 states plus the District of Columbia and Puerto Rico and is called *ch9_disability_claims*. We do not have prior knowledge about the direction of the change, and all analyses should be conducted at the 5% level of significance.

A If we wish to use a parametric test to analyze the data, which test is appropriate in this scenario?

B What are the null and alternative hypotheses for the parametric test?

C Conduct the parametric test in SAS or Stata. What do you conclude?

D Now suppose that we do not wish to make the assumptions necessary to conduct a parametric test. What is the nonparametric equivalent to use in the situation?

E What are the null and alternative hypotheses for the nonparametric test?

F Conduct the nonparametric test in SAS or Stata. What do you conclude?

G Compare the results of the parametric and nonparametric tests.

References

1. World Health Organization. Global Health Observatory Data Repository: Human resources, data by country, 2015. http://apps.who.int/gho/data/node.main.MHHR?lang=en. Updated August 5, 2015. Accessed March 11, 2016.
2. D'Agostino McGowan L, Stafford JD, Thompson VL, Johnson-Javois B, Goodman MS. Quantitative evaluation of the community research fellows training program. *Front Pblic Heal*. 2015;3(July):1–12. doi:10.3389/fpubh.2015.00179.
3. National Health and Nutrition Examination Survey. Hyattsville, MD: Centers for Disease Control and Prevention, National Center for Health Statistics. https://wwwn.cdc.gov/Nchs/Nhanes/Search/nhanes13_14.aspx. Published 2014. Accessed February 23, 2016.
4. Centers for Disease Control and Prevention. mRFEI data table. http://www.cdc.gov/obesity/downloads/2_16_mrfei_data_table.xls. Accessed October 1, 2014.
5. Social Security Administration. Data catalog: SSA disability claim data. http://catalog.data.gov/dataset/ssa-disability-claim-data. Updated September 28, 2016. Accessed April 13, 2016.

Lab D: Two-sample (parametric and nonparametric) hypothesis testing

PRACTICE PROBLEM D.1

As the demographic makeup of the United States changes, certain areas of the country are becoming minority-majorities: Places where racial and ethnic minority populations together make up a majority of the residents. We would like to look at the relationship between minority-majority status and unemployment rates. Our data uses Metropolitan Statistical Area (MSA) as the geographical unit of analysis. Specifically, we will test whether the employment rate in MSAs with a minority-majority is the same as in MSAs without a minority-majority. The data are in the file *labd_metro_areas*.[1] The variable *minority_majority* takes a value of 1 for minority-majority MSAs and 0 for non-minority-majority MSAs. The variable *unemployment_rate* is the unemployment rate in the MSA.

A What are the null and alternative hypotheses?

B Write and run the SAS or Stata code to perform the test.

C Look at the output. How many of the MSAs are minority-majorities? How many still have a population that is majority non-Hispanic white?

D What is the mean unemployment rate in minority-majority MSAs? What is the mean in MSAs without a minority-majority?

E Can we make the equal variance assumption for these data?

F What are the value and distribution of the test statistic?

G What is the p-value of the test?

H Do you reject or fail to reject the null hypothesis? What is your conclusion from the study?

PRACTICE PROBLEM D.2

The World Health Organization monitors vaccination rates for preventable diseases around the world. Table D.1 contains information on measles immunization coverage in 19 countries among children aged 1 year.[2] The percentage of coverage among the population in each country for the years 2000 and 2014 are shown. The data are also saved in the file *labd_measles_vaccinations*.

A We would like to perform a nonparametric test at the $\alpha = 0.05$ level of significance to compare the measles immunization coverage in 2000 to the coverage in 2014. What test should we use, and what are the null and alternative hypotheses of the test?

B Perform the hypothesis test in a statistical package. What is the median difference in the sample?

Table D.1 Data for Problem D.2

	Measles immunization coverage (%)	
Country	*2000*	*2014*
Argentina	91	95
Austria	75	76
Bangladesh	74	89
Belarus	98	99
Benin	70	63
Dominican Republic	85	88
Eritrea	76	96
Georgia	73	92
Guatemala	86	67
Kuwait	99	94
Luxembourg	93	99
Madagascar	57	64
Mexico	96	97
Micronesia	85	91
Nepal	71	88
Niue	99	99
Pakistan	59	63
Senegal	48	80
Serbia	89	86

BOX D.1 DESCRIPTION OF *labd_birth_weights* DATASET

The National Health and Nutrition Examination Survey (NHANES) asks caregivers of respondents aged 2 to 15 years, "Has a doctor or health professional ever told you that he/she was overweight?" Possible responses are "Yes," "No," "Don't know," or refusal to answer the question. Those who answered "Yes" to the question were coded *overweight_kid* = 1, and those who answered "No" were given a value of *overweight_kid* = 0. The caregivers are also asked, "How much did he/she weigh at birth?" Responses were recorded in pounds and ounces, and the value was converted to pounds and fractions of a pound in the variable *birth_weight*. The sample in the dataset *labd_birth_weights* is limited to those who had nonmissing birthweights and who answered "Yes" or "No" to the question about being overweight as a child.

C What is the value of the test statistic?

D What is the *p*-value?

E What do we conclude?

F It is a common mistake to assume data are independent when they are, in fact, dependent. What would happen if we did not account for the paired nature of the data? Perform a nonparametric hypothesis test for independent data. The data for this procedure are in the dataset *labd_measles_vaccinations_2*.

G What do we conclude if we assume independent samples?

PRACTICE PROBLEM D.3

We are interested in examining the association between birthweight and obesity and birthweight and overweight in childhood. Table D.2 shows birthweights from 11 children who have been classified as overweight by a health professional at some point.[3] Also, 16 birthweight measurements are included from children who have never been told that they are overweight. We do not want to assume that the underlying distributions are normally distributed. The data are in the dataset *labd_birth_weights*.

A What test is appropriate for the data?

Table D.2 Data for Problem D.3

Birthweight (pounds)		
Overweight children	*Normal weight children*	
6.50	10.50	7.38
7.63	8.31	6.44
7.00	9.25	8.00
7.56	4.69	7.00
6.44	6.56	6.00
7.81	6.69	
7.31	7.44	
8.81	8.00	
8.25	7.31	
7.25	6.31	
9.44	6.00	

B What are the null and alternative hypotheses for the test?

C What is the median birthweight among children who have been told at some point that they are overweight? What is the median birthweight among children who have never been told that they are overweight?

D What code is used to perform the hypothesis test?

E Look at the output. What is the value of the test statistic?

BOX D.2 DESCRIPTION OF *labd_vpa_pulse* DATASET

The National Health and Nutrition Examination Survey System (NHANES) asks, "Do you do any vigorous-intensity sports, fitness, or recreational activities that cause large increases in breathing or heart rate like running or basketball for at least 10 minutes continuously?" Possible responses are "Yes," "No," "Don't know," or refusal to answer the question. Those who reported engaging in a vigorous activity were coded as vpa = 1, and those who said they do not participate in VPA were coded as vpa = 0. The examination component of the survey measures the 60-second pulse rates of the respondents, and this information is contained in the variable *pulse_rate*. The data given in the problem come from a random sample of 32 adults who had measured pulse rates and answered "Yes" or "No" to the VPA question.

F What is the p-value of the test?

G What do we conclude?

H Create histograms for birthweight stratified by whether the child has ever been categorized as overweight. Upon examination of the histograms, do you feel that it would have been appropriate to use the two-sample t-test to analyze these data?

PRACTICE PROBLEM D.4

Let's return to the data presented in Practice Problem 9.2 regarding pulse rates and physical activity.[3] In that problem, we analyzed the data using the Wilcoxon rank-sum test to test the null hypothesis that the median 60-second pulse rate of the population of individuals who engage in vigorous physical activity (VPA) is equal to the median 60-second pulse rate of individuals who get no VPA. We failed to find statistically significant evidence to suggest that the difference in median 60-second pulse rate is different between those who engage in VPA and those who do not. The data are in the dataset *labd_vpa_pulse*.

Suppose that we would like to reanalyze the data, given that the assumptions for a parametric test are not violated (we will ignore the fact that the sample size is small).

A What type of hypothesis test will we use to compare the mean pulse rates among those who engage in VPA with those who do not engage in VPA?

B What are the null and alternative hypotheses?

C Can we make the equal variance assumption?

D Run the two-sample t-test and examine the output. What is the mean 60-second pulse rate for those who engage in VPA? What is the mean for those who report not engaging in VPA?

E What is the difference in means between the two groups?

F What are the value and distribution of the test statistic?

G What is the p-value?

H What do we conclude from this test?

I How do the results compare to the conclusion from the nonparametric test in Chapter 9?

PRACTICE PROBLEM D.5

The age-adjusted premature death rate, calculated as the number of deaths among residents under the age of 75 years per 100,000 population, is a measure of the health of a population. We have a sample of 200 U.S. counties and their age-adjusted premature death rates for the years 2013 and 2016.[4,5] The sample is in the dataset *labd_premature_death*. We are interested in comparing the data from the two years to look for trends in the premature death rate.

A Are the data independent or dependent?

B The value of variable *rate_difference* is the premature death rate in 2016 minus the premature death rate in 2013. Make a histogram for the difference variable, and state whether we can assume that the difference is normally distributed.

C Given the nature of the data, we would like to perform a two-sided paired t-test. What are the null and alternative hypotheses?

D Write the code to perform the test.

E Look at the output. What is the value of $\bar{d}$?

F What is the value of the test statistic? What type of distribution does it follow?

G What is the p-value? What do you conclude?

H What is the 95% confidence interval for the true difference in means?

I Say that we instead hypothesized that the mean age-adjusted premature death rate in 2016 was lower than the rate in 2013. What are the null and alternative hypotheses for this test?

J Run the test again as a one-sided test. What are the value and distribution of the test statistic?

K What is the *p*-value? What is the conclusion from the one-sided test?

L Compare the *p*-values from the two-sided and one-sided tests.

References

1. United States Census Bureau. American Community Survey: Hispanic or Latino by race, 2010–2014. http://www.socialexplorer.com/tables/ACS2014_5yr/R11256228?ReportId=R11256228. Accessed August 17, 2016.
2. World Health Organization. Global Health Observatory Data Repository: Measles (MCV), data by country, 2015. http://apps.who.int/gho/data/node.main.A826?lang=en. Updated August 25, 2016. Accessed August 18, 2016.
3. National Health and Nutrition Examination Survey, Hyattsville, MD: Centers for Disease Control and Prevention, National Center for Health Statistics. 2014. https://wwwn.cdc.gov/Nchs/Nhanes/Search/nhanes13_14.aspx. Accessed February 23, 2016.
4. County Health Rankings & Roadmaps. Years of Potential Life Lost, 2013. http://www.socialexplorer.com/tables/HD2013/R11256222?ReportId=R11256222. Accessed August 22, 2016.
5. County Health Rankings & Roadmaps. Years of Potential Life Lost, 2016. http://www.socialexplorer.com/tables/HD2016/R11256226?ReportId=R11256226. Accessed August 22, 2016.

10 Hypothesis testing with categorical data

This chapter will focus on hypothesis testing with categorical data and will include the following topics:

- Two-sample test for proportions
- The chi-squared distribution
- Odds ratios
- Sample size and power for comparing two binomial proportions

Terms

- 2 × 2 contingency table
- column marginal total (column margin)
- concordant pair
- confounder
- contingency-table method
- continuity correction
- discordant pair
- drop-out rate
- drop-in rate
- grand total
- McNemar's test
- odds ratio
- Pearson's chi-squared test (goodness of fit test)
- R × C contingency table
- row marginal total (row margin)
- type A discordant pair
- type B discordant pair
- Yates continuity correction

Introduction

In Chapters 8 and 9, we introduced two-sample tests and several different ways to compare two samples where a continuous variable is the outcome of interest. However, often the outcome variable is a categorical variable, particularly a dichotomous variable. In such a case, we can use the alternate methods discussed here to compare the two samples. We will also introduce a new probability distribution (chi-squared distribution) that is commonly used for hypothesis tests for categorical data.

Two-sample test for proportions

The two-sample test for proportions is an extension of the one-sample test for proportions that was introduced in Chapter 7. There are two approaches for testing the hypothesis: The normal theory method and the contingency-table method. The two approaches are equivalent in that they will always yield the same *p-value*, so the choice of method is usually based on convenience.

Normal theory method

It is reasonable to base the hypothesis test on the difference between the sample proportions. If this difference is very different from 0 (far in the positive or negative direction), then the null hypothesis is rejected. We assume the samples are large enough so that the normal approximation to the binomial distributions is valid (Table 10.1).

- Under the null hypothesis, $\hat{p}_1 \sim N\left(p, \frac{p(1-p)}{n_1}\right)$ and $\hat{p}_2 \sim N\left(p, \frac{p(1-p)}{n_2}\right)$.
- Therefore, the difference is $\hat{p}_1 - \hat{p}_2 \sim N\left(0, p(1-p)\left(\frac{1}{n_1} + \frac{1}{n_2}\right)\right)$.

Note that $\tilde{p}$ is the weighted average of the sample proportions $\hat{p}_1$, $\hat{p}_2$.

$$\tilde{p} = \frac{n_1\hat{p}_1 + n_2\hat{p}_2}{n_1 + n_2} \tag{10.1}$$

Intuitively, this estimate of p makes sense since each of the sample proportions is weighted by the number of people in the sample. The test statistics for proportions

Table 10.1 Two-sample test for proportions using the normal theory method

Component	*Formula*
Hypotheses	$H_0: p_1 = p_2$ $H_1: p_1 \neq p_2$
Test statistic	$Z = \frac{(\hat{p}_1 - \hat{p}_2) - (p_1 - p_2)}{\sqrt{\tilde{p}(1-\tilde{p})\left(\frac{1}{n_1} + \frac{1}{n_2}\right)}}$
Distribution of test statistic	Standard normal
Confidence interval	$\left(\hat{p}_1 - \hat{p}_2 \pm Z_{1-\alpha/2}\sqrt{\frac{\hat{p}_1(1-\hat{p}_1)}{n_1} + \frac{\hat{p}_2(1-\hat{p}_2)}{n_2}}\right)$
Assumptions	$n_1\tilde{p}(1-\tilde{p}) \geq 5$ and $n_2\tilde{p}(1-\tilde{p}) \geq 5$

Note: The two-sample test for proportions is an extension of the one-sample test for a proportion introduced in Chapter 7. In the two-sample test, we test whether or not the proportion in one group is equal to the proportion in another group.

follow a standard normal distribution, instead of a t-distribution, since only one parameter (p) needs to be estimated from the data.

Note that the estimates of standard deviation used in hypothesis testing are different from those used to construct confidence intervals. A continuity correction equal to $\left(\frac{1}{2n_1}+\frac{1}{2n_2}\right)$ may be subtracted from the numerator of the test statistic to better accommodate the normal approximation to the binomial distribution. That is, a continuous distribution may be used to approximate a discrete distribution.

EXAMPLE PROBLEM 10.1

In a yearly survey of U.S. adults,[1] information is collected on medical care and health behaviors, and we are interested in analyzing a sample of the data to determine whether having Medicare affects satisfaction with the medical care received. In particular, we want to know whether the proportions of adults who say that they are very satisfied with the care that they received are identical between those who have Medicare and those who do not. The sample has 653 adults. Of the 288 with Medicare, 213 reported being very satisfied with their medical care. Among the 365 adults not covered by Medicare, 242 were very satisfied with the medical care that they received. The dataset is called *ch10_medicare_satisfaction*.

BOX 10.1 DESCRIPTION OF *ch10_medicare_satisfaction* DATASET

The Behavioral Risk Factor Surveillance System (BRFSS) asked each participant, "Do you have Medicare? (Medicare is a coverage plan for people 65 or over and for certain disabled people.)" Respondents could answer "Yes," "No," or "Don't know," or they could refuse to answer the question. Those who reported having Medicare received a value of *medicare* = 1, while those who said that they did not have Medicare were coded as *medicare* = 0. The survey also asked, "In general, how satisfied are you with the healthcare you received?" The response had three satisfaction options, "Very satisfied," "Somewhat satisfied," and "Not at all satisfied," as well as an options for "Don't know," Not Applicable, and Refused. The variable *care_satisfied* indicates whether or not the subject was very satisfied with medical care. Those who reported being only somewhat satisfied or not at all satisfied were coded as *care_satisfied* = 0, and those who reported being very satisfied were coded as *care_satisfied* = 1. The sample in the dataset *ch10_medicare_satisfaction* is limited to those who responded "Yes" or "No" to having Medicare and who indicated a level of satisfaction with their healthcare.

A What are the point estimates of the true proportion of adults who are very satisfied with their medical care in each insurance group?

Let Group 1 be adults with Medicare and Group 2 be adults without Medicare coverage.

Then, $\hat{p}_1=\frac{x_1}{n_1}=\frac{213}{288}=0.74$ and $\hat{p}_2=\frac{x_2}{n_2}=\frac{242}{365}=0.66.$

B **What is the estimate of the true difference in population proportions?**

$$\hat{p}_1 - \hat{p}_2 = 0.74 - 0.66 - 0.08$$

C **Construct an interval estimate with 95% confidence for the true difference in population proportions. Does this interval contain 0?**

$$95\%\ \text{CI} = \left(\hat{p}_1 - \hat{p}_2 \pm Z_{1-\alpha/2} \sqrt{\frac{\hat{p}_1(1-\hat{p}_1)}{n_1} + \frac{\hat{p}_2(1-\hat{p}_2)}{n_2}} \right)$$

$$= \left(0.08 \pm 1.96 \sqrt{\frac{0.74(1-0.74)}{288} + \frac{0.66(1-0.66)}{365}} \right)$$

$$= (0.08 \pm 1.96 \times 0.04)$$

$$= (0.08 \pm 0.07) = (0.01,\ 0.15)$$

We are 95% confident that the true difference in proportions lies in the interval (0.01, 0.15). This interval does not contain the null value of 0, which would indicate that we would reject the null hypothesis $p_1 = p_2$.

D **Now we will conduct a hypothesis test to see whether the proportion of adults who are very satisfied with their medical care is the same in both populations. What are the null and alternative hypotheses?**

We wish to test the null hypothesis that the true proportion of adults with Medicare who are very satisfied with their medical care is equal to the true proportion of adults without Medicare who are very satisfied with the medical care they receive. In symbols:

$$H_0: p_1 = p_2$$

$$H_1: p_1 \neq p_2$$

E **What are the value and distribution of the test statistic?**

First, we must calculate $\tilde{p}$ to determine whether the normal approximation is appropriate.

$$\tilde{p} = \frac{n_1\hat{p}_1 + n_2\hat{p}_2}{n_1 + n_2} = \frac{288 \times 0.74 + 365 \times 0.66}{288 + 365} = \frac{454.02}{653} = 0.70$$

Thus, $n_1\tilde{p}(1 - \tilde{p}) = 288(0.70)(1 - 0.70) = 60.48 > 5$ and $n_2\tilde{p}(1 - \tilde{p}) = 365(0.70)(1 - 0.70) = 76.65 > 5$. Therefore, the normal approximation is appropriate.

$$Z = \frac{(\hat{p}_1 - \hat{p}_2) - (p_1 - p_2)}{\sqrt{\tilde{p}(1-\tilde{p})\left(\frac{1}{n_1} + \frac{1}{n_2}\right)}} = \frac{(0.74 - 0.66) - (0)}{\sqrt{0.70(1-0.70)\left(\frac{1}{288} + \frac{1}{365}\right)}} = \frac{0.08}{0.04} = 2.11$$

The test statistic has a value of 2.11 and follows a standard normal distribution.

Table 10.2 *P*-value calculation for Example Problem 10.1

Using SAS	*Using Stata*
SAS Code	**Stata Code**

```
DATA f;
pvalue = 2*(1 - PROBNORM(2.11));
RUN;

PROC PRINT DATA = f;
RUN;
```

```
di 2*(1 - (normprob(2.11)))
```

SAS Output

Obs	*p*-Value
1	0.034858

Stata Output

.03485836

Note: The *p*-value for Example Problem 10.1 can be calculated in SAS or Stata using the PROBNORM or *normprob* functions, respectively.

F What is the *p*-value of the test?

Table 10.2 demonstrates the use of statistical software to calculate the *p*-value for this test.

$$p\text{-}value = 2 \times P(Z \geq 2.11) = 0.0349$$

G Do we reject or fail to reject the null hypothesis? What do we conclude?

Because *p-value* < α, we reject the null hypothesis. We conclude that the proportion of adults with Medicare who report being very satisfied with their medical care is not equal to the proportion of adults without Medicare who are very satisfied with the care they receive. Because $\hat{p}_1 > \hat{p}_2$, we have evidence that adults with Medicare are more likely to report being very satisfied with their medical care.

H How does the interval estimate reflect the conclusion of the hypothesis test?

The interval estimate did not include 0, which matches the conclusion of the hypothesis test to reject the null hypothesis. The values in the 95% confidence interval are positive, which indicates $p_1 > p_2$.

PRACTICE PROBLEM 10.1

We are running a study to compare two regimens. The first table in our analysis will show descriptive statistics by treatment group for demographic variables and whether the characteristics differ between the treatment groups. There are 250 subjects in the trial, 130 of whom are receiving the active treatment and 120 of whom are receiving the placebo. Of the 130 subjects receiving active treatment, 76 are female.[1] In the placebo group, 67 are female. We wish to compare the percentage of female subjects in both groups using a two-sample test for proportions.

BOX 10.2 DESCRIPTION OF PRACTICE PROBLEM 10.1 DATA

The gender and race variables used in Practice problems 10.1 and 10.6 come from the Behavioral Risk Factor Surveillance System (BRFSS). However, the variable treatment is not a BRFSS variable and was randomly assigned to respondents for example purposes.

A What are the point estimates of the proportion of female subjects in each of the treatment groups?

B What is the estimate of the difference in population proportions?

C Construct an interval estimate with 99% confidence for the true difference in population proportions. Does this interval contain 0?

D Now we will conduct a hypothesis test to see whether the proportion of female subjects is the same in both treatment groups. What are the null and alternative hypotheses?

E What are the value and distribution of the test statistic?

F What is the *p*-value of the test?

G Do we reject or fail to reject the null hypothesis? What do we conclude?

Contingency table methods

An alternative to the normal theory method, a contingency table is used to examine associations between categorical variables. The table is a cross-tabulation of two variables where one variable is assigned to the rows and the other variable is assigned to the columns. Thus, each cell corresponds to a level of both of the variables. The most common form of the table has two rows and two columns, but the methods can be extended to larger dimensions. The number of rows in the table is denoted by r, and the number of columns is denoted by c. The chi-squared distribution is often used for hypothesis tests regarding contingency tables. Note that contingency tables are not used to analyze continuous variables.

Contingency-Table Method: A set of analytical methods used to determine the relationship between two categorical variables using a table matrix with one variable as the row variable and the other variable as the column variable.

The contingency table method is valid only if there is no confounding present.

Confounding: The process in which a variable that is related to both the exposure and outcome variables, called a *confounder*, affects the association between the exposure and outcome.

In this chapter, we assume no confounding is present.

2 × 2 Contingency table

2 × 2 Contingency Table: A table composed of two rows cross-classified by two columns; an appropriate way to display data that can be classified by two different binary variables, each of which has only two possible outcomes.

In a 2 × 2 contingency table, one variable is assigned to the rows, and the other variable is assigned to the columns. Each of the four cells represents the number of units with a specific value for each of the two variables. The cells are sometimes referred to by number, as labeled in Table 10.3. The row is referenced by the first number of the ordered pair, and the second number refers to the column.

The cells can also be referred to by letter, as in Table 10.4.

The observed number of units in the four cells is likewise referred to as O_{11} (observation row 1, column 1), O_{12} (observation row 1, column 2), O_{21} (observation row 2, column 1), and O_{22} (observation row 2, column 2).

Row Marginal Total (Row Margin): The total number of units in each row, displayed in the right margin; in a 2 × 2 contingency table, the row margin total is equal to a + b for the first row and c + d for the second row.

Column Marginal Total (Column Margin): The total number of units in each column, displayed in the bottom margin; in a 2 × 2 contingency table, the column marginal total is equal to a + c in the first column and b + d in the second column.

Table 10.3 Table of observed counts with number notation

	Outcome	
	Yes	*No*
Group 1	(1, 1)	(1, 2)
Group 2	(2, 1)	(2, 2)

Note: With number notation, each cell in the contingency table is labeled with an ordered pair indicating the row and column of the cell.

Table 10.4 Table of observed counts with letter notation

	Outcome		
	Yes	*No*	*Total*
Group 1	a	b	a + b
Group 2	c	d	c + d
Total	a + c	b + d	a + b + c + d

Note: With letter notation, each cell in the contingency table is labeled with a letter. In a 2 × 2 table, letters *a* through *d* are used. The grand total is the sum of *a*, *b*, *c*, and *d*.

Grand Total: The total number of units in the four cells. The grand total is displayed in the lower right corner of the table; in a 2 × 2 contingency table, the grand total is equal to a + b + c + d.

R × C contingency table

R × C Contingency Table: A table that displays the relationship between two variables using rows and columns, where the variable in the rows has $R > 2$ categories and the variable in the columns has $C > 2$ categories.

E_{ij} = the expected number of units in the cell; the product of the number of units in the ith row multiplied by the number of units in the jth column, divided by the total number of units in the table.

The sum of the expected values across any row or column must equal the corresponding row or column total, as was the case for 2 × 2 tables. This provides a good check that the expected values are computed correctly, but be aware that your numbers may be off slightly due to round-off error.

The chi-squared distribution

For tests with categorical data, we often use the chi-squared distribution. The distribution has one parameter—the number of degrees of freedom, symbolized by *k*. Random variables with such a distribution are written as $X \sim \chi^2_k$. Unlike the normal distribution, the chi-squared distribution is not symmetrical. The chi-squared distribution does not have negative values and can be thought of as the square of the normal distribution. Table 10.5 provides commands for calculating cutoffs of the chi-squared distribution using statistical software.

In SAS, *p-values* for chi-squared statistics can be calculated using the PROBCHI function. The PROBCHI function will return the probability that the observation is less than or equal to the value selected, so 1 – PROBCHI is the probability that the observation is greater than or equal to the value. The first argument in the SAS function is the value of the test statistic; the degrees of freedom constitute the second argument.

Table 10.5 Commands for calculating chi-squared distribution cutoffs

Probability	*SAS*	*Stata*
Pr (T > k)	`1 - PROBCHI(k, df)`	**`di chi2tail(df, k)`**
Pr (T < k)	`PROBCHI(k, df)`	**`di chi2(df, k)`**

Note: In SAS, the PROBCHI command calculates cutoffs of the chi-squared distribution. The analogous function in Stata is the *chi2tail* function.

In Stata, the *chi2* function will return the probability that the observation is less than or equal to the value selected, and *chi2tail* returns the probability that the observation is greater than or equal to the value. The degrees of freedom constitute the first argument in the Stata function, and the second is the value of the test statistic.

BOX 10.3 USING STATISTICAL SOFTWARE FOR THE CHI-SQUARED CONTRIBUTION

For example, if we want to calculate the p-value corresponding to a test statistic $\chi^2 = 7.5$ with 5 degrees of freedom, we could use the following code in SAS:

```
DATA;
      pvalue = 1 - PROBCHI(7.5, 5);
RUN;
```

If we would like to find the p-value using Stata, we would use the following code:

```
di chi2tail(5, 7.5)
```

Both programs return p-value = 0.1860.

METHOD 1: PEARSON'S CHI-SQUARED TEST

Pearson's Chi-Squared Test (Goodness of Fit Test): A method of analysis that is used when there are two independent groups; referred to as a "goodness of fit" test because it compares how close the observed counts are to the expected counts under the null hypothesis.

The null hypothesis of the Pearson's chi-squared test is H_0: $p_1 = p_2$ (Table 10.6), the same as in the two-sample test for proportions. An alternate way to state the null hypothesis of Pearson's chi-squared test is that there is no association between exposure and outcome.

The chi-squared test is a two-sided test although the critical region based on the chi-squared distribution is one sided. The rationale is that large values of $|O - E|$ and, correspondingly, the test statistic will be obtained under the alternative regardless of whether $p_1 < p_2$ or $p_1 > p_2$. Small values of the test statistic are evidence in favor of the null.

For a 2 × 2 table, $r = c = 2$, so the test has $(r - 1) \times (c - 1) = 1 \times 1 = 1$ degree of freedom. E_{ij} is the expected number in the ijth cell, assuming that there is no association between exposure and outcome (i.e., H_0 is true). Do not round to whole numbers. See Table 10.7 for formulas for the expected number in each cell.

Table 10.6 Pearson's chi-squared test

Component	*Formula*
Hypotheses	H_0: There is no association between exposure and outcome. H_1: There is an association between exposure and outcome. (Alternatively, $H_0: p_1 = p_2$ vs. $H_1: p_1 \neq p_2$)
Test statistic	$\chi^2 = \sum_{i=1}^{r}\sum_{j=1}^{c}\frac{(O_{ij}-E_{ij})^2}{E_{ij}}$ Adjusted: $\chi^2 = \sum_{i=1}^{r}\sum_{j=1}^{c}\frac{(\lvert O_{ij}-E_{ij}\rvert-0.5)^2}{E_{ij}}$
Distribution of test statistic	Chi-squared (χ^2) with $(r-1)(c-1)$ degrees of freedom
Assumptions	For 2 × 2 tables, none of the expected cell values are <5. For R × C tables, no more than 20% of the cell counts are <5, and no cell counts are equal to 0. Exact tests are necessary if cell counts are too small.

Note: Pearson's chi-squared test is a commonly used hypothesis test for categorical data. It can be used for both 2 × 2 tables and larger $R \times C$ tables.

Table 10.7 Expected counts in a 2 × 2 table

	Outcome		
	Yes	No	*Total*
Group 1	$E_{11} = \frac{(a+b)(a+c)}{(a+b+c+d)}$	$E_{21} = \frac{(a+c)(c+d)}{(a+b+c+d)}$	a + b
Group 2	$E_{12} = \frac{(a+b)(b+d)}{(a+b+c+d)}$	$E_{22} = \frac{(c+d)(b+d)}{(a+b+c+d)}$	c + d
Total	a + c	b + d	a + b + c + d

Note: The formulas for the expected value in each cell depend on the observed cell values (a, b, c, and d). The expected cell counts are used to calculate the chi-squared test statistic and to check assumptions for the test. If the expected cell values are too small, an exact test is necessary.

The total of the expected number of units in any row or column should be the same as the corresponding observed row and column total. This relationship provides a useful check that the expected values are computed correctly.

In some cases, we apply a continuity correction to the chi-squared test statistic by subtracting 0.5 inside the squared term in the numerator. This correction is called the Yates continuity correction. Thus, the test statistic is equal to the following:

$$\chi^2 = \sum_{i=1}^{r}\sum_{j=1}^{c}\frac{(\lvert O_{ij}-E_{ij}\rvert-0.5)^2}{E_{ij}} \qquad (10.2)$$

There is another version of the Yates-corrected statistic that is easier to calculate with a hand calculator and does not require the computation of the expected table. The formula for this test statistic follows:

$$\chi^2 = \frac{n\left(|ad - bc| - \frac{n}{2}\right)^2}{(a+b)(c+d)(a+c)(b+d)} \tag{10.3}$$

In the analysis of 2 × 2 tables, the chi-squared statistic without the Yates correction is mathematically equivalent to the square of the test statistic from the two-sample test of proportions. The *p*-values of the two tests are identical. It should be noted that statisticians disagree widely about whether a continuity correction is needed for the contingency table test. The *p*-values for test with the continuity correction are slightly larger, and the results obtained are slightly less significant. For large sample sizes, this difference should be small.

In R × C contingency tables, the Pearson's chi-squared test statistic is used for analysis just as for a 2 × 2 table. In order for the test to be valid, no more than $\frac{1}{5}$ of the cells can have expected values that are less than 5, and no cell should have an expected value less than 1. If cell counts are too small, an exact test is necessary. Although the Yates-corrected statistic can be generalized to any number of groups and outcomes, it is not commonly used in R × C situations.

Pearson's chi-squared test in SAS

PROC FREQ is the SAS procedure used to perform the Pearson's chi-squared test. If the row and column variables are specified in the TABLES statement, the CHISQ option will output both the Pearson's chi-squared result and the Yates correction.

```
PROC FREQ DATA = dataset_name;
     TABLES row_var*column_var / CHISQ;
RUN;
```

When the expected cell counts are smaller than 5, we can request the Fisher's exact chi-squared test with the EXACT option. The EXPECTED option will show the expected cell counts.

```
PROC FREQ DATA = dataset_name;
     TABLES row_var*column_var / CHISQ EXACT EXPECTED;
RUN;
```

The output includes the 2 × 2 table as well as the statistics requested.

The FREQ Procedure

Frequency Percent Row Pct Col Pct

Table of row_var by column_var

row	column 0	1	Total
0	17	11	28
	17.00	11.00	28.00
	60.71	39.29	
	29.31	26.19	
1	41	31	72
	41.00	31.00	72.00
	56.94	43.06	
	70.69	73.81	
Total	58	42	100
	58.00	42.00	100.00

Statistics for Table of row_var by column_var

Statistic	DF	Value	Prob
Chi-Square	1	0.1176	0.7316
Likelihood Ratio Chi-Square	1	0.1181	0.7311
Continuity Adj. Chi-Square	1	0.0138	0.9066
Mantel–Haenszel Chi-Square	1	0.1164	0.7329
Phi Coefficient		0.0343	
Contingency Coefficient		0.0343	
Cramer's V		0.0343	

Fisher's Exact Test	
Cell (1,1) Frequency (F)	17
Left-sided Pr <= F	0.7137
Right-sided Pr >= F	0.4555
Table Probability (P)	0.1692
Two-sided Pr <= P	0.8231

The Pearson's chi-squared test results are in the "Chi-Square" line of the "Statistics for Table of row_var by column_var" table. The "value" column is the test statistic, and "Prob" is the *p*-value. The "Continuity Adj. Chi-Square" is the chi-squared result with the Yates correction. The results from the Fisher's exact test are in the last output box; the *p*-value is in the line "Two-sided Pr < = P." Because it is an exact test, there is no test statistic value that corresponds to the *p*-value.

In addition to using individual-level data, we can also use PROC FREQ with a WEIGHT statement when we have aggregate data. The counts in the individual cells can be input by hand.

Table 10.8 Sample 2 × 2 table

	Column	
	1	0
Row 1	17	11
0	41	31

Note: The sample 2 × 2 table shows cell counts. Here, both the row variable and column variable have two possible values, 0 or 1.

For example, if we want to manually input the data shown in Table 10.8, we can use the following SAS code to read in the data. We have both a row and column variable that indicates the cell position in the table, and the variable *count* indicates the number in each cell.

```
DATA dataset_name;
        INPUT row_var column_var count;
        DATALINES;
1 1 17
0 1 11
1 0 41
0 0 31
;
RUN;
```

Then, in PROC FREQ, include a WEIGHT statement with *count* as the weight variable.

```
PROC FREQ DATA = dataset_name ORDER = DATA;
        TABLES row_var*column_var / CHISQ EXPECTED;
        WEIGHT count;
RUN;
```

The output using aggregate data looks identical to the output using individual-level data.

Pearson's Chi-Squared Test in Stata

To perform the Pearson's chi-squared test, we use the *tab* (tabulate) command. After the *tab* command, the row and column variables should be specified. Then, the *chi2* option is to be added to the end of the code.

```
tab row column, chi2
```

When the expected cell counts are smaller than 5, we can request the Fisher's exact test with the exact option. Additionally, the expected option will show the expected cell counts. To obtain the row percentages or column percentages for each cell, insert the row or column options to the side of the code after the comma.

```
tab row_var column_var, chi2 exact expected row column
```

```
+--------------------+
| Key                |
|--------------------|
|     frequency      |
| expected frequency |
|   row percentage   |
| column percentage  |
+--------------------+

           |      column_var
   row_var |         0          1 |     Total
-----------+----------------------+----------
         0 |        17         11 |        28
           |      16.2       11.8 |      28.0
           |     60.71      39.29 |    100.00
           |     29.31      26.19 |     28.00
-----------+----------------------+----------
         1 |        41         31 |        72
           |      41.8       30.2 |      72.0
           |     56.94      43.06 |    100.00
           |     70.69      73.81 |     72.00
-----------+----------------------+----------
     Total |        58         42 |       100
           |      58.0       42.0 |     100.0
           |     58.00      42.00 |    100.00
           |    100.00     100.00 |    100.00

          Pearson chi2(1) =   0.1176   Pr = 0.732
           Fisher's exact =                 0.823
   1-sided Fisher's exact =                 0.456
```

The key at the beginning of the output shows the order in which the various counts and percentages appear in each cell. In this case, the number of observations in each cell is shown on the top line, the expected count is on the second line, the row percentage is on the third line, and the column percentage is on the bottom line. The chi-squared test statistic appears on the "Pearson chi2( ) =" line, and the corresponding *p*-value is "Pr =e" The degrees of freedom for the test are shown in the parentheses on the "Pearson chi2(1) =" line. For 2 × 2 tables, there will always be 1 degree of freedom. The *p*-value for the exact test is provided on the line below the Pearson's chi-squared statistic. Both two-sided (top) and one-sided (bottom) Fisher's exact *p*-values are given.

In addition to using individual-level data, we can also use the *tabi* command when we have aggregate data rather than individual-level data. The counts in the individual cells can be input by hand. For example, if we have the 2 × 2 table shown in Table 10.8, we can use the following Stata code to read in the data.

```
tabi 17 11\41 31, chi2 expected
```

The output from the *tabi* method looks identical to the output from the *tab* command.

EXAMPLE PROBLEM 10.2

The United States Preventive Services Task Force (USPSTF) recommends screening for colorectal cancer, which involves fecal occult blood tests, sigmoidoscopies, or colonoscopies, in the general public at age 50 years and later. Suppose that we are interested in learning whether sex is associated with colorectal cancer screening. In particular, perhaps, we are interested in comparing the proportion of females and males aged 50 to 75 years who have fully met the USPSTF recommendations for screening in 2014. Sex and screening measurements were taken for a random sample of 250 subjects, and the data can be found in the dataset *ch10_crc_screening*.[1] Use these data to test the null hypothesis that the proportion of adults aged 50 to 75 years who meet the screening recommendations is the same for males and females. Use a 0.05 level of significance.

BOX 10.4 DESCRIPTION OF *chi10_crc_screening* DATASET

The Behavioral Risk Factor Surveillance System (BRFSS) asked each participant questions regarding colorectal cancer screening, from this we calculated a variable indicating whether each respondent aged 50 to 75 years had fully met the USPSTF recommendations. Those who met the screening recommendations have a value of *screened* = 1, and those who did not meet the recommendations were coded as *screened* = 0. The sex of each respondent was also recorded during the survey. The variable *female* takes a value of 1 for women and 0 for men. The dataset *ch10_crc screening* is limited to a sample of 250 men and women who had nonmissing age and screening information.

A **What is the outcome of interest? What are the two populations that we are interested in comparing?**

The outcome is the dichotomous variable of compliance with screening recommendations. We will compare males and females.

B **Tabulate the data into a 2 × 2 table. How many males and females are there? How many females met the screening guidelines? How many males met the screening guidelines?**

Using SAS, we can request a cross tabulation of the variable *female* and the variable *screened*.

```
PROC FREQ DATA = ch10_crc_screening;
      TABLES female*screened;
RUN;
```

The FREQ Procedure

Frequency
Percent
Row Pct
Col Pct

Table of Female by Screened

female(Female)	screened(Met USPSTF guidelines for colorectal cancer screening)		
	0	1	Total
0	31	67	98
	12.40	26.80	39.20
	31.63	68.37	
	41.89	38.07	
1	43	109	152
	17.20	43.60	60.80
	28.29	71.71	
	58.11	61.93	
Total	74	176	250
	29.60	70.40	100.00

In Stata, we use the tab command, specifying the two variables of interest.

```
tab female screened
```

```
           | Met USPSTF guidelines
           | for colorectal cancer
           |       screening
    Female |         0          1 |     Total
-----------+----------------------+----------
         0 |        31         67 |        98
         1 |        43        109 |       152
-----------+----------------------+----------
     Total |        74        176 |       250
```

Of the 250 subjects, 98 are male and 152 are female; 67 males and 109 females met the USPSTF screening guidelines. (See Table 10.9.)

Table 10.9 Data for Example Problem 10.2

		Met screening recommendations		
		No	*Yes*	*Total*
Sex	Male	31	67	98
	Female	43	109	152
	Total	74	176	250

Note: The 2 × 2 table shows a cross-tabulation of the data used in Example Problem 10.2. The respondents' sex is the row variable, and whether or not the respondent met the colorectal cancer screening recommendations is the column variable.

C By hand, find the expected counts for each cell in Table 10.9.

D What are the null and alternative hypotheses for the Pearson's (see Table 10.10) chi-squared test?

We want to test the following null and alternative hypotheses:

H_0: No association between sex and colorectal cancer screening compliance.
H_1: There is an association between sex and colorectal cancer screening compliance.

E What is the value of the test statistic? Do not use the Yates correction. What distribution does the test statistic follow?

The test statistic follows a chi-squared distribution with $(r-1)(c-1) = (2-1)(2-1) = 1$ degree of freedom.

$$\chi^2 = \sum_{i=1}^{r}\sum_{j=1}^{c}\frac{(O_{ij}-E_{ij})^2}{E_{ij}} = \sum_{i=1}^{2}\sum_{j=1}^{2}\frac{(O_{ij}-E_{ij})^2}{E_{ij}}$$

$$= \frac{(31-29.01)^2}{29.01} + \frac{(67-68.99)^2}{68.99} + \frac{(43-44.99)^2}{44.99} + \frac{(109-107.01)^2}{107.01}$$

$$= 0.32$$

F What is the p-value? What do you conclude?

The p-value is $P(\chi^2 \geq 0.32) = 0.5716$.

The p-value is greater than alpha, so we fail to reject the null hypothesis. We have no evidence that colorectal cancer screening rates are associated with sex for U.S. adults aged 50 to 75 years.

G Write the SAS or Stata code to perform the test.

In SAS, we request the CHISQ option in PROC FREQ. We can also include the EXPECTED option to check that the expected counts calculated in Example Problem 10.2—Part (C) are correct.

```
PROC FREQ DATA = ch10_crc_screening;
     TABLES female*screened / EXPECTED CHISQ;
RUN;
```

In Stata, we add the *chi2* option to the tab command to request the Pearson's chi-squared test. The expected option can also be inserted to get the expected counts.

```
tab female screened, chi2 expected
```

Table 10.10 Expected counts for Example Problem 10.2

	Met screening recommendations		
	No	*Yes*	*Total*
Male	$\frac{(a+b)(a+c)}{(a+b+c+d)} = \frac{(31+67)(31+43)}{(31+67+43+109)} = 29.01$	$\frac{(a+b)(b+d)}{(a+b+c+d)} = \frac{(31+67)(67+109)}{(31+67+43+109)} = 68.99$	a + b = 31 + 67 = 98
Female	$\frac{(a+c)(c+d)}{(a+b+c+d)} = \frac{(31+43)(43+109)}{(31+67+43+109)} = 44.99$	$\frac{(c+d)(b+d)}{(a+b+c+d)} = \frac{(43+109)(67+109)}{(31+67+43+109)} = 107.01$	c + d = 43 + 109 = 152
Total	a + c = 31 + 43 = 74	b + d = 67 + 109 = 176	a + b + c + d = 31 + 67 + 43 + 109 = 250

Note: The expected counts for each cell are calculated from the observed cell counts presented in Table 10.9.

H Does the output match the hand calculation?

SAS:

The FREQ Procedure

Frequency Expected Percent Row Pct Col Pct

Table of Female by Screened

female(Female)	screened(Met USPSTF guidelines for colorectal cancer screening)		
	0	1	Total
0	31	67	98
	29.008	68.992	
	12.40	26.80	39.20
	31.63	68.37	
	41.89	38.07	
1	43	109	152
	44.992	107.01	
	17.20	43.60	60.80
	28.29	71.71	
	58.11	61.93	
Total	74	176	250
	29.60	70.40	100.00

Statistics for Table of Female by Screened

Statistic	DF	Value	Prob
Chi-Square	1	0.3196	0.5719
Likelihood Ratio Chi-Square	1	0.3182	0.5727
Continuity Adj. Chi-Square	1	0.1793	0.6720
Mantel–Haenszel Chi-Square	1	0.3183	0.5726
Phi Coefficient		0.0358	
Contingency Coefficient		0.0357	
Cramer's V		0.0358	

Fisher's Exact Test	
Cell (1,1) Frequency (F)	31
Left-Sided Pr <= F	0.7609
Right-Sided Pr >= F	0.3348
Table Probability (P)	0.0957
Two-sided Pr <= P	0.5739

The "chi-square" line of the output provides the Pearson's chi-squared test result, and we can see that the test statistic has a value of 0.3196 with 1 degree of freedom. The corresponding *p*-value is 0.5719. These numbers are within rounding error of the hand calculations.

Stata:

```
+--------------------+
| Key                |
|--------------------|
|     frequency      |
| expected frequency |
+--------------------+

           | Met USPSTF guidelines
           | for colorectal cancer
           |       screening
    Female |         0          1 |     Total
-----------+----------------------+----------
         0 |        31         67 |        98
           |      29.0       69.0 |      98.0
-----------+----------------------+----------
         1 |        43        109 |       152
           |      45.0      107.0 |     152.0
-----------+----------------------+----------
     Total |        74        176 |       250
           |      74.0      176.0 |     250.0

          Pearson chi2(1) =   0.3196   Pr = 0.572
```

The bottom line of the output provides the Pearson's chi-squared test, and we can see that the test statistic has a value of 0.3196 with 1 degree of freedom. The corresponding p-value is 0.572. These numbers are within rounding error of the hand calculations.

PRACTICE PROBLEM 10.2

We are concerned that people with lower education levels have limited access to healthcare resources, and we would like to see whether there is an association between education level and having a routine place for healthcare. A sample of 349 adults were asked whether there is a place that they usually go when they are sick or need advice about health.[2] Their education level was also recorded. The dataset is called *ch10_edu_healthcare*.

BOX 10.5 DESCRIPTION OF *ch10_edu_healthcare* DATASET

The National Health and Nutrition Examination Survey (NHANES) asked respondents, "Is there a place that you usually go when you are sick or need advice about your health?" Possible responses included "Yes," "There is no place," "There is more than one place," or "Don't know," or participants could refuse to answer the question. Those who indicated having at least 1 place were coded as *routine_healthcare* = 1, whereas those who reported not having a place to go when sick or for health advice were coded as *routine_healthcare* = 0. The survey also asked adults aged 20 and older, "What is the highest grade or level of school you have completed or the highest degree you have received?" Possible responses ranged from "Less than 9th grade" to "College graduate or above" with a refusal option and a "Don't know" option. In the dataset *ch10_edu_healthcare*, the variable *education* has four levels: (1) less than high school, (2) high school graduate or GED, (3) some college or associate degree, or (4) college graduate or above. Those who did not answer the education question or did not know their education level are excluded from the sample in the dataset.

A What are the null and alternative hypotheses for the test?

B Write the code to perform the test in a statistical package. Is an exact test necessary?

C What is the value of the test statistic? What distribution does the test statistic follow?

D What is the *p*-value? What do you conclude?

E Which education group has the highest percentage of subjects with a routine place for healthcare?

F Which education group has the lowest percentage of subjects with a routine place for healthcare?

METHOD 2: MCNEMAR'S TEST

McNemar's Test: A contingency table method used for paired (dependent), dichotomous data.

In a McNemar's 2 × 2 contingency table, the entries represent a single pair, as opposed to the entries in a Pearson's chi-squared 2 × 2 table for independent data where each entry represents one subject. The pair can be concordant or discordant (Table 10.11).

Concordant Pair: A matched pair in which the outcome is the same for each member of the pair.

Discordant Pair: A matched pair in which the outcomes differ for the members of the matched pair.

Table 10.11 Table setup for McNemar's test

		Control	
		Exposed	*Unexposed*
Case	Exposed	Concordant	Discordant (*r*)
	Unexposed	Discordant (*s*)	Concordant

Note: The table setup for McNemar's test is different from the typical 2 × 2 table setup. Each entry in a cell represents a pair, which is either concordant or discordant.

Concordant pairs provide no information about the differences between treatment groups and are not used in the assessment. Instead, we focus on discordant pairs, which can be divided into two types: type A and type B.

Type A Discordant Pair: A discordant pair in which the treatment A member of the pair has the event and the treatment B member of the pair does not.

Type B Discordant Pair: A discordant pair in which the treatment B member of the pair has the event and the treatment A member does not.

Let p = probability that a discordant pair is of type A. If the treatments are equally effective, then about an equal number of type A and type B discordant pairs would be expected, and p should equal $\frac{1}{2}$. If treatment A is more effective than treatment B, then fewer type A than type B discordant pairs would be expected. Thus, p should be less than $\frac{1}{2}$. However, if treatment B is more effective than treatment A, then more type A than type B discordant pairs would be expected, and p should be greater than $\frac{1}{2}$. Therefore, we wish to test the following hypotheses:

$$H_0: p = \frac{1}{2}$$

$$H_1: p \neq \frac{1}{2}$$

Another way to phrase the null hypothesis is that there is no association between the exposure and outcome; the alternative is that there is an association between exposure and outcome.

Like the Pearson's chi-squared test, McNemar's test is a two-sided test despite the one-sided nature of the critical region. When cell counts are small, the test statistic can be adjusted by subtracting 1 from the numerator before taking the square in order to approximate the exact binomial p-value. See Table 10.12.

McNemar's Test in SAS

In SAS, we run McNemar's test with PROC FREQ. The AGREE option in the tables statement will request the output from McNemar's test. For small counts, the exact

Table 10.12 McNemar's test

Component	*Formula*
Hypotheses	H_0: There is no association between exposure and outcome. H_1: There is an association between exposure and outcome. $\left(\text{Alternatively, } H_0: p = \frac{1}{2} \text{ vs. } H_1: p \neq \frac{1}{2}\right)$
Test statistic	$\chi^2 = \frac{(r-s)^2}{r+s}$ Continuity corrected estimate: $\chi^2 = \frac{(\lvert r-s \rvert - 1)^2}{r+s}$
Distribution of test statistic	Chi-squared (χ^2) with 1 degree of freedom
Assumptions	Normal approximation to the binomial holds if $r + s \geq 20$

Note: McNemar's test is used for paired, dichotomous data. The null and alternative hypotheses are the same as in the Pearson's chi-squared test. The number of discordant pairs determines the test statistic, which follows a chi-squared distribution.

p-value for McNemar's test can be requested by adding an EXACT line with the MCNEM option. It will appear in the output in the "Exact Pr >= S" line.

```
PROC FREQ DATA = dataset_name;
      TABLES row_var*column_var / AGREE;
      EXACT MCNEM;
RUN;
```

The FREQ Procedure

Frequency Expected Percent Row Pct Col Pct

Table of row_var by column_var

row_var	column_var		
	0	1	Total
0	405	88	493
	321.82	171.18	
	62.50	13.58	76.08
	82.15	17.85	
	95.74	39.11	
1	18	137	155
	101.18	53.819	
	2.78	21.14	23.92
	11.61	88.39	
	4.26	6089	
Total	423	225	648
	65.28	34.72	100.00

Statistics for Table of row_var by column_var

McNemar's Test	
Statistic (S)	46.2264
DF	1
Asymptotic Pr > S	<.0001
Exact Pr >= S	<.0001

Simple Kappa Coefficient	
Kappa	0.6108
ASE	0.0331
95% Lower Conf Limit	0.5459
95% Upper Conf Limit	0.6757

McNemar's Test in Stata

We use the *mcc* command in Stata to conduct McNemar's test for paired data. The two categorical variables should be specified after the *mcc* statement. The exact p-value is given by default.

```
mcc row_var column_var
```

```
                 | Controls              |
Cases            |  Exposed   Unexposed  |      Total
-----------------+-----------------------+------------
         Exposed |       137          18 |        155
       Unexposed |        88         405 |        493
-----------------+-----------------------+------------
           Total |       225         423 |        648

McNemar's chi2(1) =  46.23    Prob > chi2 = 0.0000
Exact McNemar significance probability      = 0.0000

Proportion with factor
        Cases       .2391975
        Controls    .3472222     [95% Conf. Interval]
                   ---------     --------------------
        difference -.1080247     -.1395771  -.0764722
        ratio       .6888889      .6183318   .7674971
        rel. diff. -.1654846     -.2169854  -.1139838

        odds ratio  .2045455       .115896    .342342   (exact)
```

If we do not have the data set but have cell counts, we can use the McNemar's calculator command (mcci) in Stata.

```
mcci a b c d
```

If we input the cell values from the table in the example Stata output for McNemar's test above, we will see the resulting output is the same.

```
mcci 137 18 88 405
```

```
                 | Controls                  |
Cases            |   Exposed   Unexposed     |       Total
-----------------+------------------------+------------
         Exposed |       137          18     |         155
       Unexposed |        88         405     |         493
-----------------+------------------------+------------
           Total |       225         423     |         648

McNemar's chi2(1) = 46.23     Prob > chi2 = 0.0000
Exact McNemar significance probability       = 0.0000

Proportion with factor
        Cases        .2391975
        Controls     .3472222       [95% Conf. Interval]
                     ---------      --------------------
        difference -.1080247       -.1395771  -.0764722
        ratio        .6888889        .6183318   .7674971
        rel. diff. -.1654846       -.2169854  -.1139838

        odds ratio   .2045455         .115896    .342342    (exact)
```

The value of the test statistic appears in the "McNemar's chi2( ) =" line, with the degrees of freedom in parentheses. The *p*-value of the test is in the "Prob > chi2 =" line of the output. The "Exact McNemar significance probability =" line shows the exact *p*-value. The last line of the output will be covered later in this chapter in the section Method 3: Odds Ratio Methods.

EXAMPLE PROBLEM 10.3

We have data from 500 subjects enrolled in a study at an outpatient care center.[3] Each subject was asked, "Has a doctor (or other health professional) ever told you that you have diabetes?" Subsequently, information on their personal history of diabetes was obtained from their medical record. There is concern that there is a fair amount of inconsistency between the self-reported measure and the medical record measure. Each entry in the table corresponds to the paired response of a single individual (See Table 10.13). The data are also in the dataset *ch10_diabetes*.

Table 10.13 Data for Example Problem 10.3

		Medical record		
		Has diabetes	*No diabetes*	*Total*
Self-Reported	Has Diabetes	183	20	203
	No Diabetes	12	285	297
	Total	195	305	500

Note: The 2×2 table shows a cross-tabulation of the data used in Example Problem 10.3. The row indicates whether or not the subject self-reported having diabetes. The column indicates if the medical record showed a history of diabetes.

A What type of test is appropriate?

Because we have paired, dichotomous data, McNemar's test is appropriate.

B Write the appropriate null and alternative hypotheses.

H_0: There is no association between the self-reported diabetes indicator and the medical record diabetes indicator.
H_1: There is an association between the self-reported diabetes indicator and the medical record diabetes indicator.

C What are the value and distribution of the test statistic?

The test statistic follows a χ^2 distribution with 1 degree of freedom.

We should also note that the normal approximation to the binomial holds since

$$r + s = 20 + 12 = 32 > 20.$$

$$\chi^2 = \frac{(|r - s|)^2}{(r + s)} = \frac{(|20 - 12|)^2}{(20 + 12)} = \frac{64}{32} = 2$$

D What is the p-value? What can we conclude from this?

$$p\text{-value} = P(\chi_1^2 \geq 2)$$

We can either use a statistical package or the chi-square distribution table. Using the chi-square table (Appendix Table A.5), we get $p > 0.10$. Using SAS or Stata (Table 10.14), we get $p = 0.1573$.

Because $0.1573 > \alpha = 0.05$, we fail to reject the null hypothesis. We do not have evidence of an association between the self-reported diabetes measure and the medical record diabetes indicator.

Table 10.14 *P*-value calculation for Example Problem 10.3

Using SAS	*Using Stata*
SAS Code	Stata Code
```DATA d; pvalue = 1 - PROBCHI(2, 1); RUN; PROC PRINT DATA = d; RUN;```	```di chi2tail(1, 2)```
SAS Output	Stata Output
Obs: 1; *p-value*: 0.15730	.15729921

SAS Code:

```
DATA d;
     pvalue = 1 - PROBCHI(2, 1);
RUN;

PROC PRINT DATA = d;
RUN;
```

Stata Code:

```
di chi2tail(1, 2)
```

SAS Output:

Obs	*p-value*
1	0.15730

Stata Output: .15729921

Note: The *p*-value for Example Problem 10.3 can be calculated in SAS or Stata using the PROBCHI or *chi2tail* functions, respectively. Note that the *p*-value is two-sided, there is no need to multiply the function by 2.

E Check the hand calculation results against SAS or Stata results.

The variable *self_diabetes* is coded such that a value of 1 indicates a response of "yes" to the question, "Has a doctor (or other health professional) ever told you that you have diabetes?" A value of 0 indicates a response of "no." The variable *mr_diabetes* takes a value of 1 if the medical record indicated a personal history of diabetes and a value of 0 if it did not.

In SAS, we use PROC FREQ with the AGREE option. Selected output boxes are shown after the code.

```
PROC FREQ DATA = ch10_diabetes;
      TABLES self_diabetes*mr_diabetes / AGREE;
RUN;
```

Frequency
Percent
Row Pct
Col Pct

The FREQ Procedure

Table of self_diabetes by mr_diabetes

self_diabetes(Self-Reported Having Diabetes)	mr_diabetes(Medical Record Indicates Diabetes) 0	1	Total
0	285	12	297
	57.00	2.40	59.40
	95.96	4.04	
	93.44	6.15	
1	20	183	203
	4.00	36.60	40.60
	9.85	90.15	
	6.56	93.85	
Total	305	195	500
	61.00	39.00	100.00

Statistics for Table of self_diabetes by mr_diabetes

McNemar's Test	
Statistic (S)	2.0000
DF	1
Pr > S	0.1573

SAS calculates a test statistic of $2 \sim \chi_1^2$. The corresponding p-value is 0.1573, which is within rounding error of the p-value from the hand calculation.

In Stata, we use the *mcc* command and specify *self_diabetes* and *mr_diabetes* as the two binary variables.

```
mcc self_diabetes mr_diabetes
```

```
                 | Controls                |
Cases            |   Exposed    Unexposed  |        Total
-----------------+-------------------------+------------
         Exposed |       183           20  |          203
       Unexposed |        12          285  |          297
-----------------+-------------------------+------------
           Total |       195          305  |          500

McNemar's chi2(1) =        2.00    Prob > chi2 = 0.1573
Exact McNemar significance probability       = 0.2153

Proportion with factor
        Cases            .406
        Controls          .39     [95% Conf. Interval]
                    ---------     --------------------
        difference       .016     -.0081301    .0401301
        ratio        1.041026      .9846002    1.100685
        rel. diff.   .0262295     -.0096422    .0621012

        odds ratio   1.666667      .7759543    3.739329   (exact)
```

The output from Stata shows a test statistic of $2 \sim \chi_1^2$. The corresponding p-value is 0.1573, which is within rounding error of the hand calculation.

METHOD 3: ODDS RATIO METHODS

If p is the probability of the outcome, then $\frac{p}{1-p}$ equals the odds of the outcome.

Odds Ratio (OR): A ratio that compares the odds of a given outcome in two groups; a measure of the strength of association between the outcome and membership in one of two groups (e.g., esposed/unexposed, case/control).

The OR is a valid measure of association for cohort as well as case-control studies. Recall that the risk ratio is not valid for case-control studies. The OR is interpreted in slightly different ways, depending on the type of study. When the OR is greater than 1, we say that one group has X times the odds of the other group, where X = OR.

For cohort or cross-sectional studies, we interpret the OR as the odds of having the outcome. We might say that those exposed have X times the odds of the outcome compared with those unexposed. For case-control studies, the odds refer to the odds of being exposed rather than having the outcome. Thus, the interpretation is that those with the outcome have X times the odds of being exposed compared with those who do not have the outcome. For example, if the OR = 1.20, then those with the outcome have 1.20 times the odds of being exposed compared with those who do not have the outcome.

If the OR is less than 1, we often interpret the OR in terms of reduced odds. For a cohort or cross-sectional study, this means that those exposed have X reduced odds of having the outcome compared with those who are not exposed, where X = (1 – OR)100%. In a case-control study, we say that those with the outcome have X reduced odds of being exposed compared to those who do not have the outcome. For example, if the OR = 0.70 in a cohort study, those exposed have 30% reduced odds of having the outcome compared with those who are not exposed.

The estimated OR is calculated as

$$\widehat{\text{OR}} = \frac{\dfrac{\hat{p}_1}{(1-\hat{p}_1)}}{\dfrac{\hat{p}_2}{(1-\hat{p}_2)}} = \frac{ad}{bc} \qquad (10.4)$$

When there is no association, the OR = 1. This means that the odds of the outcome (or exposure) are the same in both groups. Table 10.15 shows the hypotheses and formulas for ORs and confidence intervals for both independent and paired data. The standard error and confidence interval for ORs are calculated by first finding the standard error and confidence interval for the natural log of the OR and then exponentiating (taking the antilogarithm) the result. Note that $e^{\ln(X)} = X$, and thus $e^{\ln(OR)} = OR$.

Odds ratio methods in SAS

We can obtain ORs in PROC FREQ using the RELRISK option. The EXPECTED option can also be inserted if we want to see the expected cell counts.

```
PROC FREQ DATA = dataset_name;
    TABLES row_var*column_var / RELRISK;
RUN;
```

Table 10.15 Odds ratio and confidence intervals

Component	*Independent data*	*Paired data*
Hypotheses	H_0: OR = 1 H_1: OR $\neq$ 1 (Alternatively, H_0: There is no association between exposure and outcome vs. H_1: There is an association between exposure and outcome)	
Estimated OR	$\widehat{OR} = \dfrac{\frac{\hat{p}_1}{(1-\hat{p}_1)}}{\frac{\hat{p}_2}{(1-\hat{p}_2)}} = \dfrac{ad}{bc}$	$\widehat{OR} = \dfrac{r}{s}$
$\widehat{se}\left[\ln(\text{OR})\right]$	$\sqrt{\dfrac{1}{a}+\dfrac{1}{b}+\dfrac{1}{c}+\dfrac{1}{d}}$	$\sqrt{\dfrac{r+s}{rs}}$
CI for ln(OR)	$\ln\left(\widehat{OR}\right) \pm Z_{1-\alpha/2}\sqrt{\dfrac{1}{a}+\dfrac{1}{b}+\dfrac{1}{c}+\dfrac{1}{d}}$	$\ln\left(\widehat{OR}\right) \pm Z_{1-\alpha/2}\sqrt{\dfrac{r+s}{rs}}$
CI for OR	$e^{\left[\ln\left(\widehat{OR}\right) \pm Z_{1-\alpha/2}\sqrt{\frac{1}{a}+\frac{1}{b}+\frac{1}{c}+\frac{1}{d}}\right]}$	$e^{\left[\ln\left(\widehat{OR}\right) \pm Z_{1-\alpha/2}\sqrt{\frac{r+s}{rs}}\right]}$
Assumptions	All expected cell counts should be ≥ 5 for the normal approximation to be reasonable.	

Note: The hypothesis test for the odds ratio uses the same hypothesis as in the Pearson's and McNemar's tests, but the null and alternative hypotheses can also be stated in terms of the odds ratio. The assumptions and hypotheses are the same for independent and dependent data, but the other aspects of the test are not.

The FREQ Procedure

Frequency Percent Row Pct Col Pct

Table of row_var by column_var

row_var	column_var: 0	column_var: 1	Total
0	17 17.00 60.71 29.31	11 11.00 39.29 26.19	28 28.00
1	41 41.00 56.94 70.69	31 31.00 43.06 73.81	72 72.00
Total	58 58.00	42 42.00	100 100.00

Statistics for Table of row_var by column_var

Odds Ratio and Relative Risks			
Statistic	Value	95% Confidence Limits	
Odds Ratio	1.1685	0.4797	2.8466
Relative Risk (Column 1)	1.0662	0.7444	1.5272
Relative Risk (Column 2)	0.9124	0.5362	1.5527

The output gives the 2 × 2 table as well as the OR, the relative risk, and their confidence intervals. The OR appears on the "Odds Ratio" line under the "Value" column. The 95% confidence interval for the OR is also given.

Note that if we are interested in the relative risk, the correct output depends on the order of the levels of the binary variables in the table. If the table is set up with 1/yes in the first column/row and 0/no in the second column/row, then the "Relative Risk (Column 1)" is the correct relative risk. Tables set up with 0/no in the first column/row and 1/yes in the second column row have a relative risk equal to the inverse of "Relative Risk(Column 2)."

Odds Ratio Methods in Stata

To calculate an OR in Stata, specify the two variables to be tabulated in the *cc* command. The *woolf* option requests that the Woolf approximation (most similar to hand calculations) is used to calculate the standard error and confidence interval for the OR. By default, Stata calculates the exact confidence intervals if the *woolf* option is left out. The exact option can also be specified if the cell counts are small. This will request the Fisher's exact test p-value in the output.

```
cc row_var column_var, woolf
```

```
                       | column_var           |        Proportion
                       | Exposed Unexposed    |    Total      Exposed
-----------------+----------------------+----------------------
           Cases |     31          41    |      72       0.4306
        Controls |     11          17    |      28       0.3929
-----------------+----------------------+----------------------
       Total           |     42          58    |     100        0.4200
                       |                      |
                       |     Point estimate   |   [95% Conf. Interval]
                       |----------------------+----------------------
Odds ratio (Woolf)     |      1.168514        |   .4796675    2.846609
Attr. frac. ex. (Woolf)|      .1442125        |  -1.084777    .6487049
Attr. frac. pop        |      .0620915        |
                 +---------------------------------------------
                          chi2(1) =      0.12  Pr>chi2 = 0.7316
```

The output shows the 2 × 2 table as well as the OR, 95% confidence intervals, and results from the Pearson's chi-squared test. The OR appears in the second half of the table under the "Point Estimate" column. The 95% confidence interval for the OR is also given on the same line. The bottom line of the output, "chi2( ) =", shows the test statistic and *p*-value for the Pearson's chi-squared test for the 2 × 2 table. The degrees of freedom for the test are shown in parentheses.

If we have aggregate cell counts rather than an individual-level dataset, we can use the *cci* command to input the 2 × 2 table and obtain an OR. We list all four cell counts: a, b, c, and d.

```
cci a b c d, woolf
```

The output from the *cci* command is identical in structure to the output from the *cc* command.

EXAMPLE PROBLEM 10.4

A total of 450 U.S. high school students were asked whether, in the past year, they had been bullied on school property and whether they felt so sad or hopeless almost every day for two weeks or more in a row that they were prevented from doing some usual activities.[4] Of the 86 high schoolers who reported being bullied on school property, 45 indicated that they felt so sad or hopeless almost every day for two or more weeks in a row that they were prevented from doing some usual activities. Of the 450 high schoolers surveyed, 364 did not report being bullied on school property, but 84 of the 364 did indicate feeling so sad or hopeless almost every day for two or more weeks in a row that their feeling interfered with participation in usual activities. The corresponding dataset is called *ch10_mh_bullying*.

BOX 10.6 DESCRIPTION OF *ch10_mh_bullying* DATASET

The Youth Risk Behavior Surveillance System (YRBSS) asked each student, "During the past 12 months, have you ever been bullied on school property?" Those who responded "Yes" received a value of 1 for the variable *bullied*. If the student reported not having been bullied, he or she was coded as *bullied* = 0. The survey also asked, "During the past 12 months, did you ever feel so sad or hopeless almost every day for two weeks or more in a row that you stopped doing some usual activities?" The variable *sad* indicates the response to this question, with a value of 1 indicating "Yes" and 0 indicating "No." The dataset *ch10_mh_bullying* contains a sample of 450 students.

A What are the null and alternative hypotheses?

The null hypothesis is that the odds of feeling so sad or hopeless almost every day for two or more weeks in a row that it affected participation in usual activities were equal for high school students who reported being bullied on school grounds and for those who did not report being bullied on school grounds. The alternative hypothesis is that the odds of feeling so sad or hopeless almost every day for two or more weeks in a row that it affected participation in usual activities were not the same for high school students who reported being bullied on school grounds and for those who did not report being bullied on school grounds. In symbols,

$$H_0\text{: OR} = 1$$

$$H_1\text{: OR} \neq 1$$

B Make a 2 × 2 table for the data.

C What were the odds of feeling so sad or hopeless (see Table 10.16) almost every day for two or more weeks in a row that it affected participation in usual activities for those who reported being bullied on school property? What were the odds for high schoolers who did not report bullying?

The odds of feeling sad or hopeless among high schoolers who have been bullied:

$$\frac{\hat{p}_1}{1-\hat{p}_1} = \frac{\frac{45}{86}}{1-\frac{45}{86}} = 1.10$$

The odds of feeling sad or hopeless among high schoolers who did not indicate any bullying:

$$\frac{\hat{p}_1}{1-\hat{p}_1} = \frac{\frac{84}{364}}{1-\frac{84}{364}} = 0.30$$

Table 10.16 Data for Example Problem 10.4

		Felt sad or hopeless		
		No	*Yes*	*Total*
Report Bullying	No	280	84	364
	Yes	41	45	86
	Total	321	129	450

Note: The 2 × 2 table shows a cross-tabulation of the data used in Example Problem 10.4. The row variable indicates whether or not the subject reported being bullied on school property, and the column variable indicates whether the student felt so sad or hopeless almost every day for two or more weeks in a row that it affected participation in usual activities.

D What was the OR?

$$\widehat{OR} = \frac{\dfrac{\hat{p}_1}{(1-\hat{p}_1)}}{\dfrac{\hat{p}_2}{(1-\hat{p}_2)}} = \frac{ad}{bc} = \frac{280 \times 45}{84 \times 41} = 3.66$$

High schoolers who reported being bullied on school property in the past year had 3.66 times the odds of feeling so sad or hopeless almost every day for two or more weeks in a row that it affected participation in usual activities compared to those who reported not being bullied.

E Do we meet the assumption about small cell counts?

We need to calculate the expected counts in each cell (see Table 10.17).

All of the expected counts are greater than 5, so the normal approximation is valid.

F Calculate a 95% confidence interval around the OR. What can we conclude from the interval?

We will use $Z_{1-\alpha/2} = 1.96$ to calculate the confidence interval around the OR since $\alpha = 0.05$.

$$e^{\left[\ln\left(\widehat{OR}\right) \pm Z_{1-\alpha/2}\sqrt{\frac{1}{a}+\frac{1}{b}+\frac{1}{c}+\frac{1}{d}}\right]}$$

$$= e^{\left[\ln(3.66) \pm 1.96\sqrt{\frac{1}{280}+\frac{1}{84}+\frac{1}{41}+\frac{1}{45}}\right]}$$

$$= e^{1.30 \pm 0.49} = (2.24,\ 5.96)$$

Table 10.17 Expected counts for Example Problem 10.4

		Felt sad or hopeless		
		No	*Yes*	*Total*
Report Bullying	No	$\frac{364 \times 321}{450} = 259.65$	$\frac{364 \times 129}{450} = 104.35$	364
	Yes	$\frac{86 \times 321}{450} = 61.35$	$\frac{86 \times 129}{450} = 24.65$	86
	Total	321	129	450

Note: The expected counts for each cell are calculated from the observed cell counts presented in Table 10.16.

We are 95% confident that the true OR lay in the interval (2.24, 5.96). As this interval does not conclude the null value of 1, we reject the null hypothesis that the odds ratio was equal to 1. Compared with high school students who were not bullied, high school students who reported being bullied had higher odds of feeling so sad or hopeless almost every day for two or more weeks in a row that it affected participation in usual activities.

G Use SAS or Stata to check the OR and confidence interval (CI).

We can obtain the OR and CI in SAS using PROC FREQ with the RELRISK option. We will include the EXPECTED option so that we can check the expected cell count calculations we made in Example Problem 10.4—Part (E).

```
PROC FREQ DATA = ch10_mh_bullying;
      TABLES bullied*sad / EXPECTED RELRISK;
RUN;
```

The FREQ Procedure

Frequency / Expected / Percent / Row Pct / Col Pct

Table of Bullied by Sad

bullied(Bullied on school property in the past year)	sad(Felt so sad or hopeless almost every day for two weeks or more in a row in the past year that you stopped doing some usual activities) 0	1	Total
0	280	84	364
	259.65	104.35	
	62.22	18.67	80.89
	76.92	23.08	
	87.23	65.12	
1	41	45	86
	61.347	24.653	
	9.11	10.00	19.11
	47.67	52.33	
	12.77	34.88	
Total	321	129	450
	71.33	28.67	100.00

Statistics for Table of bullied by sad

Odds Ratio and Relative Risks

Statistic	Value	95% Confidence Limits	
Odds Ratio	3.6585	2.2450	5.9622
Relative Risk (Column 1)	1.6135	1.2840	2.0276
Relative Risk (Column 2)	0.4410	0.3348	0.5809

The first table in the output is the 2 × 2 table with the expected frequencies. The "Statistics for Table of bullied by sad" table shows an OR of 3.66 and a 95% confidence interval of (2.25, 5.96). These match the hand calculations done in Example Problem 10.4—Part (D) and (F).

In Stata, we will use the *cc* command with the *woolf* option to obtain the OR and confidence interval.

```
cc bullied sad, woolf
```

Alternatively, we could input the cell counts by hand using the *cci* command. The output from the *cci* command is identical to the output produced by the *cc* command.

```
cci 45 41 84 280, woolf
```

```
                 | sad                    |              Proportion
                 | Exposed Unexposed      |    Total      Exposed
-----------------+------------------------+------------------------
           Cases |      45          41    |       86       0.5233
        Controls |      84         280    |      364       0.2308
-----------------+------------------------+------------------------
           Total |     129         321    |      450       0.2867
                 |                        |
                 |   Point estimate       |  [95% Conf. Interval]
                 |------------------------+------------------------
Odds ratio (Woolf)     |    3.658537      |     2.244959    5.962198
Attr. frac. ex. (Woolf)|     .7266667     |     .5545576    .8322766
Attr. frac. pop        |     .3802326     |
                 +-------------------------------------------------
                          chi2(1) =      29.10  Pr>chi2 = 0.0000
```

The OR appears on the first line under the "Point estimate" column. The OR is 3.66, with a 95% confidence interval (2.24, 5.96). These estimates match the hand calculations done in Example Problem 10.4—Parts (D) and (F).

PRACTICE PROBLEM 10.3

The following data are taken from an investigation regarding an outbreak of *Salmonella* enteritidis infections.[5] Of the 85 people who became ill during the outbreak, 62 reported eating bean sprouts in the week prior to becoming sick. In a survey of healthy people, six people reported eating bean sprouts in the week prior to the interview. The number of *Salmonella* enteritidis infections in each group is shown in Table 10.18.

Table 10.18 Data for Practice Problem 10.3

	Ate bean sprouts		
	Yes	*No*	*Total*
Ill	62	23	85
Not Ill	6	94	100
Total	68	117	185

Note: The 2 × 2 table shows a cross-tabulation of the data used in Practice Problem 10.3. The row variable indicates whether or not the subject became ill with a *Salmonella* enteritidis infection, and the column variable indicates whether or not the subject ate bean sprouts.

A Perform a chi-square test without the Yates correction to test the association between consumption of bean sprouts and the onset of gastroenteritis. What are the null and alternative hypotheses?

B Fill in the expected counts in Table 10.19.

C What are the value and distribution of the test statistic?

D What is the p-value? Do we reject or fail to reject the null hypothesis? What is your conclusion?

E What are the estimated odds of becoming ill among those who ate bean sprouts?

Table 10.19 Expected counts for Practice Problem 10.3

	Ate bean sprouts		
	Yes	*No*	*Total*
Ill			85
Not Ill			100
Total	68	117	185

Note: Fill in the expected counts for each cell using the observed cell counts presented in Table 10.18.

F What are the estimated odds of becoming ill among those who did not eat bean sprouts?

G What is the estimated OR of becoming ill, comparing those who ate bean sprouts to those who did not? Interpret the OR in words.

H Check the results in a statistical package.

I By hand, construct a 95% confidence interval for the true OR. Check that the confidence interval matches the SAS or Stata output.

Sample size and power for comparing two binomial proportions

INDEPENDENT SAMPLES

To estimate the sample size and power needed for a two-sided test comparing binomial proportions, we must first have a sense of the projected true probabilities of success in the two groups, symbolized by p_1 and p_2. The absolute value of the difference of the projected true probabilities of success is delta. In symbols, $\Delta = |p_2 - p_1|$. We also must calculate $\bar{p}$ as in Equation 10.5:

$$\bar{p} = \frac{p_1 + kp_2}{1 + k} \tag{10.5}$$

The sample size needed to compare two binomial proportions using a two-sided test with significance level α and power $1 - \beta$, where 1 sample (n_2) is k times as large as the other sample (n_1), is shown in Table 10.20. The table also shows the power achieved in comparing two binomial proportions with significance level α and samples of size n_1 and n_2 for the specific alternative Δ. To do calculations for a one-sided test, replace $\frac{\alpha}{2}$ with α.

PAIRED SAMPLES

Before calculating sample size and power for McNemar's test for correlated proportions, we need to establish the projected proportion of discordant pairs among all pairs, p_D, and the projected proportion of discordant pairs of type A among discordant pairs, p_A. The sample size and power needed to compare two binomial proportions using a two-sided McNemar's test with significance level α and power $1 - \beta$ are shown in Table 10.21.

For the power calculation, note that n is the number of matched pairs. Replace $\frac{\alpha}{2}$ with α to calculate values for a one-sided test. Note that the crucial element in calculating sample size and power for matched-pair studies based on binomial proportions is the knowledge of the probability of discordance between outcomes for members of a

Table 10.20 Sample size and power for independent two-sided, two-sample proportions test

Term	*Formula*
Δ	$\Delta = \lvert p_2 - p_1 \rvert$
$\bar{p}$	$\bar{p} = \dfrac{p_1 + kp_2}{1+k}$
Sample size	$n_1 = \dfrac{\left[Z_{1-\alpha/2}\sqrt{\bar{p}(1-\bar{p})\left(1+\frac{1}{k}\right)} + Z_{1-\beta}\sqrt{p_1(1-p_1)+\frac{p_2(1-p_2)}{k}} \right]^2}{\Delta^2}$ $n_2 = kn_1$
Power	$\text{power} = \phi\left[\dfrac{\Delta}{\sqrt{\frac{p_1(1-p_1)}{n_1}+\frac{p_2(1-p_2)}{n_2}}} - Z_{1-\alpha/2}\dfrac{\sqrt{\bar{p}(1-\bar{p})\left(\frac{1}{n_1}+\frac{1}{n_2}\right)}}{\sqrt{\frac{p_1(1-p_1)}{n_1}+\frac{p_2(1-p_2)}{n_2}}} \right]$

Note: Before calculating the sample size and power for an independent two-sided, two-sample test for proportions, we calculate the quantities Δ and $\bar{p}$. The allocation ratio, k, also influences the sample size calculation.

Table 10.21 Sample size and power for paired two-sided, two-sample proportions test

Term	*Formula*
p_D	p_D = projected proportion of discordant pairs among all pairs
p_A	p_A = projected proportion of discordant pairs of type A among discordant pairs
Sample size (matched pairs)	$n = \dfrac{\left[Z_{1-\alpha/2} + 2Z_{1-\beta}\sqrt{p_A(1-p_A)} \right]^2}{4(p_A - 0.5)^2 p_D}$
Sample size (individuals)	$n = \dfrac{\left[Z_{1-\alpha/2} + 2Z_{1-\beta}\sqrt{p_A(1-p_A)} \right]^2}{2(p_A - 0.5)^2 p_D}$
Power	$\text{power} = \phi\left[\dfrac{1}{2p_A(1-p_A)}\left(Z_{\alpha/2} + 2\lvert p_A - 0.5 \rvert \sqrt{np_D} \right) \right]$

Note: The sample size and power for a paired two-sided, two-sample binomial proportions test depend on the projected proportions of discordant pairs.

matched pair. This probability depends on the strictness of the matching criteria and how strongly related the matching criteria are to the outcome variable.

Sample size and power for two binomial proportions in SAS

INDEPENDENT SAMPLES

To perform a sample size or power calculation for a two-sample binomial proportions test or the Pearson's chi-squared test in SAS, we use PROC POWER with the TWOSAMPLE FREQ and TEST = PCHI options. We specify p_1 and p_2 in the GROUPPROPORTIONS statement. By default, the NULLPROPORTIONDIFF is set to 0, and ALPHA is set to 0.05.

If both groups have the same size, $n_1 = n_2$, then we can either request the sample size in each group (n_1) using the NPERGROUP statement, or we can get the total sample size ($n_{total} = 2n_1$) using the NTOTAL statement. Similar to other power calculations we have seen, the SIDES = U or SIDES = L options may be used to request a one-sided test.

```
PROC POWER;
        TWOSAMPLEFREQ TEST = PCHI
        GROUPPROPORTIONS = (0.45 0.60)
        NULLPROPORTIONDIFF = 0
        ALPHA = 0.05
        POWER = 0.80
        NPERGROUP =.;
        *NTOTAL =.;
RUN;
```

The POWER Procedure
Pearson Chi-Squared Test for Proportion Difference

Fixed Scenario Elements	
Distribution	Asymptotic normal
Method	Normal approximation
Null Proportion Difference	0
Alpha	0.05
Group 1 Proportion	0.45
Group 2 Proportion	0.6
Nominal Power	0.8
Number of Sides	2

Computed N per Group	
Actual Power	N per Group
0.800	173

The output gives a table summarizing the input parameters and then a table with the sample size per group ("Computed N per Group"). If we use the NTOTAL option instead, the output shows the "Computed N Total" in the final output box. If the groups are not the same size, this is specified in the GROUPWEIGHTS statement. For example, if Group 1 is twice as large as Group 2 ($n_1 = 2n_2$), then the GROUPWEIGHTS statement should be written as it is in the following code. (Note that if GROUPWEIGHTS is used, only the total sample size can be requested. Also, note that the NPERGROUP option will not work with unbalanced groups.)

```
PROC POWER;
        TWOSAMPLEFREQ TEST = PCHI
        GROUPPROPORTIONS = (0.45 0.60)
        GROUPWEIGHTS = (2 1)
        POWER = 0.80
        NTOTAL =.;
RUN;
```

The POWER Procedure
Pearson Chi-Squared Test for Proportion Difference

Fixed Scenario Elements	
Distribution	Asymptotic normal
Method	Normal approximation
Group 1 Proportion	0.45
Group 2 Proportion	0.6
Group 1 Weight	2
Group 2 Weight	1
Nominal Power	0.8
Number of Sides	2
Null Proportion Difference	0
Alpha	0.05

Computed N per Group	
Actual Power	N Total
0.801	390

The output gives the total sample size, so the allocation ratio must be used to obtain the sample size in each of the groups. For power calculations, leave the power option blank. Either the NTOTAL or NPERGROUP options can be used with a balanced design, but only the NTOTAL option is available if $n_1 \neq n_2$.

```
PROC POWER;
        TWOSAMPLEFREQ TEST = PCHI
        GROUPPROPORTIONS = (0.45 0.60)
        NULLPROPORTIONDIFF = 0
        ALPHA = 0.05
        POWER = .
        NTOTAL = 400;
RUN;
```

The POWER Procedure
Pearson Chi-Squared Test for Proportion Difference

Fixed Scenario Elements	
Distribution	Asymptotic normal
Method	Normal approximation
Null Proportion Difference	0
Alpha	0.05
Group 1 Proportion	0.45
Group 2 Proportion	0.6
Total Sample Size	400
Number of Sides	2
Group 1 Weight	1
Group 2 Weight	1

Computed Power
Power
0.854

The final output box gives the power of the test given the input parameters.

PAIRED SAMPLES

To do the calculations in SAS, we use the PAIREDFREQ statement in PROC POWER. The DIST = NORMAL and METHOD = CONNOR options request a normal approximation McNemar's test; the default DIST option requests an exact test. The DISCPROPORTIONS statement is where we specify the two discordant proportions (p_r and p_s) with a vertical bar between them.

```
PROC POWER;
        PAIREDFREQ DIST = NORMAL METHOD = CONNOR
        DISCPROPORTIONS = 0.10 | 0.15
        POWER = 0.80
        NPAIRS = .;
RUN;
```

The POWER Procedure
McNemar Normal Approximation Test

Fixed Scenario Elements	
Distribution	Asymptotic normal
Method	Connor normal approximation
Success–Failure Proportion	0.1
Failure–Success Proportion	0.15
Nominal Power	0.8
Number of Sides	2
Alpha	0.05

Computed N Pairs	
Actual Power	N Pairs
0.800	783

The "Computed N Pairs" output box gives the number of pairs needed to achieve the specified level of power. For the sample code, 783 pairs are needed to have 80% power when the discordant proportions are 0.10 and 0.15, and $\alpha = 0.05$. If we want a power calculation rather than a sample size calculation, we set the POWER option to missing and fill in the NPAIRS option.

```
PROC POWER;
      PAIREDFREQ DIST = NORMAL METHOD = CONNOR
      DISCPROPORTIONS = 0.10 | 0.15
      POWER = .
      NPAIRS = 900;
RUN;
```

The power of the test appears in the final output box.

The POWER Procedure
McNemar Normal Approximation Test

Fixed Scenario Elements	
Distribution	Asymptotic normal
Method	Connor normal approximation
Success–Failure Proportion	0.1
Failure–Success Proportion	0.15
Nominal Power	900
Number of Sides	2
Alpha	0.05

Computed Power
Power
0.852

Sample size and power for two binomial proportions in stata

INDEPENDENT SAMPLES

To perform a sample size or power calculation for a two-sample binomial proportions test or the Pearson's chi-squared test in Stata, we use the power command with the *twoproportions* option. Next, we specify the proportions in the two groups, p_1 and p_2. The alpha and power levels are specified after the comma in order to request a sample size calculation. The default alpha level is 0.05, and the default power level is 0.80. The *onesided* option requests the calculation corresponding to a one-sided test. This assumes balanced groups.

```
power twoproportions 0.45 0.60, test(chi2) alpha(0.05) power(0.8)
```

```
Estimated sample sizes for a two-sample proportions test
Pearson's chi-squared test
Ho: p2 = p1  versus  Ha: p2 != p1

Study parameters:

        alpha =     0.0500
        power =     0.8000
        delta =     0.1500   (difference)
           p1 =     0.4500
           p2 =     0.6000

Estimated sample sizes:

            N =        346
  N per group =        173
```

With balanced groups, the total sample size is shown on the "N =" line, and the "N per group=" line shows that many subjects are needed in each group. If the groups are not the same size, insert the *nratio* option. The value is the ratio of n_2 to n_1. For example, if Group 1 is twice as large as Group 2 ($n_1 = 2n_2$), then the sample size ratio would be 0.5.

```
power twoproportions 0.45 0.60, test(chi2) nratio(0.5)
```

```
Estimated sample sizes for a two-sample proportions test
Pearson's chi-squared test
Ho: p2 = p1  versus  Ha: p2 != p1

Study parameters:

        alpha =     0.0500
        power =     0.8000
        delta =     0.1500   (difference)
```

```
        p1 =      0.4500
        p2 =      0.6000
     N2/N1 =      0.5000

Estimated sample sizes:

         N =         390
        N1 =         260
        N2 =         130
```

The "N =" line shows the total sample size, and the "N1 =" and "N2 =" lines show the sample sizes needed in the first and second groups, respectively. To request a power calculation rather than a sample size calculation, drop the *power* option and insert the *n* option showing the total sample size. Insert the *nratio* option if the groups are not balanced. The *onesided* option performs a power calculation for a one-sided test.

```
power twoproportions 0.45 0.60, test(chi2) alpha(0.05) n(400)
```

```
Estimated power for a two-sample proportions test
Pearson's chi-squared test
Ho: p2 = p1   versus  Ha: p2 != p1

Study parameters:

     alpha =      0.0500
         N =         400
 N per group =       200
     delta =      0.1500   (difference)
        p1 =      0.4500
        p2 =      0.6000
Estimated power:

     power =      0.8545
```

The "power =" line shows the power of the test.

PAIRED SAMPLES

For paired samples, we use the *power* command with the *pairedproportions* option. The two discordant proportions, p_r and p_s, are specified next. The alpha and power levels are specified after the comma, although they can be omitted if the default level is acceptable. The *onesided* option can be inserted at the end of the code line to request a calculation for a one-sided test.

```
power pairedproportions 0.10 0.15, alpha(0.05) power(0.8)
```

```
Estimated sample size for a two-sample paired-proportions test
Large-sample McNemar's test
Ho: p21 = p12  versus  Ha: p21 != p12

Study parameters:

        alpha =    0.0500
        power =    0.8000
        delta =    0.0500   (difference)
          p12 =    0.1000
          p21 =    0.1500

Estimated sample size:

            N =       783
```

The output shows the estimated number of pairs needed to achieve the given level of power. To request a power calculation, the *power* option is dropped, and the *n* option, specifying the sample size, is inserted.

```
power pairedproportions 0.10 0.15, n(900)
```

```
Estimated power for a two-sample paired-proportions test
Large-sample McNemar's test
Ho: p21 = p12  versus  Ha: p21 != p12

Study parameters:

        alpha =    0.0500
            N =       900
        delta =    0.0500   (difference)
          p12 =    0.1000
          p21 =    0.1500

Estimated power:

        power =    0.8521
```

The power of the test appears on the last line of the output.

Sample size and power in a clinical trial setting

In the previous estimations of power and sample size, we have assumed perfection in the compliance (ability to follow) treatment regimens. To be more realistic, we should examine how these estimates will change if compliance is not perfect.

Suppose that we are planning a clinical trial comparing an active treatment versus a placebo. There are two types of noncompliance to consider:

- ***Drop-out Rate* (λ_1):** The proportion of participants in the active-treatment group who do not actually receive the active treatment.
- ***Drop-in Rate* (λ_2):** The proportion of participants in the placebo group who actually receive the active treatment outside of the study protocol.

In the presence of noncompliance, sample size and power estimates should be based on the compliance-adjusted rates $\left(p_1^*, p_2^*\right)$ rather than on the perfect compliance rates (p_1, p_2). Table 10.22 shows the sample sizes for each group, accounting for drop-out and drop-in rates. To adjust the sample size in each group for noncompliance in a clinical trial setting, we replace p_1, p_2, Δ, and $\bar{p}$ with p_1^*, p_1^*, Δ^*, and $\bar{p}^*$, respectively. If noncompliance rates are low (λ_1, λ_2 each ≤ 0.10), then the approximate sample size formula can be used. In the approximate formula, $n_{perfectcompliance}$ is the sample size in each group under the assumption of perfect compliance.

EXAMPLE PROBLEM 10.5

We are interested in racial disparities in hypertension and would like to compare the prevalence of hypertension among black patients to the prevalence among white patients. Before we collect the sample, we need to conduct sample size calculations to know how many subjects to enroll. From national estimates, we think that reasonable estimates are $p_{1(black)} = 0.39$ and $p_{2(white)} = 0.32$ for the proportion with hypertension.[2]

A **What is the value of Δ?**

Delta is the absolute value of the difference of the projected true probabilities of success.

$$\Delta = |p_2 - p_1| = |0.32 - 0.39| = |-0.07| = 0.07$$

B **If we plan to enroll equal numbers of black and white participants, what is the value of $\bar{p}$?**

To calculate $\bar{p}$, we need to know k. Because we plan to enroll equal numbers of black and white subjects, $n_1 = n_2$; thus, $k = 1$.

$$\bar{p} = \frac{p_1 + kp_2}{1+k} = \frac{0.39 + 1(0.32)}{1+1} = \frac{0.71}{2} = 0.355$$

C **How many subjects are necessary to achieve 90% power if we perform a two-sided test with $\alpha = 0.05$?**

We have $p_1 = 0.39$, $p_2 = 0.32$, $\Delta = 0.07$, $\bar{p} = 0.355$, $k = 1$, $\alpha = 0.05$, $Z_{1-\alpha/2} = 1.96$, $\beta = 0.20$, and $Z_{1-\beta} = 1.28$.

Table 10.22 Sample size adjusted for drop-out and drop-in rates

Term	*Formula*
p_1^*	$p_1^* = (1-\lambda_1)p_1 + \lambda_1 p_2$
p_2^*	$p_2^* = (1-\lambda_2)p_1 + \lambda_2 p_2$
$\bar{p}*$	$\bar{p}^* = \left(p_1^* + p_2^*\right)$
$\Delta*$	$\Delta* = \left\|p_1^* + p_2^*\right\| = (1-\lambda_1-\lambda_2)\left\|p_1 - p_2\right\| = (1-\lambda_1-\lambda_2)\Delta$
Sample size	$n_1 = n_2 = \frac{\left[Z_{1-\alpha/2}\sqrt{2\bar{p}(1-\bar{p})} + Z_{1-\beta}\sqrt{p_1^*\left(1-p_1^*\right) + p_2^*\left(1-p_2^*\right)}\right]}{\Delta*^2}$
Approximate sample size (λ_1, λ_2 each ≤ 0.10)	$n_{1,approx} = n_{2,approx} = \frac{1}{(1-\lambda_1-\lambda_2)^2} \times \frac{\left[Z_{1-\alpha/2}\sqrt{2\bar{p}(1-\bar{p})} + Z_{1-\beta}\sqrt{p_1(1-p_1) + p_2(1-p_2)}\right]^2}{\Delta^2} = \frac{n_{perfectcompliance}}{(1-\lambda_1-\lambda_2)^2}$

Note: Sample size calculations for a two-sided, two-sample binomial proportions test with drop-ins and drop-outs.

$$n_1 = \frac{\left[Z_{1-\alpha/2}\sqrt{\bar{p}(1-\bar{p})\left(1+\frac{1}{k}\right)} + Z_{1-\beta}\sqrt{p_1(1-p_1)+\frac{p_2(1-p_2)}{k}}\right]^2}{2}$$

$$= \frac{\left[1.96\sqrt{0.355(0.645)(1+1)} + 1.28\sqrt{0.39(0.61)+\frac{0.32(0.68)}{1}}\right]^2}{0.07^2}$$

$$= \frac{\left[1.96\sqrt{0.46}+128\sqrt{0.46}\right]^2}{0.0049} = \frac{(1.33+0.86)^2}{0.0049} = \frac{4.80}{0.0049} = 979.02$$

Because $n_1 = n_2$, 980 subjects are needed in each group. The total number of participants needed to achieve 90% power assuming no drop-out is $n_{total} = 2n_1 = 2 \times 980 = 1960$.

D Using SAS or Stata, perform the sample size calculation in Example Problem 10.5—Part (C).

To do the sample size calculation in SAS, we use PROC POWER with the TWOSAMPLEFREQ option. Because we have a situation where $n_1 = n_2$, we can either use the NPERGROUP option and then multiply the output by 2 to obtain the total sample size, or we can use the NTOTAL option to obtain the total sample size. The GROUPWEIGHTS option is not necessary since we plan to enroll equal numbers of black and white participants. Thus, both groups have weight = 1.

```
PROC POWER;
        TWOSAMPLEFREQ TEST = PCHI
        GROUPPROPORTIONS = (0.32 0.39)
        NULLPROPORTIONDIFF = 0
        POWER = 0.90
        NPERGROUP =.;
RUN;
```

The POWER Procedure
Pearson Chi-Squared Test for Proportion Difference

Fixed Scenario Elements	
Distribution	Asymptotic normal
Method	Normal approximation
Null Proportion Difference	0
Group 1 Proportion	0.32
Group 2 Proportion	0.39
Nominal Power	0.9
Number of Sides	2
Alpha	0.05

Computed N per Group	
Actual Power	N per Group
0.900	980

The "Computed N per Group" output box gives the required sample size per group. To achieve 90% power, 980 subjects in each group are necessary; 980 is the number that we calculated by hand in Example Problem 10.5—Part (C).

Using Stata, we run the *power* command with the *twoproportions* option. We have a balanced design since we plan to enroll equal numbers of black and white participants. Thus, the *nratio* option is not needed. We can also drop the *alpha* option since $\alpha = 0.05$ is the default.

```
power twoproportions 0.32 0.39, test(chi2) power(0.9)
```

```
Estimated sample sizes for a two-sample proportions test
Pearson's chi-squared test
Ho: p2 = p1  versus  Ha: p2 != p1

Study parameters:

       alpha =    0.0500
       power =    0.9000
       delta =    0.0700  (difference)
          p1 =    0.3200
          p2 =    0.3900

Estimated sample sizes:

           N =      1960
 N per group =       980
```

The total sample size and the sample size in each group appear at the bottom of the output. To achieve 90% power, 1960 total subjects or 980 subjects in each group are necessary; 980 is the number that we calculated by hand in Example Problem 10.5—Part (C).

PRACTICE PROBLEM 10.4

Select which methods are appropriate for the type of data. See Table 10.23.

Table 10.23 Practice Problem 10.4

Method	*Independent*	*Dependent*
Two-Sample Test for Proportions		
Pearson's Chi-Squared Test		
McNemar's Test		
Odds Ratio		

Table 10.24 Data for Practice Problem 10.5

	Met screening recommendations		
	No	*Yes*	*Total*
Men	31	67	98
Women	43	109	152
Total	74	176	250

PRACTICE PROBLEM 10.5

Let's return to the data presented in Example Problem 10.3 regarding sex category and colorectal cancer screening. Table 10.24 is a 2 × 2 table with the counts, and the corresponding dataset is *ch10_crc_screening*.

A Comparing females with males, what is the estimated OR for meeting screening recommendations? Interpret the OR in words.

B What is the 95% confidence interval for the OR? How do you interpret this?

C Does there appear to be an association between sex category and meeting colorectal cancer screening recommendations? Why or why not?

PRACTICE PROBLEM 10.6

Let's return to the data presented in Practice Problem 10.1 regarding the study comparing two regimens. There are 250 subjects in the trial, 130 of whom are on the active treatment and 120 of whom are on the placebo. The corresponding dataset is *ch10_demographics*.

A Sex is the first variable of interest. We already analyzed sex using a two-sample test for proportions in Practice Problem 10.1, but we will now try a slightly different approach. Using SAS or Stata, determine how many males and females are in the active treatment group. How many males and females are in the placebo group?

B To see whether there is a difference in sex composition between the two regimens, we wish to conduct a Pearson's chi-squared test. What are the null and alternative hypotheses?

C Write the code to run the test.

D What are the values for the test statistic and the degrees of freedom?

E What is the p-value?

F Do we reject or fail to reject the null hypothesis? What is the conclusion?

G Compare the test statistic and p-value with the calculations in Practice Problem 10.1.

H Next, we would like to know whether there is a difference in race of the subjects on the two regimens. What type of test is appropriate for the data?

I What are the null and alternative hypotheses for the appropriate test?

J Perform the test using SAS or Stata. What are the value and distribution of the test statistic?

K What is the p-value, and what can we conclude?

References

1. Behavioral Risk Factor Surveillance System (BRFSS). Atlanta, GA: Centers for Disease Control and Prevention; 2014. http://www.cdc.gov/brfss/annual_data/annual_data.htm. September 11, 2015. Accessed February 23, 2016.
2. National Health and Nutrition Examination Survey. Hyattsville, MD: Centers for Disease Control and Prevention, National Center for Health Statistics. 2014. https://wwwn.cdc.gov/Nchs/Nhanes/Search/nhanes13_14.aspx. Accessed February 23, 2016.
3. Fan JH, Lyons S, Goodman MS, Blanchard MS, Kaphingst KA. Relationship between health literacy and unintentional and intentional medication nonadherence in medically underserved patients with type 2 diabetes. *Diabetes Educ*. 2016;42(2):199–208. doi:10.1177/0145721715624969.
4. Youth Risk Behavior Surveillance System (YRBSS). Atlanta, GA: Centers for Disease Control and Prevention. 2013. www.cdc.gov/yrbs. Updated August 11, 2016. Accessed March 11, 2016.
5. Centers for Disease Control and Prevention. Multistate outbreak of *Salmonella* enteritidis infections linked to bean sprouts. http://www.cdc.gov/salmonella/enteritidis-11-14/index.html. Update January 23, 2015. Accessed October 27, 2016.

11 Analysis of variance (ANOVA)

This chapter will focus on one-way analysis of variance and will include the following topics:

- Within- and between-group variation
- ANOVA assumptions
- Testing for significance
- Multiple comparisons

Terms

- ANOVA
- between-group variation
- grand mean
- one-way
- within-group variation

Introduction

An analysis of variance (ANOVA) is appropriate when we seek to compare the means of three or more groups.

ANOVA: Compares the means of three or more independent groups used with a continuous outcome and categorical factor of interest that distinguishes the independent groups from each other.

It is an extension of the two-sample t-test when there are more than two groups ($k > 2$). For example, suppose that we have a weight loss trial where one group is randomized to nutrition counseling, one group is randomized to a group exercise program, and a third control group is randomized to no intervention. After several weeks, the study staff records the body fat percentage of each participant. We would calculate the mean body fat percentage of each group and use an ANOVA to compare those means.

The null hypothesis of an ANOVA is that all k means are equal. The alternate hypothesis (H_1) is that at least one group mean is different from the others. This does not mean that all group means are necessarily different from each other. As long as one of the group means is unequal to at least one of the others, the null hypothesis is rejected.

$$H_0: \mu_1 = \mu_2 = \ldots = \mu_k$$

In this chapter, we will focus on the one-way ANOVA.

One-Way ANOVA: A reference to the single factor or characteristic that distinguishes the populations from each other.

In the weight loss trial example, we assume that the only difference between the groups is the intervention type. If we wanted to look at more than one factor between the groups at the same time (e.g., intervention type and race), we would use a two-way ANOVA (not covered in this book).

Within- and between-group variation

ANOVA is dependent on estimates of spread or dispersion. In other words, the procedure analyzes the variances of the data. There are two sources of variation in the data: Within-group and between-group.

Within-Group Variation: The variation of individual values around their group mean (Figure 11.1).

Recall from Chapter 8, the chapter on two-sample *t*-tests, that s_p^2 is the pooled variance (σ^2). The within-group variance $\left(s_W^2\right)$ is an extension of s_p^2 to *k* groups. It is calculated as the weighted (by sample size) average of the variances of the *k* groups (Equation 11.1). It can also be thought of as the mean square error (MS_E), or the within-group (error) sum of squares divided by the within-group degrees of freedom.

$$s_W^2 = \frac{SS_E}{df_E} = \frac{(n_1-1)s_1^2+(n_2-1)s_2^2+\ldots+(n_k-1)s_k^2}{n_1+n_2+\ldots+n_k-k} \tag{11.1}$$

Between-Group Variation $\left(s_B^2\right)$*:* The variation of the group means around the grand mean; an estimate of the common variance (σ^2); see Figure 11.2.

The between-group variance is calculated as the average of the squared deviations of the sample means $\bar{x}_i$ from the grand mean $\bar{x}$ (Equation 11.2). It can also be thought of as the mean square model (MS_M), or the between-group (model) sum of squares divided by the between-group degrees of freedom.

$$s_B^2 = \frac{SS_M}{df_M} = \frac{(\bar{x}_1-\bar{x})^2 n_1+\ldots+n_k(\bar{x}_k-\bar{x})^2}{k-1} \tag{11.2}$$

Grand Mean: The overall average of the $N = n_1+n_2+\ldots+n_k$ observations that make up the *k* different samples (Equation 11.3).

$$\bar{x} = \frac{n_1\bar{x}_1+n_2\bar{x}_2+\ldots+n_k\bar{x}_k}{n_1+n_2+\ldots+n_k} \tag{11.3}$$

In the case that the null hypothesis is true and the means of the groups are all equal, then the variability within the *k* different populations should be the same as the variability among their respective means. In other words, the ANOVA procedure analyzes

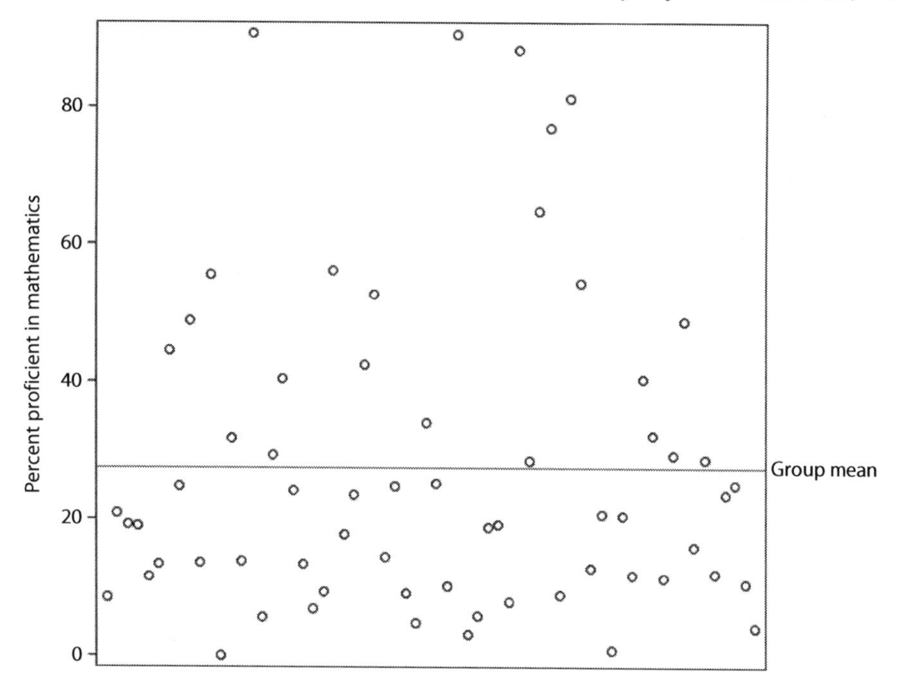

Figure 11.1 **Visualization of variation of individual values around the group mean.** Each school's percent proficiency in mathematics is plotted as an open dot. These are the individual values. The group mean is illustrated by the horizontal line. Some individual values are closer to the group mean than others are.

the variances of the groups in the context of the variance of the whole dataset. Under the null hypothesis, we would expect $s_W^2 \approx s_B^2$.

If the value of s_B^2 is large relative to the value of s_W^2, then at least one of the means is different from the others (a rejection of the null hypothesis). When the variability within the *k* different populations is small relative to the variability of their respective means, this suggests that the population means are, in fact, different.

ANOVA assumptions

To perform an ANOVA, we make three assumptions about the underlying data. If any of the assumptions do not hold, then an ANOVA might not be the most appropriate way to analyze the data at hand. It is important to note that the ANOVA is a fairly robust procedure and will tolerate some minor violations of the following assumptions.

1 Samples from the *k* populations are independent.
2 Samples from the *k* populations are normally distributed.
3 Variances in the *k* populations are equal (i.e., $\sigma_1 = \sigma_2 = \ldots \sigma_k$).

Independence

The independence assumption requires that samples from the *k* populations are independent. The design of the study is a good indicator of whether the data meet this

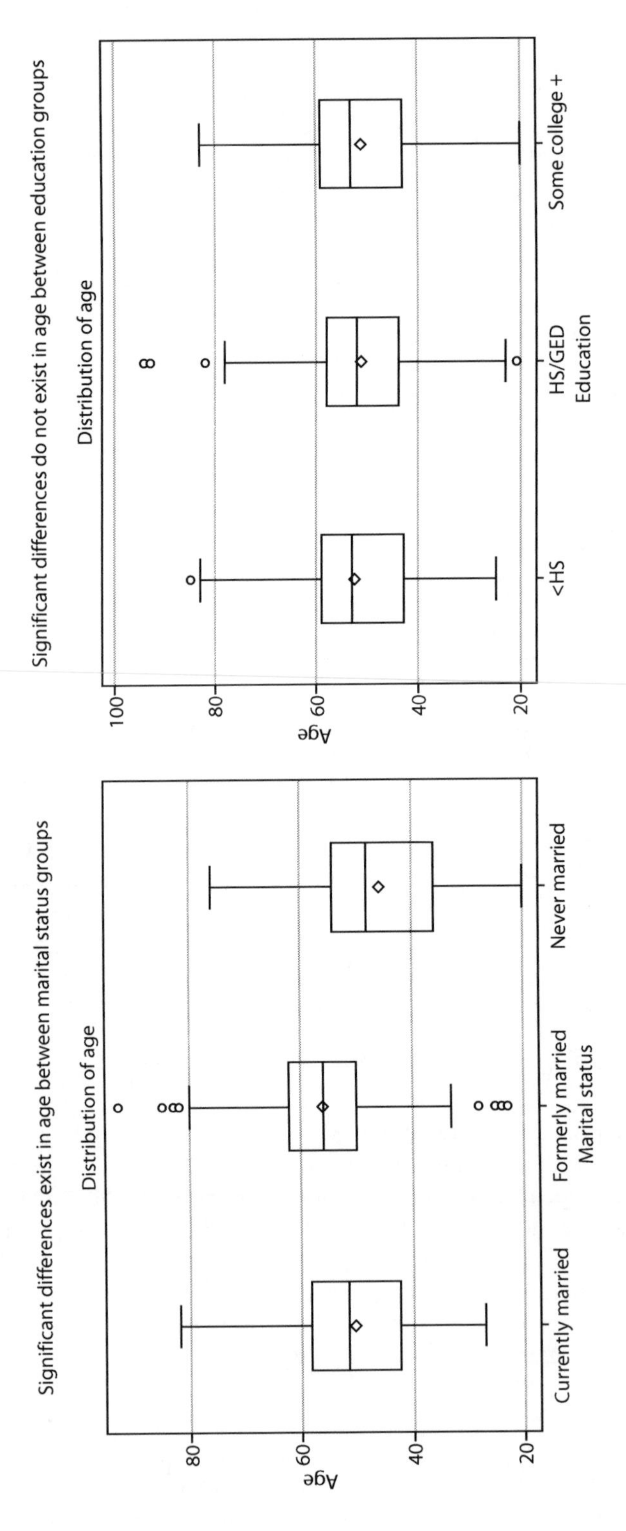

Figure 11.2 **Example of failing to reject and rejecting the null hypothesis of an ANOVA.** The left-most box plot displays the case where the between-group variance $\left(s_B^2\right)$ is large relative to the within-group variance $\left(s_W^2\right)$. The right-most box plot displays the case where the between-group and within-group variances are approximately the same. HS represents high school, and GED represents general education diploma.

assumption. For example, ascertaining differences in the mean resting heart rate of those who exercise vigorously, moderately, or lightly would be an appropriate case for which to use an ANOVA. Ascertaining differences in the mean heart rate of a population before, during, and after exercise would not be a good candidate for an ANOVA because the same participants are in each of the three populations (dependent data).

Normality

To meet the normality assumption, the outcome variable should be normally distributed in each of the k populations. We can check this assumption by plotting the data in a histogram using the HISTOGRAM statement of PROC UNIVARIATE in SAS or the histogram command in Stata.

Equal variance

The third assumption specifies that the variances in the k populations are equal. We can compare the variances of the k different groups using PROC MEANS or PROC UNIVARIATE in SAS or the *summarize* command in Stata. To be thorough, however, we should statistically test the differences in the variance.

In SAS, the HOVTEST option in PROC GLM requests the Levene test for homogeneity of variance. In Stata, the Bartlett test for equal variances is included by default when using the *oneway* command.

The null hypothesis for both of these tests is that the variances of all k groups are equal. If the null hypothesis is rejected and we find that there is a difference in the variances between the k groups, we can use the Welch's ANOVA in SAS (output included when WELCH is requested as an option in the MEANS statement of PROC GLM) or the W test in Stata (the *wtest* command is part of the *wtest* package and must be downloaded using *findit wtest*), which are robust to the homogeneity of variance assumption but beyond the scope of this book.

Testing for significance

Once we have established that our analysis meets the three assumptions, we are ready to test the null hypothesis that the means of the k populations are all equal. To do this, we use an F-statistic (Equation 11.4).

$$F = \frac{s_B^2}{s_W^2} \tag{11.4}$$

We want to know whether the group means vary around the grand mean more than the individual observations vary around the group means. Under the null hypothesis, both the between- and within-groups variation will estimate the common variance (σ^2); therefore, F will be close to 1. If there is a difference among populations, the between-groups variance exceeds the within-groups variance, and F will be greater than 1.

The F-statistic cannot assume negative values, so we do not double the final p-value. In the case in which we are only comparing two independent samples, the F-test reduces to a two-sample t-test. The F-statistic is drawn from the F distribution, which has two types

Table 11.1 ANOVA table and equations

Source	*DF*	*Sum of squares*	*Mean square*	*F-value*
Model (Between-group)	$k - 1$	SS_M	$s_B^2 = MS_M = \frac{SS_M}{k-1}$	$\frac{MS_M}{MS_E}$
Error (Within-group)	$n - k$	SS_E	$s_W^2 = MS_E = \frac{SS_E}{n-k}$	
Total	$n - 1$	SS_T		

of degrees of freedom. There are numerator degrees of freedom which correspond to the degrees of freedom between groups (the *Model df* in SAS output and *Between-group df* in Stata output) and denominator degrees of freedom, which correspond to the degrees of freedom within the groups (the *Error df* in SAS output and the *Within-group df* in Stata output). To determine the critical value of the F-statistic, we can use a table of the F distribution (see the Appendix, Table A6). Table 11.1 shows the information provided in an ANOVA table.

Multiple comparisons

If the null hypothesis is rejected, we conclude that at least one of the means is different from the others. The F-test indicates that there is a difference, but in order to discover which mean is different from the others, we should perform pairwise comparisons.

We must perform all $\binom{k}{2}$ pairwise comparisons of the means with a series of two-sample t-tests to detect which groups are different. Performing multiple tests, however, increases the probability of making a type I error. To compensate for this issue, we must be more conservative in each of the individual comparisons. If we reduce the α level for each of the pairwise tests, we ensure that the overall level of significance is kept at a predetermined level. Because these tests are not independent, we will adjust the overall significance level using a Bonferroni correction (α^*) as shown in Equation 11.5.

$$\alpha^* = \frac{\alpha}{\binom{k}{2}} \tag{11.5}$$

The adjusted significance level for the individual comparisons depends on the number of tests being conducted. As the number of tests increases, the corrected significance level will decrease. The Bonferroni correction is highly conservative, meaning that it reduces statistical power. Thus, it may fail to reject a difference between means when one actually exists.

Instead of using the pooled variance estimate $\left(s_P^2\right)$ when conducting the t-test, we use the within-groups variation $\left(s_W^2\right)$ to take advantage of the additional information that is available by estimating the pooled variance of all k samples instead of just the two samples being tested. The degrees of freedom for each t-test will be $n–k$. Don't forget to double the p-value for two-sided tests.

Using SAS to conduct an ANOVA

In this chapter, we rely on PROC GLM to conduct an ANOVA. PROC ANOVA can handle only balanced designs (equal number of observations in each group), whereas PROC GLM can handle both balanced and unbalanced designs. To run an ANOVA, we need a continuous outcome and a categorical grouping variable. The following SAS code will run an ANOVA on the data.

```
PROC GLM DATA=dataset;
        CLASS group_variable;
        MODEL outcome_variable = group_variable;
RUN;
```

The MODEL statement is where we will specify the continuous variable whose mean we are interested in comparing between the groups (*outcome_variable*). We will also specify the categorical variable (*group_variable*) in the MODEL statement, after the equal sign. The grouping variable (*group_variable*) must also go in a CLASS statement so that it is treated as a categorical variable and not as a continuous variable.

Results from this procedure include the overall ANOVA table, model fit statistics, and the type I and III sum of squares ANOVA tables. Because we are running a one-way ANOVA, these tables will be identical to the overall ANOVA. A histogram is also presented.

Homogeneity of variance in SAS

The MEANS statement will give us a summary of the mean and standard deviation of each of the levels and also allows us to request the test for homogeneity of variance (the HOVTEST option) so that we can check the assumption for the equality of variance.

```
PROC GLM DATA=dataset;
        CLASS group_variable;
        MODEL outcome_variable = group_variable;
        MEANS group_variable / HOVTEST;
RUN;
```

Running this procedure will output the same results as the previous code, with the addition of a table containing the results of the Levene test for homogeneity of variance.

Multiple comparisons in SAS

In the event that we detect a significant difference between groups, we could subset the data and run individual PROC TTEST analyses, or we could request the multiple comparisons and the Bonferroni correction from SAS by adding the BON option to the MEANS statement.

```
PROC GLM DATA=dataset;
        CLASS group_variable;
        MODEL outcome_variable = group_variable;
        MEANS group_variable / BON;
RUN;
```

SAS will not give the actual Bonferroni-corrected *p*-values in the associated output. Instead, it denotes which pairs are significant by marking the significant pairs with asterisks in the final column of the output table.

Using Stata to conduct an ANOVA

To run an ANOVA in Stata, we use the *oneway* command. This command reports one-way ANOVA models and has the capacity to perform multiple comparison tests. For more complicated ANOVAs, we would use the *anova* command. In the command, the continuous outcome variable (*outcome_variable*) is specified first, followed by the categorical grouping variable (*group_variable*)

```
oneway outcome_variable group_variable
```

Results from the *oneway* command include the overall ANOVA table and the results from the Bartlett test for equal variances.

Multiple comparisons in stata

In the event that we detect a significant difference between groups, we could subset the data and run individual *t*-test analyses, or we could request the multiple comparisons and the Bonferroni correction from Stata by adding the *bonferroni* option to the *oneway* command.

```
oneway outcome_variable group_variable, bonferroni
```

Stata returns a *k* by *k* table containing the difference in means between each pair of levels and the Bonferroni-corrected *p*-value.

EXAMPLE PROBLEM 11.1

Suppose that we are interested in comparing the hemoglobin HbA1c levels (%) of people who have diabetes and who are either taking no medication, taking just insulin, taking just diabetic pills, or who are taking both insulin and diabetic pills. The outcome is the A1c level (measured continuously), and the categorical variable is the participant's medication group. A random sample of 200 people who have diabetes was taken from the National Health and Nutrition Examination Survey (NHANES).[1] Use the *diabetics* dataset to answer the questions.

A What are the null and alternate hypotheses of an ANOVA?

$$H_0: \mu_{Both\ medications} = \mu_{Insulin\ only} = \mu_{Pills\ only} = \mu_{No\ medication}$$

BOX 11.1 DESCRIPTION OF DIABETES DATASET

The National Health and Nutrition Examination Survey (NHANES) assesses the health and nutritional status of adults and children in the United States. Participants included in our sample self-identified as having diabetes (responded "yes" to "Other than during pregnancy, have you ever been told by a doctor or other health professional that you have diabetes or sugar diabetes?"). The continuous variable is hemoglobin A1c levels (*A1c*) and the categorical variable is medication group (*medication_group*). The medication group variable was created from the responses to two questions on the survey: (1) Are you taking insulin now? and (2) Are you now taking diabetic pills to lower your blood sugar? *Medication_group* has four levels: (1) participants who are taking both insulin and diabetic pills to lower their blood sugar; (2) participants who are only taking insulin; (3) participants who are only taking diabetic pills; and (4) participants who are taking neither.

The alternate hypothesis is that at least one group's mean is different from the others.

Use the code in Table 11.2 to conduct an ANOVA.

First, we will investigate the homogeneity of variance assumption. We are interested in whether the variance in mean HbA1c level is different in the four medication groups.

Levene's Test for Homogeneity of A1c Variance ANOVA of Squared Deviations from Group Means

Source	DF	Sum of Squares	Mean Square	F Value	Pr > F
medication_group	3	74.5895	24.8632	1.21	0.3073
Error	196	4027.2	20.5469		

```
Bartlett's test for equal variances:  chi2(3) =   7.2750
Prob>chi2 = 0.064
```

B Are the variances in the populations equal?

Using the Levene test, we fail to reject the null hypothesis that the variances are equal because $p = 0.3073$, which is larger than our cutoff of 0.05.

Table 11.2 Code for ANOVA (Example Problem 11.1)

SAS code	*Stata code*

`PROC GLM DATA=diabetics;`
`CLASS medication_group;`
`MODEL A1c = medication_group;`
`MEANS medication_group / HOVTEST;`
`RUN;`
	`oneway a1c medication_group`

Using the Bartlett test, we fail to reject the null hypothesis that the variances are equal because $p = 0.064$, which is larger than our cutoff of 0.05.

On the basis of these results, we assume that the equal variance assumption is not violated, and we proceed with our ANOVA. We examine the ANOVA table that was output when we ran the code in Table 11.2.

Source	DF	Sum of Squares	Mean Square	F Value	Pr > F
Model	3	30.8547264	10.2849088	4.89	0.0027
Error	196	412.2088236	2.1031062		
Corrected Total	199	443.0635500			

```
                     Analysis of Variance
    Source              SS         df        MS            F        Prob > F
------------------------------------------------------------------------
Between groups    30.8547264      3     10.2849088     4.89       0.0027
Within groups     412.208824    196     2.10310624
------------------------------------------------------------------------
    Total         443.06355     199     2.22645
```

C What is the estimate of the within-groups variance?

The ANOVA output tables display the within-group variation as the Mean Square Error (SAS) or Within groups MS (Stata). The within-group variation is 2.10.

D What is the estimate of the between-groups variance?

The ANOVA output tables display the between-group variation as the Model Mean Square (SAS) or Between groups MS (Stata). The between-group variation is 10.28.

E What are the value and distribution of the test statistic?

The F-statistic is 4.89. It is distributed with three numerator degrees of freedom (the *Model df* in SAS output and *Between-groups df* in Stata output) and 196 denominator degrees of freedom (the *Error df* in SAS output and the *Within-groups df* in Stata output).

F What is your conclusion for the hypothesis test from Example Problem 11.1—Part (A)?

The p-value of the test is 0.0027. Therefore, we can reject the null hypothesis and conclude that at least one of the means is significantly different from the others.

We now know that there is a significant difference in the mean A1c, but we are not sure between which medication groups the difference lies. To figure this out, we will perform multiple pairwise two-sample t-tests comparing each medication group with all of the others.

Table 11.3 Code for multiple pairwise tests (Example Problem 11.1)

SAS code	*Stata code*

`PROC GLM DATA=diabetics;`
`CLASS medication_group;`
`MODEL A1c = medication_group;`
`MEANS medication_group / BON;`
`RUN;`
	`oneway a1c medication_group,`
	`bonferroni`

G How many pairwise tests should you perform?

There are four levels in the medication regimen category variable, so we should perform $\binom{k}{2} = \binom{4}{2} = 6$ *t*-tests.

H What type I error rate should you use?

The adjusted significance level, using the Bonferroni correction (Equation 11.5), is the following:

$$\alpha^* = \frac{\alpha}{\binom{k}{2}} = \frac{0.05}{6} = 0.008$$

In order to reject the null hypothesis that both groups' means are the same, the *p*-value obtained from the *t*-test would need to be less than 0.008.

To perform the multiple pairwise tests, we run our ANOVA again and adjust the syntax as follows (Table 11.3).

BOX 11.2 FORMATTING VARIABLES

Temporarily Formatting Variables in SAS:
To make our output easier to interpret, we can format our variables within a PROC statement. This assigns temporary formats to the variables, but will not permanently format them in the dataset.

First, we assign the format class using PROC FORMAT. Use the VALUE statement to name your format (e.g., *formatname*), and assign a formatted label to each value of the variable. Refer to Lab A for more information.

```
PROC FORMAT;
      VALUE formatname 1 = "First Format" 2 = "Second Format";
RUN;
```

Then, assign the format within the PROC GLM for nicely formatted output. Do not forget the period after the format name; this tells SAS that it is a format, not a variable.

```
PROC GLM DATA=diabetics;
       CLASS medication_group;
       MODEL A1c = medication_group;
       MEANS medication_group / BON;
       FORMAT medication_group formatname.;
RUN;
```

Formatting Variables in Stata:

Use the *label define* command to state the labels associated with each level of the variable.

```
label define formatname 1 "First Format" 2 "Second Format"
```

Then, assign that label to a specific variable using the *label values* command.

```
label values medication_group formatname
```

When you run your ANOVA again for multiple pairwise testing, the labels will be displayed automatically.

```
oneway a1c medication_group, Bonferroni
```

If you wish to suppress the label in further analyses, add the *nolabel* option to your *oneway* command. Refer to Lab A for more information.

```
oneway a1c medication_group, bonferroni nolabel
```

Comparisons significant at the 0.05 level are indicated by *.**

medication_group Comparison	Difference between Means	Simultaneous 95% Confidence Limits		
Insulin only—Both medications	0.5670	–0.2774	1.4115	
Insulin only—No medication	0.7943	–0.5216	2.1103	
Insulin only—Diabetic pills only	1.0144	0.2962	1.7326	***
Both medications—Insulin only	–0.5670	–1.4115	0.2774	
Both medications—No medication	0.2273	–1.0757	1.5302	
Both medications—Diabetic pills only	0.4474	–0.2468	1.1415	
No medication—Insulin only	–0.7943	–2.1103	0.5216	

No medication—Both medications	–0.2273	–1.5302	1.0757	
No medication—Diabetic pills only	0.2201	–1.0049	1.4450	
Diabetic pills only—Insulin only	–1.0144	–1.7326	–0.2962	***
Diabetic pills only—Both medications	–0.4474	–1.1415	0.2468	
Diabetic pills only—No medication	–0.2201	–1.4450	1.0049	

```
            Comparison of a1c by medication~p
                       (Bonferroni)
Row Mean-|
Col Mean |    Both med    Insulin    Pills on
---------+--------------------------------
Insulin  |     .567045
         |       0.450
         |
Pills on |    -.447359    -1.0144
         |       0.525      0.001
         |
No medic |    -.227273    -.794318    .220087
         |       1.000      0.656      1.000
```

I What is your conclusion after the pairwise testing?

In the SAS output, we can see that there is a statistically significant difference between the "Insulin only" (2) and "Diabetic pills only" (3) groups. Conversely, there is no difference between the other pairwise tests. For example, the difference between the mean HbA1c levels in the "Insulin only" (2) and "Both medications" (4) groups is not statistically significant.

The table output by the BON option assesses twice as many pairwise tests as are necessary based on our calculation in Example Problem 11.1—Part (H). This is because it allows for both directions of the relationship between groups. For instance, the difference and confidence limits of "Insulin only" (2) versus "Both medications" (4) are the inverse of that of "Both medications" (4) versus "Insulin only" (2). The doubling of the output allows us to easily choose which direction is most meaningful to report, without having to manipulate the code to give us the directionality that we desire.

In the Stata output, we can see that there is a statistically significant difference (p = 0.001) between the "Insulin only" (2) and "Diabetic pills only" (3) groups. Conversely, there is no statistically significant difference between the other pairwise tests. For example, the difference between the mean HbA1c levels in the "Insulin only" (2) and "Both medications" (4) groups is not statistically significant.

EXAMPLE PROBLEM 11.2

We selected a random sample of 1000 adults from the NHANES dataset.[1] The sample of 306 average-weight (or less than average-weight) participants had an average total cholesterol of 181.2 mg/dL and standard deviation of 39.6 mg/dL. The sample of 316 overweight participants had an average total cholesterol of 191.9 mg/dL and a standard deviation of 43.7 mg/dL. Finally, the sample of 378 participants who were obese had an average total cholesterol of 193.3 mg/dL with a standard deviation of 40.6 mg/dL. Data for this problem are stored in the *cholbmi* dataset.

BOX 11.3 DESCRIPTION OF THE *cholbmi* DATASET

The *cholbmi* dataset contains a random sample of 1000 adults from the National Health and Nutrition Examination Survey (NHANES). The continuous variable is cholesterol level (*cholesterol*), measured in mg/dL. The group variable (*bmi_cat*) was created from the continuous value of each participant's reported BMI. The group variable has three levels: (1) average weight or less (BMI < 25); (2) overweight (BMI ≥ 25 and BMI < 30); and (3) obese (BMI of 30 or greater).

A Why is an ANOVA an appropriate method for analyzing these data?

We are interested in comparing the means of three independent groups (i.e., average or less-than-average weight, overweight, or obese). Using a *t*-test would not be appropriate because we have more than two groups that we are interested in comparing.

Before we proceed, we need to check that the three assumptions for an ANOVA are met.

Assumption 1: Samples from k populations are independent.

This is true. We know that the observations are independent from the structure of our dataset. Each participant can be in only one of the groups, and we have no reason to believe that the participants are correlated with each other.

Assumption 2: Samples from the k populations are normally distributed.

We will check this assumption by creating a histogram of the outcome (cholesterol) for each BMI group. Use the code in Table 11.4, as appropriate.

Table 11.4 Code to check normal distribution assumption (Example Problem 11.2)

SAS code	*Stata code*

`PROC SORT DATA= cholbmi;`
`BY bmi_cat;`
`RUN;`
 	
`PROC UNIVARIATE DATA= cholbmi;`
`VAR cholesterol;`
`HISTOGRAM cholesterol;`
`BY bmi_cat;`
`RUN;`
	`twoway histogram cholesterol,`
	`by(bmi_cat)`

Examining the histograms by eye (Figure 11.3), we can see that the distribution of total cholesterol for each group is approximately normal. By comparing the means and medians to see whether they are relatively close to each other for each group, we also conclude that our outcome variable is approximately normally distributed in each of the three groups.

Assumption 3: Variances in the *k* populations are equal.

We want the standard deviation of total cholesterol to be approximately equal in each of our three groups. We can check the standard deviations of each group and see whether they are relatively close (Figures 11.3 and 11.4), but a more objective way is to perform a homogeneity of variance test. We include the HOVTEST option in the MEANS statement of PROC GLM in SAS and examine the Levene test table in the output. In Stata, we examine the Bartlett test *p*-value.

Levene's Test for Homogeneity of cholesterol Variance ANOVA of Squared Deviations from Group Means

Source	DF	Sum of Squares	Mean Square	F Value	Pr > F
bmi_cat	2	20493888	10246944	1.46	0.2336
Error	997	7.0154E9	7036543		

```
Bartlett's test for equal variances:  chi2(2) =   3.4197
Prob>chi2 = 0.181
```

Per the Levene test in SAS, the *p*-value is 0.2336; thus, we fail to reject the null hypothesis that the variances are equal. Per the Bartlett test in Stata, the *p*-value is 0.181; therefore, we fail to reject the null hypothesis that the variances are equal. We can proceed with the ANOVA.

B **What are the null and alternative hypotheses for this ANOVA?**

Our null hypothesis is that the average total cholesterol is the same in each of the three BMI categories.

$H_0: \mu_{avg\ wgt} = \mu_{overwgt} = \mu_{obese}$

Our alternative hypothesis is that the average total cholesterol for at least one of the BMI categories is different from the others (at least one group mean is different).

H_1: at least one mean is different

C **What is the estimate of the within-groups variance $\left(s_W^2\right)$? Calculate by hand.**

The within-groups variance is the weighted average of the three BMI categories' sample variances. Use Equation 11.1.

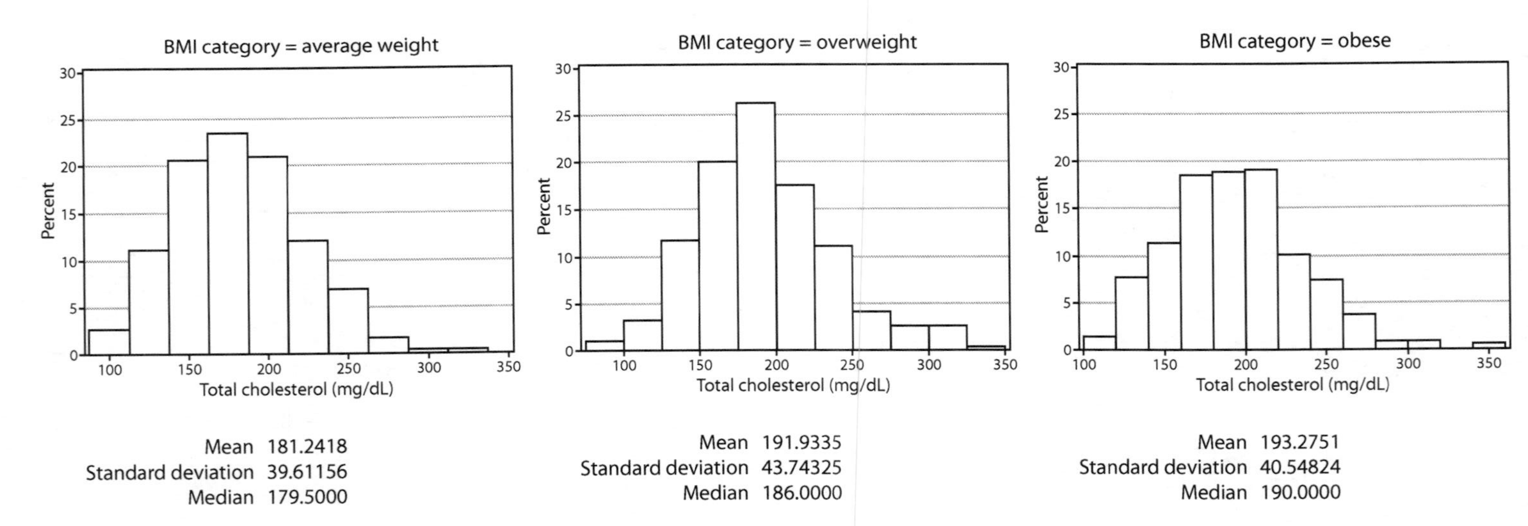

Figure 11.3 **Histogram and statistics for distribution of cholesterol for each BMI group from Example Problem 11.2, using SAS.** This figure displays histograms representing the distribution of cholesterol for each of the three BMI groups. Relevant statistics are reported below the histogram of each group for comparison. This information will help to decide whether we can accept the assumption that the samples from the three populations are normally distributed. "Percent" on the *y*-axis refers to the portion of the sample that has a certain cholesterol level, summing to 100.

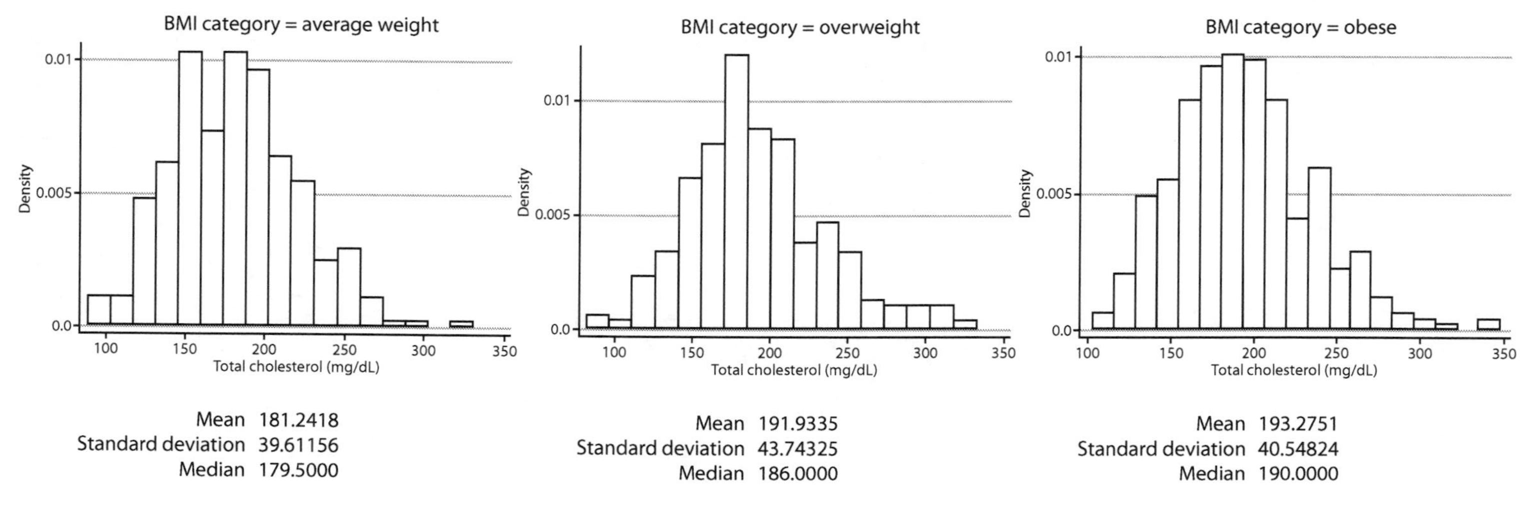

Figure 11.4 **Histogram and statistics for distribution of cholesterol for each BMI group from Example Problem 11.2, using Stata.** This figure displays histograms representing the distribution of cholesterol for each of the three BMI groups. Relevant statistics are reported below the histogram of each group for comparison. This information will help to decide whether we can accept the assumption that the samples from the three populations are normally distributed. "Density" on the *y*-axis refers to the portion of the sample that has a certain cholesterol level, summing to 1.

$$s_W^2 = \frac{(n_{avg\ wgt} - 1)s_{avg\ wgt}^2 + (n_{overwgt} - 1)s_{overwgt}^2 + (n_{obese} - 1)s_{obese}^2}{n_{avg\ wgt} + n_{overwgt} + n_{obese} - k}$$

$$= \frac{(306-1)(39.61156)^2 + (316-1)(43.74325)^2 + (378-1)(40.58424)^2}{306+316+378-3}$$

$$= \frac{478568.08412 + 602743.65498 + 620949.36221}{997}$$

$$= \frac{1702261.10131}{997}$$

$$= 1707.383$$

We can check this calculation using the code in Table 11.5.

Source	DF	Sum of Squares	Mean Square	F-Value	Pr > F
Model	2	28017.344	14008.672	8.20	0.0003
Error	997	1702261.095	1707.383		
Corrected Total	999	1730278.439			

```
                    Analysis of Variance
    Source           SS          df        MS            F      Prob > F
------------------------------------------------------------------------
Between groups   28017.3438       2    14008.6719     8.20     0.0003
Within groups     1702261.1     997    1707.38324
------------------------------------------------------------------------
    Total        1730278.44     999    1732.01045
```

In SAS, the within-groups variance can be found in the ANOVA table, as the mean square error. The mean square (MS) is 1707.383, which is the same as the within-groups variance that we obtained by hand.

Table 11.5 Code for ANOVA (Example Problem 11.2)

SAS code	*Stata code*

`PROC GLM DATA=cholbmi;`
`CLASS bmi_cat;`
`MODEL cholesterol = bmi_cat;`
`RUN;`
	`oneway cholesterol bmi_cat`

In Stata, the within-groups variance can be found in the ANOVA table, as the within-groups mean square (MS). This is 1707.383, which is the same as the within-groups variance that we obtained by hand.

D **What is the estimate of the between-groups variance $\left(s_B^2\right)$? Calculate by hand.**

The between-groups variance is the variation of each BMI category's group mean away from the grand mean.

First, we calculate the grand mean (Equation 11.3), which is the overall average of the 1000 observations.

$$\bar{x} = \frac{(n_{avg\ wgt})\bar{x}_{avg\ wgt} + (n_{overwgt})\bar{x}_{overwgt} + (n_{obese})\bar{x}_{obese}}{n_{avg\ wgt} + n_{overwgt} + n_{obese}}$$

$$= \frac{(306)(181.2418) + (316)(191.9335) + (378)(193.2751)}{306 + 316 + 378}$$

$$= \frac{55459.9908 + 60650.986 + 73057.9878}{1000}$$

$$= \frac{189168.9646}{1000}$$

$$= 189.16896$$

Then, we calculate the variation between each BMI category's mean from the grand mean (Equation 11.2).

$$s_B^2 = \frac{(n_{avg\ wgt})(\bar{x}_{avg\ wgt} - \bar{x})^2 + (n_{overwgt})(\bar{x}_{overwgt} - \bar{x})^2 + (n_{obese})(\bar{x}_{obese} - \bar{x})^2}{k-1}$$

$$= \frac{(306)(181.2418 - 189.16896)^2 + (316)(191.9335 - 189.16896)^2 + (378)(193.2751 - 189.16896)^2}{3-1}$$

$$= \frac{306 \times (-7.92716)^2 + 316 \times (2.76454)^2 + 378 \times (4.10614)^2}{2}$$

$$= \frac{19228.99890 + 2415.08733 + 6373.22580}{2}$$

$$= \frac{28017.31203}{2}$$

$$= 14008.656$$

We can check this calculation using the same ANOVA table output from Example Problem 11.2—Part (C).

In SAS, the between-groups variance can be found in the ANOVA table, as the model mean square. This is 14008.672. This is similar to the between-groups variance that we obtained by hand.

In Stata, the between-groups variance can be found in the ANOVA table, as the between-groups MS. This is 14008.672. This is similar to the between-groups variance that we obtained by hand.

E What is the value of the test statistic? Calculate by hand.

The appropriate test statistic for an ANOVA is the F-statistic.

$$F = \frac{s_B^2}{s_W^2} = \frac{14008.7}{1707.4} = 8.20$$

Referring back to our ANOVA table, we see that in both SAS and Stata that the F-statistic is also 8.20.

F What is the p-value for the test? Draw a conclusion for the test.

The p-value can be obtained from the ANOVA output and is 0.0003.

Alternately, we can approximate the p-value from the F distribution table in the Appendix, Table A.6. There are 2 numerator degrees of freedom (k–1) and 997 denominator degrees of freedom (n–k). From the table, we can use 2 as our numerator degrees of freedom and 120 as our denominator degrees of freedom. The F-statistic that we obtained by hand is between the critical values of 8.18 and 11.38. Therefore, our p-value falls between 0.005 and 0.001.

The p-value, obtained through either method, is less than 0.05 and indicates that we should reject the null hypothesis that the mean total cholesterol is the same for all three BMI categories. At least one group mean is different.

G Given your conclusion, should other tests be conducted? Explain.

If we are interested in which mean is different from the others, we should perform pairwise tests to compare the population means. We will have to perform $\binom{k}{2}$ pairwise tests. Since we have three groups, we will need to perform three pairwise tests and also adjust the α level to correct for multiple testing errors.

H What is the new type I error rate after adjusting for multiple tests?

To adjust for multiple tests, we will use the Bonferroni correction to calculate the new type I error rate (Equation 11.5).

$$\alpha^* = \frac{\alpha}{\binom{k}{2}} = \frac{0.05}{3} = 0.017$$

This result means that in order to reject the null hypothesis that a pairwise difference is statistically significant, the p-value for that t-test must be less than 0.017.

I Perform the pairwise tests. What is your conclusion after the pairwise testing?

To determine which groups are significantly different from each other, we could subset the data and perform a series of t-tests using PROC TTEST (SAS) or *ttest* (Stata). We have previously shown that the equal variances assumption holds, so we would use the pooled method of estimation to obtain the p-values (in SAS). We would, then, compare these p-values to our new type I error rate of 0.017, which we calculated in Example Problem 11.2—Part (H).

Run the following code for each pairwise comparison. There should be three totals: average weight versus overweight, average weight versus obese, and overweight versus obese. First, we compare the "Average weight" and "Overweight"

Table 11.6 SAS code and output for multiple t-tests (Example Problem 11.2)

SAS code / *SAS output*

"Average vs. Overweight"

```
PROC TTEST DATA=cholbmi;
WHERE bmi_cat IN (1,2);
VAR cholesterol;
CLASS bmi_cat;
RUN;
```

Equality of Variance

Method	Num DF	Den DF	F Value	Pr > F
Folded F	315	305	1.22	0.0815

Method	Variances	DF	t Value	Pr > |t|
Pooled	Equal	620	–3.19	0.0015
Satterwaithe	315	305	–3.20	0.0015

"Average vs. Obese"

```
PROC TTEST DATA=cholbmi;
WHERE bmi_cat IN (1,3);
VAR cholesterol;
CLASS bmi_cat;
RUN;
```

Equality of Variance

Method	Num DF	Den DF	F Value	Pr > F
Folded F	377	305	1.05	0.6593

Method	Variances	DF	t Value	Pr > |t|
Pooled	Equal	620	–3.19	0.0015
Satterwaithe	315	305	–3.20	0.0015

"Overweight vs. Obese"

```
PROC TTEST DATA=cholbmi;
WHERE bmi_cat IN (2,3);
VAR cholesterol;
CLASS bmi_cat;
RUN;
```

Equality of Variance

Method	Num DF	Den DF	F Value	Pr > F
Folded F	315	377	1.16	0.1635

Method	Variances	DF	t Value	Pr > |t|
Pooled	Equal	692	–0.42	0.6757
Satterwaithe	Unequal	650.16	–0.42	0.6777

groups. In SAS (Table 11.6), we compare the pooled p-value of 0.0015 to the adjusted type I error rate of 0.017. In Stata (Table 11.7), we compare the p-value (0.0015) for the alternate hypothesis that the difference is not equal to zero (H_a: diff !=0) to the adjusted type I error rate of 0.017. The "Average weight" and "Obese" groups are also significantly different, with a p-value of 0.0015.
Conversely, we could adjust for multiple testing within PROC GLM (SAS) or the *oneway* command (Stata); see code provided in Table 11.8.

Comparisons significant at the 0.05 level are indicated by *.**

bmi_cat Comparison	Difference Between Means	Simultaneous 95% Confidence Limits		
Obese—Overweight	1.342	–6.211	8.894	
Obese—Average weight	12.033	4.414	19.653	***
Overweight—Obese	–1.342	–8.894	6.211	
Overweight—Average weight	10.692	2.745	18.639	***
Average weight—Obese	–12.033	–19.653	–4.414	***
Average weight—Overweight	–10.692	–18.639	–2.745	***

```
Row Mean-|
Col Mean |    Average    Overweig
---------+---------------------
Overweig |     10.6917
         |       0.004
         |
   Obese |     12.0333     1.34159
         |       0.000       1.000
```

Again, we see that the difference between the mean total cholesterol for the overweight and obese groups is not statistically significant, but the mean total cholesterol in the average or less than average-weight group is significantly different from both the overweight and obese groups.

EXAMPLE PROBLEM 11.3

Suppose that we are interested in comparing the HbA1c levels (%) of a sample of patients who receive treatment for their diabetes in a primary safety net clinic.[2] The outcome is the HbA1c level (measured continuously), and the categorical variable is the participant's education status. The analytic sample is made up of the 261 participants who had nonmissing HbA1c levels and education status values. Use the *coh_a1c* dataset to answer the questions. From the study design, we know that the observations are independent. Assume that the HbA1c level is normally distributed in each of the education groups.

Table 11.7 Stata code and output for multiple *t*-tests (Example Problem 11.2)

Stata code and output

"Average vs. Overweight"

```
ttest cholesterol if bmi_cat == 1 | bmi_cat == 2, by(bmi_cat)
                        Two-sample t test with equal variances
   ------------------------------------------------------------------------------
      Group |     Obs        Mean    Std. Err.   Std. Dev.   [95% Conf. Interval]
   ---------+--------------------------------------------------------------------
   Average  |     306    181.2418    2.264442    39.61156    176.7859    185.6977
   Overweig |     316    191.9335     2.46075    43.74325     187.092    196.7751
   ---------+--------------------------------------------------------------------
   combined |     622    186.6736    1.686841     42.0697     183.361    189.9862
   ---------+--------------------------------------------------------------------
       diff |           -10.69171    3.349427               -17.26931   -4.114117
   ------------------------------------------------------------------------------
       diff = mean(Average) - mean(Overweig)                         t =  -3.1921
   Ho: diff = 0                                     degrees of freedom =      620
       Ha: diff < 0                 Ha: diff != 0                 Ha: diff > 0
    Pr(T < t) = 0.0007         Pr(|T| > |t|) = 0.0015          Pr(T > t) = 0.9993
```

"Average vs. Obese"

```
ttest cholesterol if bmi_cat == 1 | bmi_cat == 3, by(bmi_cat)
                        Two-sample t test with equal variances
   ------------------------------------------------------------------------------
      Group |     Obs        Mean    Std. Err.   Std. Dev.   [95% Conf. Interval]
   ---------+--------------------------------------------------------------------
   Average  |     306    181.2418    2.264442    39.61156    176.7859    185.6977
      Obese |     378    193.2751    2.087428    40.58424    189.1707    197.3796
   ---------+--------------------------------------------------------------------
   combined |     684    187.8918     1.55112    40.56706    184.8463    190.9374
   ---------+--------------------------------------------------------------------
       diff |            -12.0333    3.087666               -18.09578   -5.970829
   ------------------------------------------------------------------------------
       diff = mean(Average) - mean(Obese)                            t =  -3.8972
   Ho: diff = 0                                     degrees of freedom =      682
       Ha: diff < 0                 Ha: diff != 0                 Ha: diff > 0
    Pr(T < t) = 0.0001         Pr(|T| > |t|) = 0.0001          Pr(T > t) = 0.9999
```

"Overweight vs. Obese"

```
ttest cholesterol if bmi_cat == 2 | bmi_cat == 3, by(bmi_cat)
                        Two-sample t test with equal variances
   ------------------------------------------------------------------------------
      Group |     Obs        Mean    Std. Err.   Std. Dev.   [95% Conf. Interval]
   ---------+--------------------------------------------------------------------
   Overweig |     316    191.9335     2.46075    43.74325     187.092    196.7751
      Obese |     378    193.2751    2.087428    40.58424    189.1707    197.3796
   ---------+--------------------------------------------------------------------
   combined |     694    192.6643    1.595309    42.02663     189.532    195.7965
   ---------+--------------------------------------------------------------------
       diff |           -1.341588    3.205335               -7.634937    4.951761
   ------------------------------------------------------------------------------
       diff = mean(Overweig) - mean(Obese)                           t =  -0.4185
   Ho: diff = 0                                     degrees of freedom =      692
       Ha: diff < 0                 Ha: diff != 0                 Ha: diff > 0
    Pr(T < t) = 0.3378         Pr(|T| > |t|) = 0.6757          Pr(T > t) = 0.6622
```

Table 11.8 Code for bonferroni correction (Example Problem 11.2)

SAS code	*Stata code*
PROC GLM DATA=cholbmi; CLASS bmi_cat; MODEL cholesterol = bmi_cat; MEANS bmi_cat / BON; RUN;	oneway *cholesterol bmi_cat*, Bonferroni

BOX 11.4 DESCRIPTION OF *coh_a1c* DATASET

The Center for Outpatient Health survey took place in the waiting room of a primary care safety net clinic affiliated with an urban teaching hospital. Eligible participants were 18 years of age or older and English speaking. A researcher abstracted hemoglobin A1c levels (*hba1c*) from consenting participants' medical records. Education was self-reported on the written survey, and the categories were collapsed into three categories for analytic purposes: (1) less than high school degree; (2) high school degree or equivalent; and (3) some college or more education.

We still need to check that the variances in the k populations are equal. We include the HOVTEST option in the MEANS statement of PROC GLM in SAS and examine the Levene test table in the output. In Stata, we examine the Bartlett test p-value. Use the code in Table 11.9 to determine whether the assumption of homogeneity of variances is valid.

A **What is the result of a test for homogeneity of variance in these data?**

Levene's Test for Homogeneity of HbA1c Variance ANOVA of Squared Deviations from Group Means

Source	DF	Sum of Squares	Mean Square	F Value	Pr > F
education	2	571.3	285.6	3.20	0.0423
Error	258	23022.3	89.2336		

```
B Bartlett's test for equal variances:  chi2(2) =  13.3921
Prob>chi2 = 0.001
```

Using the Levene test in SAS, we reject the null hypothesis that the variances are equal because the p-value = 0.0423, which is less than 0.05. Using the Bartlett test in Stata, we reject the null hypothesis that the variances are equal because the p-value = 0.001, which is less than 0.05.

Therefore, we should not proceed with an ANOVA and must use a more robust test. In SAS, we will request the Welch's test by adding the WELCH option to the MEANS statement. In Stata, we will request the W test by first downloading the *wtest* package and then running the *wtest* command. See Table 11.10 for the code.

Table 11.9 Code for testing homogeneity of variance (Example Problem 11.3)

SAS code	*Stata code*

`PROC GLM DATA=coh_a1c;`
`CLASS education;`
`MODEL a1c = education;`
`MEANS education / HOVTEST;`
`RUN;`
	`oneway a1c education`

Table 11.10 Code for welch ANOVA / W test (Example Problem 11.3)

SAS code	*Stata code*

`PROC GLM DATA=coh_a1c;`
`CLASS education;`
`MODEL a1c = education;`
`MEANS education / WELCH;`
`RUN;`
	`findit wtest`
	`Download the wtest package`
	`wtest a1c education`

Welch's ANOVA for HbA1C			
Source	**DF**	**F Value**	**Pr > F**
education	2.0000	0.87	0.4209
Error	129.9		

```
-----------------------------------------------------------------
Dependent Variable is hba1c and Independent Variable is
education
WStat(  2, 129.92) =   0.871, p= 0.4209
-----------------------------------------------------------------
```

B **What is the value of the test statistic, and what is your conclusion for your test? State your *p*-value in your answer.**

The Welch's ANOVA output table displays the adjusted F-statistic and its p-value. The F-statistic is 0.87, with a p-value = 0.4209. The Wtest output displays the adjusted F-statistic and its p-value. The F-statistic is 0.87, with a p-value = 0.4209. Therefore, we fail to reject the null hypothesis and conclude that we do not have evidence to show that any of the means are significantly different from the others.

C **Should you perform multiple pairwise tests? If so, what type I error rate should you use?**

No, you should not perform multiple pairwise tests because you failed to reject the null hypothesis.

PRACTICE PROBLEM 11.1

A What distribution does an ANOVA test statistic follow?

B List the assumptions for an ANOVA.

PRACTICE PROBLEM 11.2

Evaluate the following scenarios, determine whether an ANOVA would be a suitable procedure to analyze the data, and state why or why not.

A We are interested in the rate of incidents that are due to driving while intoxicated (DWI) in a particular city. Researchers would like to know whether these rates differ by educational attainment. A representative sample of citizens are surveyed and divided into four educational attainment groups (i.e., less than high school, high school/GED, some college, college degree or greater). Most participants reported no drunk-driving incidents.

B Researchers would like to investigate the difference in colorectal cancer incidence between men and women in the United States.

C Researchers are conducting a three-arm clinical trial for the treatment of depression. Participants are randomized to one of three treatments (i.e., Drug A, Drug B, or placebo). After six weeks of taking the prescribed treatment, they are assessed for depression severity using a validated continuous scale.

D A sample of patients in an emergency room reported their distress level before seeing a healthcare professional, after seeing the triage nurse, and after being discharged. Researchers would like to compare the mean distress level of these three time points.

PRACTICE PROBLEM 11.3

Birth data can be obtained from the Centers for Disease Control and Prevention.[3] The *National Vital Statistics Report* of the fertility rates in the 50 states in 2014 is summarized by region in Table 11.11.[4] We are interested in comparing fertility rates across the four regions. Use Table 11.11 and the *birthdeath_byregion* dataset to answer the questions.

BOX 11.5 DESCRIPTION OF *birthdeath_byregion* DATASET

The United States Department of Health and Human Services releases annual statistics on births and fetal deaths. The data are reported on the state level and aggregated to the region level. The fertility rate (*fertilityrate*) is the estimated number of births over a woman's lifetime, per 1000 women. The number of deaths (*deaths*) is the estimated number of resident deaths in the 1000s.

Table 11.11 Fertility rate per 1000 women by region (Practice Problem 11.3)

Region	*n*	*Mean*	*Standard deviation*
Midwest	12	67.50	6.30
Northeast	9	54.74	3.60
South	16	63.68	3.58
West	13	67.38	6.30

A State the null and alternate hypotheses.

B Construct 95% confidence intervals for the mean fertility rate per region (refer back to Chapter 6—Equation 6.4). Do you notice anything that suggests that the regions' means may not be the same?

C What is the value of the within-groups variance?

D What is the value of the between-groups variance?

E What are the value and distribution of the test statistic?

F What is your conclusion for your test? State your p-value in your answer.

G Fill in the ANOVA table (Table 11.12).

H Should you perform multiple pairwise tests? If so, what type I error rate should you use?

Table 11.12 Blank ANOVA table for Practice Problem 11.3

Source	*DF*	*Sum of squares*	*Mean square*	*F-value*	*Pr > F*
Model (Between-group)					
Error (Within-group)					
Total					

PRACTICE PROBLEM 11.4

Data on deaths can also be obtained from the Centers for Disease Control and Prevention.[5] The *National Vital Statistics Report* of the number of resident deaths in the 50 states in 2014 is summarized by region in Table 11.13.[4] We are interested in comparing the number of resident deaths across the four regions. Use the *birthdeath_byregion* dataset to answer the questions.

A State the null and alternate hypotheses.

B Construct 95% confidence intervals for the mean number of deaths per region (refer to Chapter 6—Equation 6.4). Do you notice anything that suggests that the regions' means may not be the same?

C What is the value of the within-groups variance?

D What is the value of the between-groups variance?

E What are the value and distribution of the test statistic?

F What is your conclusion for your test? State your p-value in your answer.

G Fill in the ANOVA table (Table 11.14).

H Should you perform multiple pairwise tests? If so, what type I error rate should you use?

PRACTICE PROBLEM 11.5

We selected a random sample of 2000 adults from the NHANES dataset.[1] We categorized the adults into three groups: Those who had never been told they had high blood pressure (n = 1466), those who had been told once (n = 124), and those who had been

Table 11.13 Number of resident deaths in the 1000s by region (Practice Problem 11.4)

Region	n	*Mean*	*Standard deviation*
Midwest	12	50.78	37.30
Northeast	9	52.80	54.03
South	16	63.78	51.16
West	13	39.74	64.03

Table 11.14 Blank ANOVA table for Practice Problem 11.4

Source	*DF*	*Sum of squares*	*Mean square*	*F-value*	*Pr > F*
Model (Between-group)					
Error (Within-group)					
Total					

told two or more times (n = 404). We are interested in how long these adults spend doing sedentary activities in any given day. The sample of participants who had normal blood pressure spent, on average, 409 minutes per day doing sedentary activities, with a standard deviation of 193 minutes. Those who had been told once that they had high blood pressure spent about 410 minutes per day doing sedentary activities, with a standard deviation of 191 minutes. The participants who had been told at least twice that they had high blood pressure engaged in sedentary activities about 447 minutes per day, with a standard deviation of 201 minutes. Use the *anova_pa_htn* dataset to answer the following questions. You may assume that the data are normally distributed.

BOX 11.6 DESCRIPTION OF *anova_pa_htn* DATASET

The *anova_pa_htn* dataset comes from a random sample of 2000 adults who participated in the NHANES. The outcome is minutes of sedentary activity (*sedentary*) in one day, and the grouping variable is how often a participant has been told that he or she has high blood pressure (*bloodpressure*). The grouping variable was created from responses to two questions in the survey: "Have you ever been told by a doctor or other professional that you had high blood pressure?" and "Were you told on two or more different visits that you had high blood pressure?" *Bloodpressure* has three levels: (0) never told had high blood pressure, (1) told once that had high blood pressure, and (2) told at least twice had high blood pressure.

A What code should be specified to test the assumption for homogeneity of variance?

B Conduct an ANOVA, and fill in the ANOVA table using Table 11.15.

C What code did you use to run the ANOVA in Practice Problem 11.5—Part (B)?

D What are the null and alternative hypotheses?

E What are the value and distribution of the test statistic?

Table 11.15 Blank ANOVA table for Practice Problem 11.5

Source	*DF*	*Sum of squares*	*Mean square*	*F-value*	*Pr > F*
Model (Between-group)					
Error (Within-group)					
Total					

F What is your conclusion for your test? State your p-value in your answer.

G Should any additional test be conducted? If so, what test and how many?

H What option should be specified to obtain the adjusted significance of pairwise tests?

I What is the significance level of these tests?

J What is the distribution of the test statistic?

References

1. National Health and Nutrition Examination Survey. Hyattsville, MD: Centers for Disease Control and Prevention, National Center for Health Statistics. 2014. https://wwwn.cdc.gov/Nchs/Nhanes/Search/nhanes13_14.aspx. Accessed August 1, 2016.
2. Fan JH, Lyons S, Goodman MS, Blanchard MS, Kaphingst KA. Relationship between health literacy and unintentional and intentional medication nonadherence in medically underserved patients with type 2 diabetes. *Diabetes Educ*. 2016;42(2):199–208. doi:10.1177/0145721715624969.
3. Hamilton BE, Martin JA, Osterman MJK, Curtin SC, Mathews TJ. *National Vital Statistics Reports: Births: Final Data for 2014*. Hyattsville, MD: National Center for Health Statistics; 2015:64(12). http://www.cdc.gov/nchs/data/nvsr/nvsr64/nvsr64_12.pdf.
4. State and territorial data. Centers for Disease Control and Prevention website. http://www.cdc.gov/nchs/fastats/state-and-territorial-data.htm. Updated October 6, 2016. Accessed October 10, 2016.
5. Kochanek K, Murphy SL, Xu J, Tejada-Vera B. *National Vital Statistics Reports: Deaths: Final Data for 2014*. Hyattsville, MD: National Center for Health Statistics; 2016:65(4). http://www.cdc.gov/nchs/data/nvsr/nvsr65/nvsr65_04.pdf.

12 Correlation

This chapter will focus on linear correlation between two continuous variables and will include the following topics:

- Population correlation coefficient (ρ)
- Pearson correlation coefficient (r)
- Spearman rank correlation coefficient (r_s)

Term

- correlation

Introduction

In Chapter 10, we used the odds ratio (OR) to measure the strength of association between two dichotomous variables. In this chapter, we will use a correlation coefficient to measure the strength of a linear association between two continuous variables.

Population correlation coefficient (ρ)

The population correlation coefficient quantifies the true strength of the linear association between two continuous variables, X and Y. It is denoted using the Greek letter rho (ρ) and is a dimensionless number, meaning that it has no units of measurement. The values for the population correlation coefficient can fall between -1 and 1. A ρ of 0 indicates no linear correlation between the two continuous variables. A positive correlation coefficient indicates a positive linear relationship, whereas a negative correlation coefficient indicates a negative linear relationship. The strength of the correlation ranges from negligible to very high, as shown in Table 12.1.[1]

It is important to note that a ρ of 0 does not imply a lack of a relationship between the two variables; the relationship is just not a linear one (e.g., quadratic as in Figure 12.1c). However, a ρ of 1 or -1 implies that if all the pairs of outcomes (x_i, y_i) were plotted, they would fall on a straight line (an exact linear relationship).

Keep in mind that a strong correlation does not imply causation. In fact, a significant correlation of any magnitude does not necessarily imply causation between the two

Table 12.1 Interpreting the correlation coefficient

Absolute value of correlation coefficient	*Interpretation*
0.90 to 1.00	Very high correlation
0.70 to 0.90	High correlation
0.50 to 0.70	Moderate correlation
0.30 to 0.50	Low correlation
0.00 to 0.30	Negligible correlation

Source: Mukaka, M. M., *Malawi Med J.*, 24(3), 69–71, 2012. doi:10.1016/j.cmpb.2016.01.020.

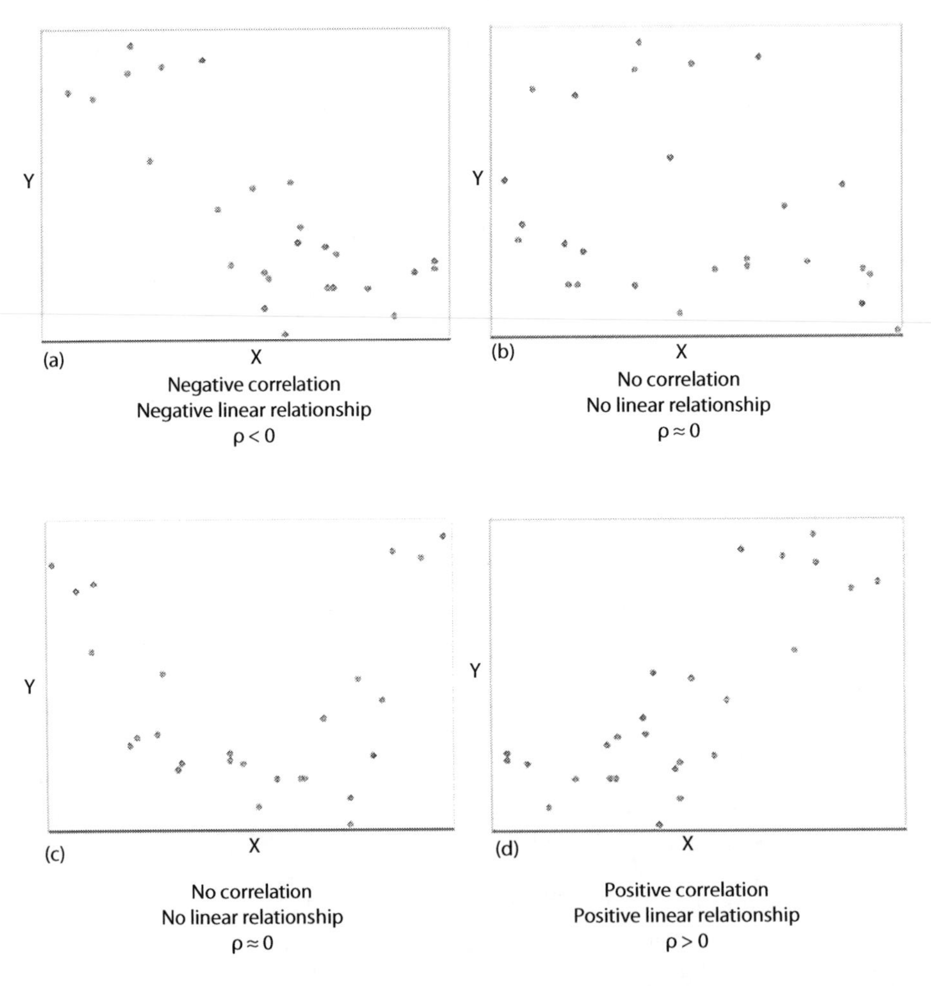

Figure 12.1 **Four correlation coefficients and their implied linear relationships.** Graph (a) shows a negative correlation ($\rho < 0$) between X and Y, implying a negative linear relationship between the X and Y variables. Graph (b) shows no correlation ($\rho \approx 0$), implying no linear relationship between the X and Y variables. Graph (c) also shows no correlation ($\rho \approx 0$), implying no linear relationship between the X and Y variables. The relationship in Graph (c) appears to be quadratic. Graph (d) shows a positive correlation ($\rho > 0$) between X and Y, implying a positive linear relationship between the X and Y variables.

continuous variables X and Y. Correlation will only quantify the association between the two variables; it cannot be used to claim that one variable causes another. Therefore, even when we do observe correlation between two variables, we do not assume the association extends beyond the range of the observed data.

Visualizing correlated data

It is useful to plot the variables to get a quick idea of how the data in the sample are associated. We can see whether the association between our X and Y variables is approximately linear and whether there appears to be a positive or negative correlation present.

We use PROC SGPLOT in SAS with the SCATTER statement or the *scatter* command in Stata to get a visualization of the relationship between the variables in our data (see Table 12.2 for sample code).

Pearson correlation coefficient (r)

To estimate the population correlation, we will calculate a correlation coefficient for a sample of the population. This estimate is known as the Pearson correlation coefficient (r) and can be thought of as the average of the product of the standard normal deviations. In other words, it is calculated using the difference between each pair of outcomes (x_i, y_i) and the respective means $(\bar{x}, \bar{y})$ of the continuous variables X and Y. See Equation 12.1 for the formula:

$$r = \frac{\sum_{i=1}^{n}(x_i - \bar{x})(y_i - \bar{y})}{\sqrt{\sum_{i=1}^{n}(x_i - \bar{x})^2 \sum_{i=1}^{n}(y_i - \bar{y})^2}} \tag{12.1}$$

Like the population correlation, this estimation will quantify only the strength of the linear association. If the relationship between X and Y is nonlinear, correlation will not be a valid measure of the association.

The estimated correlation cannot be extrapolated beyond the observed range of the X and Y variables. The relationship between X and Y may change outside of our observed region, and we, therefore, must limit our conclusions to the observed range of the variables.

We can, then, use the sample correlation coefficient to test the null hypothesis that no correlation exists in the population. Our null hypothesis is that the true population correlation is equal to zero.

Table 12.2 Code for scatterplot to visualize correlated data

SAS code	*Stata code*

`PROC SGPLOT DATA = dataset;`
`SCATTER Y = var_1 X = var_2;`
`RUN;`
	`scatter` *`var_1 var_2`*

H_0: $\rho = 0$

H_1: $\rho \neq 0$

To test the null hypothesis, we must meet two assumptions:

1 The pairs of observations X and Y are obtained randomly.
2 The pairs of observations X and Y are normally distributed.

We use a test statistic (Equation 12.2) that follows a t-distribution with $n - 2$ degrees of freedom.

$$t = r\sqrt{\frac{n-2}{1-r^2}} \tag{12.2}$$

Once we obtain the critical value t, we can compare it to the t table in Appendix Table A.4 to find our p-value and determine whether we should reject or fail to reject our null hypothesis. A failure to reject the null hypothesis (and conclude that the population correlation is not different from 0) would not imply that our variables X and Y are independent. A rejection of the null hypothesis only implies that the nature of the relationship between the two variables is linear.

Using SAS to calculate the Pearson correlation coefficient

We use PROC CORR to calculate the Pearson correlation coefficient for pairs of variables. When k variables are specified in the VAR statement, SAS will display a $k \times k$ table with the correlation coefficients and p-values for each pair of variables.

When using the following code, the output will be a 2 × 2 table with the Pearson correlation coefficient and significance for the association between two variables (*var_1* and *var_2*).

```
PROC CORR DATA = dataset;
    VAR var_1 var_2;
RUN;
```

The first output table (Simple Statistics) is a summary statistics table of each of the input variables. This table contains useful statistics such as the mean, standard deviation, minimum, and maximum for each variable.

Simple Statistics						
Variable	N	Mean	Std Dev	Sum	Minimum	Maximum
var_1	10	0.52135	0.26692	5.21346	0.07968	0.96353
var_2	10	0.48251	0.26385	4.82505	0.16525	0.95988

The second table (Pearson Correlation Coefficients) is the $k \times k$ table of the Pearson correlation coefficient and, below that, the p-value addressing the test of the null hypothesis that there is no correlation. The values are symmetric along the diagonal. For example, the correlation coefficient between *var_1* and *var_2* is −0.17587, and the p-value is 0.6270. We can conclude that there is a negligible and nonsignificant relationship between *var_1* and *var_2*.

Pearson Correlation Coefficients, N = 10
Prob > |r| under H0: Rho = 0

	var_1	var_2
var_1	1.00000	−0.17587
		0.6270
var_2	−0.17587	1.00000
	0.6270	

The following table is an extension of the 2 × 2 table, to include four variables. The first row of the table shows the relationship between *var_1* and the other variables (including itself), the second row shows the relationship between *var_2* and all of the other variables (including itself), and so on.

Pearson Correlation Coefficients, N = 10
Prob > |r| under H0: Rho = 0

	var_1	var_2	var_3	var_k
var_1	1.00000	−0.17587	0.09700	−0.20123
		0.6270	0.7898	0.5772
var_2	−0.17587	1.00000	0.12614	−0.24910
	0.6270		0.7284	0.4877
var_3	0.09700	0.12614	1.00000	−0.13877
	0.7898	0.7284		0.7022
var_k	−0.20123	−0.24910	−0.13877	1.00000
	0.5772	0.4877	0.7022	

Testing a different "Null" hypothesis about the Pearson correlation coefficient, using SAS

Occasionally, we are interested in determining whether the correlation in our data is similar to an established correlation in the literature. In this case, testing the correlation of our data against the population correlation coefficient of 0 is not as useful. To change the null population correlation coefficient to a different value, use the option of the Fisher Z transformation with RHO0 = *value*. The value must be between −1 and 1. This option can be used only when calculating a Pearson correlation coefficient.

To investigate whether the correlation in the data is significantly different from 0.7, we would run the following code:

```
PROC CORR DATA = dataset FISHER(RHO0=0.7);
     VAR var_1 var_2;
RUN;
```

Pearson Correlation Statistics (Fisher's z Transformation)

Variable	With Variable	N	Sample Correlation	Fisher's z	Bias Adjustment	Correlation Estimate	95% Confidence Limits		H0:Rho = Rho0 Rho0	p-Value
var_1	var_2	10	–0.17587	–0.17771	–0.00977	–0.16638	–0.720527	0.517452	0.7	0.0041

From the output, we look at the last two columns to see whether we should reject or fail to reject our null hypothesis that the correlation in the data is significantly different from the population correlation coefficient of 0.7. The last column shows that the *p*-value for Rho0 is 0.0041, which is less than 0.05. We can reject the null hypothesis and determine that the correlation in our data is significantly different from 0.7.

Using Stata to calculate the Pearson correlation coefficient

We use the *pwcorr* command with the *sig* option to calculate the Pearson correlation coefficient for pairs of variables. If *k* variables are specified in the variable list, Stata will display a $k \times k$ table with the correlation coefficients and *p*-values for each pair of variables.

When using the following code, the output will be a 2×2 table with the Pearson correlation coefficient and significance for the association between two variables (*var_1* and *var_2*).

```
pwcorr var_1 var_2, sig
```

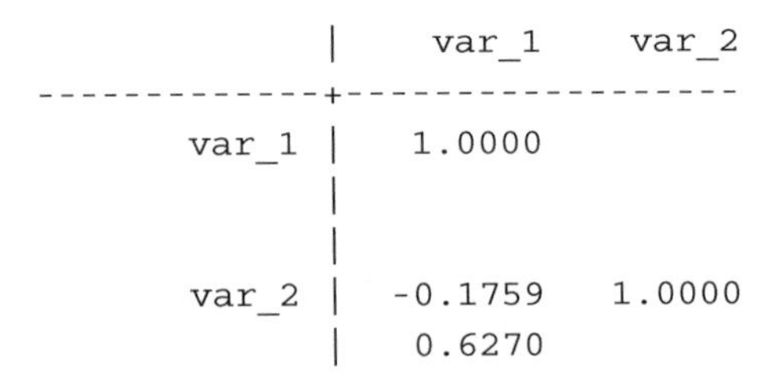

```
             |    var_1     var_2
-------------+------------------
       var_1 |   1.0000
             |
             |
       var_2 |  -0.1759    1.0000
             |   0.6270
```

The top value in the table is the Pearson correlation coefficient and, below that, the *p*-value addressing the null hypothesis that there is no correlation. For example, the correlation coefficient between *var_1* and *var_2* is –0.1759, and the *p*-value is 0.6270. We can conclude that there is a negligible and nonsignificant relationship between *var_1* and *var_2*.

The following Stata output table is an extension of the 2×2 table, to include four variables. The first column of the table shows the relationship between *var_1* and the other variables (including itself), the second column shows the relationship between *var_2* and all of the other variables (including itself), and so on.

```
             |    var_1      var_2      var_3      var_k
-------------+----------------------------------------
       var_1 |   1.0000
             |
             |
       var_2 |  -0.1759     1.0000
             |   0.6270
             |
       var_3 |   0.0970     0.1261     1.0000
             |   0.7898     0.7284
             |
       var_k |  -0.2012    -0.2491    -0.1388     1.0000
             |   0.5772     0.4877     0.7022
```

EXAMPLE PROBLEM 12.1

Suppose that we wish to examine the relationship between weight and the HbA1c levels of adults.[2] The values for a random sample of 15 adults appear in Table 12.3, as well as scatterplots of the data (Figure 12.2). Assume the data are approximately normally distributed.

BOX 12.1 DESCRIPTION OF EXAMPLE PROBLEM 12.1 DATA

The Center for Outpatient Health survey took place in the waiting room of a primary care safety net clinic affiliated with an urban teaching hospital. Eligible participants were aged 18 years or older and English speaking. A researcher abstracted hemoglobin A1c (*hba1c*) and weight (*weight*) from consenting participants' medical records. This dataset contains a random sample of 15 adult participants with reported values for HbA1c and weight.

We can see from the scatterplots (Figures 12.2a,b) that there is a decrease in HbA1c that corresponds to an increase in weight. There appears to be a negative correlation. The distribution looks approximately linear.

To determine the correlation of our sample, we calculate the Pearson correlation coefficient. First, we will calculate the mean of our X variable (*weight*) and our Y variable (*HbA1c*). This is displayed in the last row of Table 12.4 (columns 2 and 5). Then, we will calculate $x_i - \bar{x}$ and $y_i - \bar{y}$ for each observation, as shown in columns 3 and 6 of Table 12.4.

Next, we will take the product of $x_i - \bar{x}$ and $y_i - \bar{y}$, as shown in Table 12.4, column 8. To get the numerator for the Pearson correlation coefficient, we sum that calculated product over all observations (last row of column 8).

The final component is the calculation of each observation's squared deviation from the mean (Table 12.4, columns 4 and 7).

Table 12.3 HbA1c and weight in an adult sample

ID	*Weight (pounds)*	*HbA1c level (%)*
126	269	7.3
177	120	12.1
193	224	7.5
207	223	9.4
283	211	5.9
308	307	5.5
354	296	7.2
362	111	7.8
368	162	6.9
703	187	7.4
728	230	6.5
810	238	6.8
871	252	7.6
967	163	10.3
994	341	6.6

We now have all the components to calculate the Pearson correlation coefficient, using Equation 12.1.

$$r = \frac{\sum_{i=1}^{n}(x_i - \bar{x})(y_i - \bar{y})}{\sqrt{\sum_{i=1}^{n}(x_i - \bar{x})^2 \sum_{i=1}^{n}(y_i - \bar{y})^2}} = \frac{-934.2}{\sqrt{61447 * 41.8}} = \frac{-934.2}{1601.7} = -0.58 \quad (12.3)$$

We can, then, test our hypothesis that no correlation exists in the total population using our test statistic, calculated from Equation 12.2.

$$t = r\sqrt{\frac{n-2}{1-r^2}} = -0.58\sqrt{\frac{15-2}{1-(-0.58)^2}} = -2.59 \quad (12.4)$$

Because the t-distribution is symmetrical, we know that the probability of falling below a critical value of −2.59 corresponds to the probability of falling above a critical value of 2.59. Using the t table in Appendix Table A.4, with $n - 2 = 13$ degrees of freedom, we can see that our test statistic of 2.59 is between 2.160 ($p = 0.025$) and 2.650 ($p = 0.01$). Because these are the p-values for the upper tail, we double them and determine that p is between 0.05 and 0.02. These values are below our cutoff of 0.05. We, therefore, reject the null hypothesis that there is no correlation ($\rho = 0$) and conclude that weight and HbA1c levels are significantly correlated. We can check our work using the code in Table 12.5 and the *corr_hba1c* dataset.

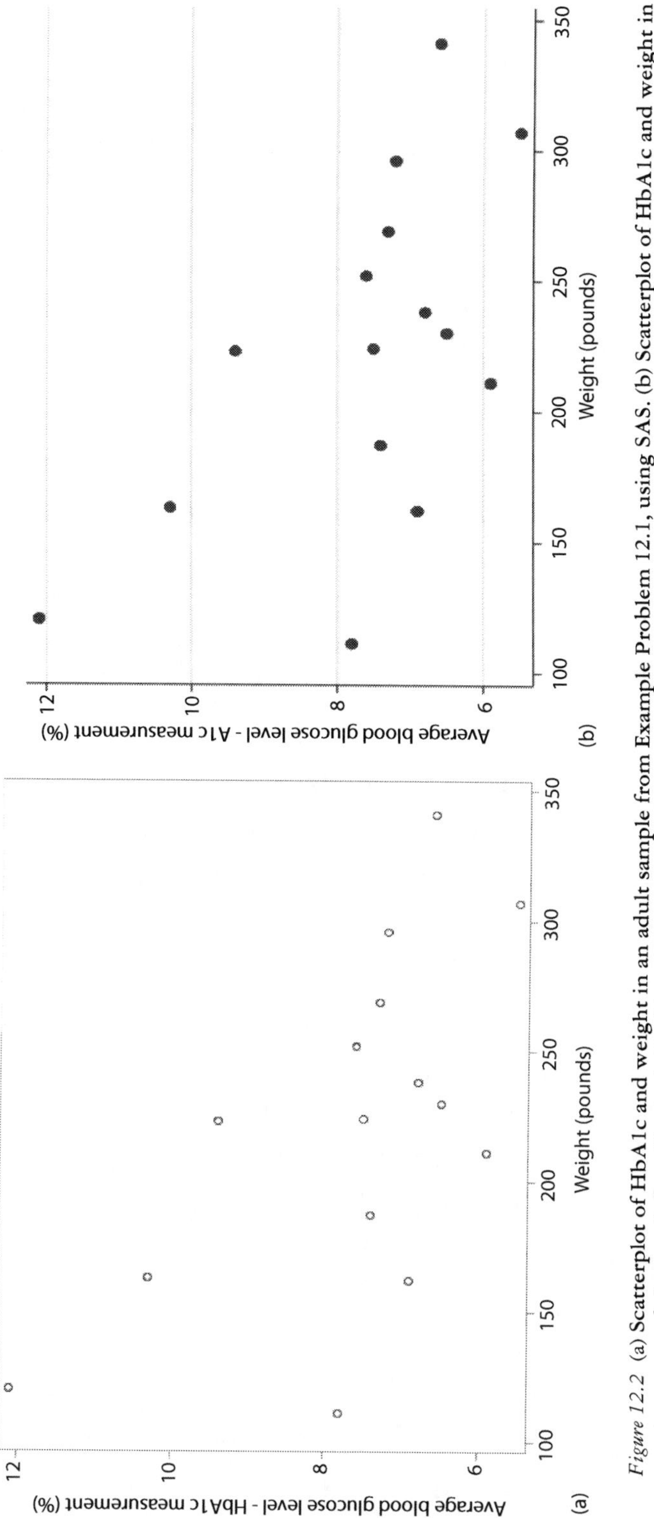

Figure 12.2 **(a) Scatterplot of HbA1c and weight in an adult sample from Example Problem 12.1, using SAS. (b) Scatterplot of HbA1c and weight in an adult sample from Example Problem 12.1, using Stata.** The scatterplot shows the relationship between the HbA1c and weight of the subjects.

Table 12.4 Hand calculation of Pearson correlation coefficient

ID	*Weight (X)*	$(x_i - \bar{x})$	$(x_i - \bar{x})^2$	*HbA1c (Y)*	$(y_i - \bar{y})$	$(y_i - \bar{y})^2$	$(x_i - \bar{x})*(y_i - \bar{y})$
126	269	46.7	2180.9	7.3	–0.4	0.2	–18.7
177	120	–102.3	10465.3	12.1	4.4	19.4	–450.1
193	224	1.7	2.9	7.5	–0.2	0.0	–0.3
207	223	0.7	0.5	9.4	1.7	2.9	1.2
283	211	–11.3	127.7	5.9	–1.8	3.2	20.3
308	307	84.7	7174.1	5.5	–2.2	4.8	–186.3
354	296	73.7	5431.7	7.2	–0.5	0.3	–36.9
362	111	–111.3	12387.7	7.8	0.1	0.0	–11.1
368	162	–60.3	3636.1	6.9	–0.8	0.6	48.2
703	187	–35.3	1246.1	7.4	–0.3	0.1	10.6
728	230	7.7	59.3	6.5	–1.2	1.4	–9.2
810	238	15.7	246.5	6.8	–0.9	0.8	–14.1
871	252	29.7	882.1	7.6	–0.1	0.0	–3.0
967	163	–59.3	3516.5	10.3	2.6	6.8	–154.2
994	341	118.7	14089.7	6.6	–1.1	1.2	–130.6
	$\bar{x}$ = 222.3		Σ = 61447.0	$\bar{y}$ = 7.7		Σ = 41.8	Σ = –934.2

Table 12.5 Code for calculating the Pearson correlation coefficient (Example Problem 12.1)

SAS code	*Stata code*

`PROC CORR DATA = corr_hba1c;`
`VAR weight hba1c;`
`RUN;`
	`pwcorr weight hba1c, sig`

We get the following 2 × 2 correlation table (output table), depending on which software you use.

Pearson Correlation Coefficients, N = 15 Prob > |r| under H0: Rho = 0		
	Weight	**HbA1C**
Weight Subject's Weight, pounds	1.00000	–0.58350 0.0224
HbA1C Average Blood Glucose Level—HbA1c measurement, %	–0.58350 0.0224	1.00000

```
             |   weight    hba1c
-------------+------------------
      weight |   1.0000
             |
             |
       hba1c |  -0.5835   1.0000
             |   0.0224
             |
```

The Pearson correlation coefficient is −0.58, which is equal to our hand-calculated coefficient. The p-value is 0.0224, which falls within our calculated p-value range.

EXAMPLE PROBLEM 12.2

A random sample of countries was taken from the World Health Organization's Global Health Observatory (GHO) data repository.[3,4] We are interested in the association between the availability of family planning and the total fertility rate in rural residence areas of these sampled countries. Our X variable is a percent of demand for family planning that has been satisfied, and our Y variable is the total fertility rate per woman (Table 12.6). Use the *familyplanning* dataset (Box 12.2).

BOX 12.2 DESCRIPTION OF THE *familyplanning* DATASET

The Global Health Observatory (GHO) is a repository of health-related data from over 194 countries. The *familyplanning* dataset contains data on reproductive health in rural areas of 13 countries in 2012. Demand for family planning satisfied (*familyplan*) is the percent of women of reproductive age who are sexually active and who have their need for family planning satisfied with modern methods. This is a measure of contraception coverage. Total fertility rate per woman (*fertilityrate*) is the number of children who would be born per woman during her childbearing years if she kept to a schedule of age-specific fertility rates.

First, we visualize the data to get an idea of the association between our variables (Figure 12.3). See Table 12.7 for code.

BOX 12.3 LABEL DATA VALUES

In SAS, using the DATALABEL= option allows us to see which countries are at the low or high end of our data.

In Stata, the mlabel (*variable_name*) allows us to see which countries are at the low or high end of our data. This is not a necessary option, but produces graphs that allow for interpretation in context of the data.

Table 12.6 Family planning and fertility rate in rural residential areas

Country	*Demand for family planning satisfied (%)*	*Total fertility rate (per woman)*
Comoros	29.1792	4.84204
Gabon	39.8277	5.89397
Guinea	16.6430	6.07371
Haiti	48.2659	4.38506
Indonesia	88.9133	2.68521
Jordan	87.2955	3.87219
Kyrgyzstan	65.5658	3.88812
Mali	24.7210	6.78738
Niger	42.3201	8.23990
Pakistan	60.1399	4.44694
Peru	88.8425	3.58494
Senegal	25.8924	6.49117
Tajikistan	53.1131	3.76948

We can see a slight negative trend in our data but cannot draw any statistical conclusions or quantify the relationship.

Next, we will calculate the Pearson correlation coefficient using the code in Table 12.8.

Pearson Correlation Coefficients, N = 13
Prob > |r| under H0: Rho = 0

	FamilyPlan	**FertilityRate**
FamilyPlan	1.00000	–0.75185
Demand for Family Planning Satisfied, %		0.0030
FertilityRate	–0.75185	1.00000
Total Fertility Rate, children per woman	0.0030	

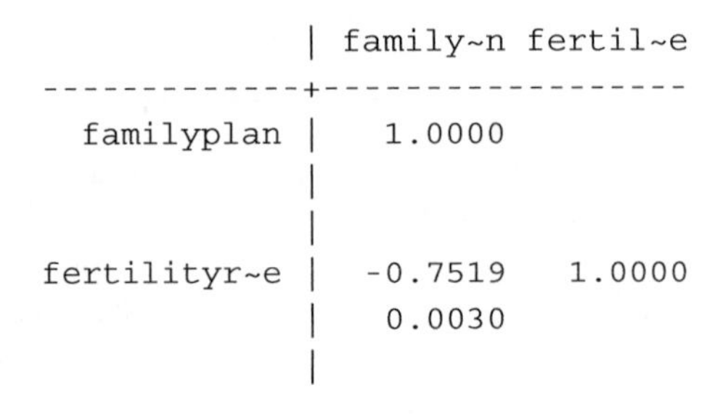

```
             | family~n fertil~e
-------------+------------------
  familyplan |   1.0000
             |
             |
fertilityr~e |  -0.7519   1.0000
             |   0.0030
             |
```

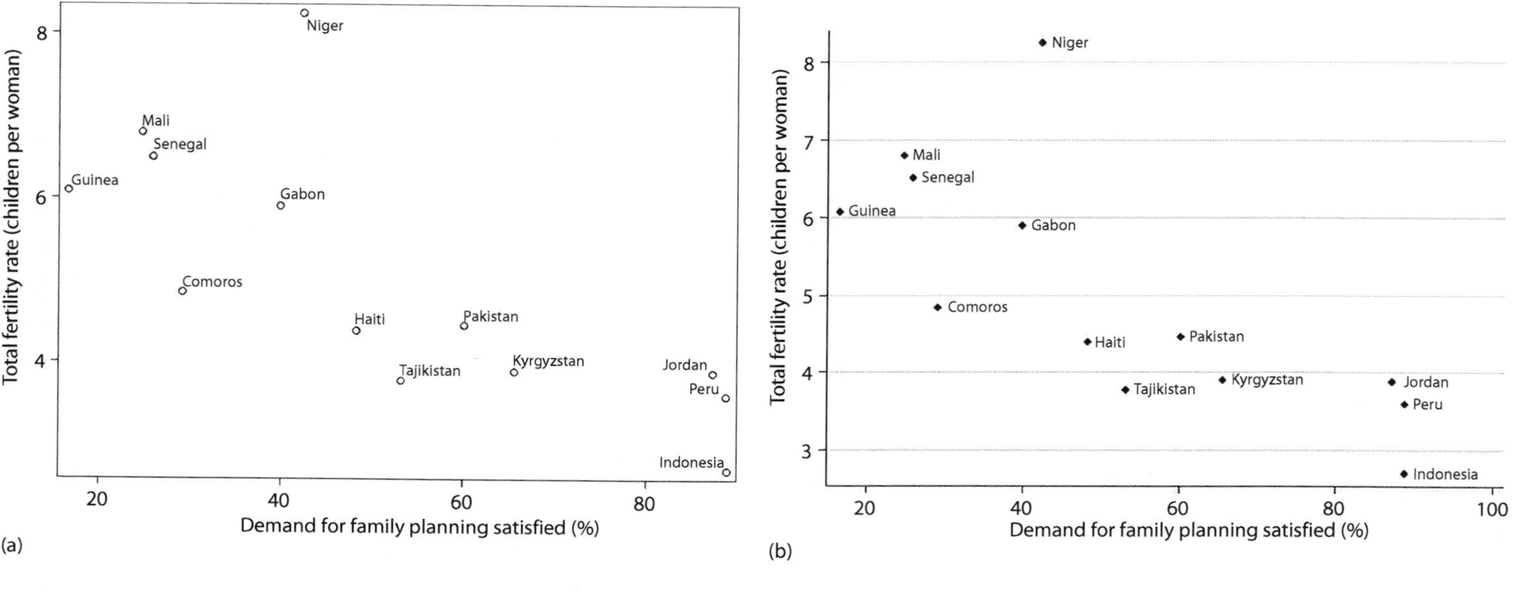

Figure 12.3 **(a) Scatterplot of satisfied demand for family planning and total fertility rate from Example Problem 12.2, using SAS. (b) Scatterplot of satisfied demand for family planning and total fertility rate from Example Problem 12.2, using Stata.** The scatterplot shows the relationship between the percent of demanded family planning that was satisfied and the total fertility rate of each country.

Table 12.7 Code for scatterplot (Example Problem 12.2)

SAS code	*Stata code*

`PROC SGPLOT DATA = familyplanning;`
`SCATTER Y = fertilityrate X =`
`familyplan / DATALABEL=country;`
`RUN;`
	`scatter fertilityrate`
	`familyplan, mlabel(country)`

Table 12.8 Code to calculate the Pearson correlation coefficient (Example Problem 12.2)

SAS code	*Stata code*

`PROC CORR DATA = familyplanning;`
`VAR familyplan fertilityrate;`
`RUN;`
	`pwcorr familyplan`
	`fertilityrate, sig`

From the output table, we can see that the Pearson correlation coefficient is −0.75. This implies a strong, negative correlation between satisfied demand for family planning and total fertility rate. This conclusion corresponds to our observations from the scatterplot. The *p*-value is 0.0030 for the test to determine whether there is correlation between our two variables in the population. The *p*-value is less than 0.05, so we reject our null hypothesis and determine that satisfied demand for family planning and total fertility rate are significantly correlated.

PRACTICE PROBLEM 12.1

During the diagnosis and treatment of renal and liver diseases, doctors frequently use creatinine and albumin measurements. A battery of measurements was taken using serum specimens on a probability sample of the civilian noninstitutionalized population of the United States as part of the National Health and Nutrition Examination Survey (NHANES).[5] Using a random sample of 250 respondents (the *biochem* dataset, see Box 12.4), answer the questions.

BOX 12.4 DESCRIPTION OF *biochem* DATASET

The laboratory component of the 2014 National Health and Nutrition Examination Survey (NHANES) collects a standard biochemistry profile. Albumin (*albumin*) is a continuous variable and is measured in g/dL. Creatinine (*creatinine*) is a continuous variable and is measured in mg/dL.

A What can you say about the relationship between the two serum measurements (creatinine and albumin) based on the scatterplots in Figure 12.4?

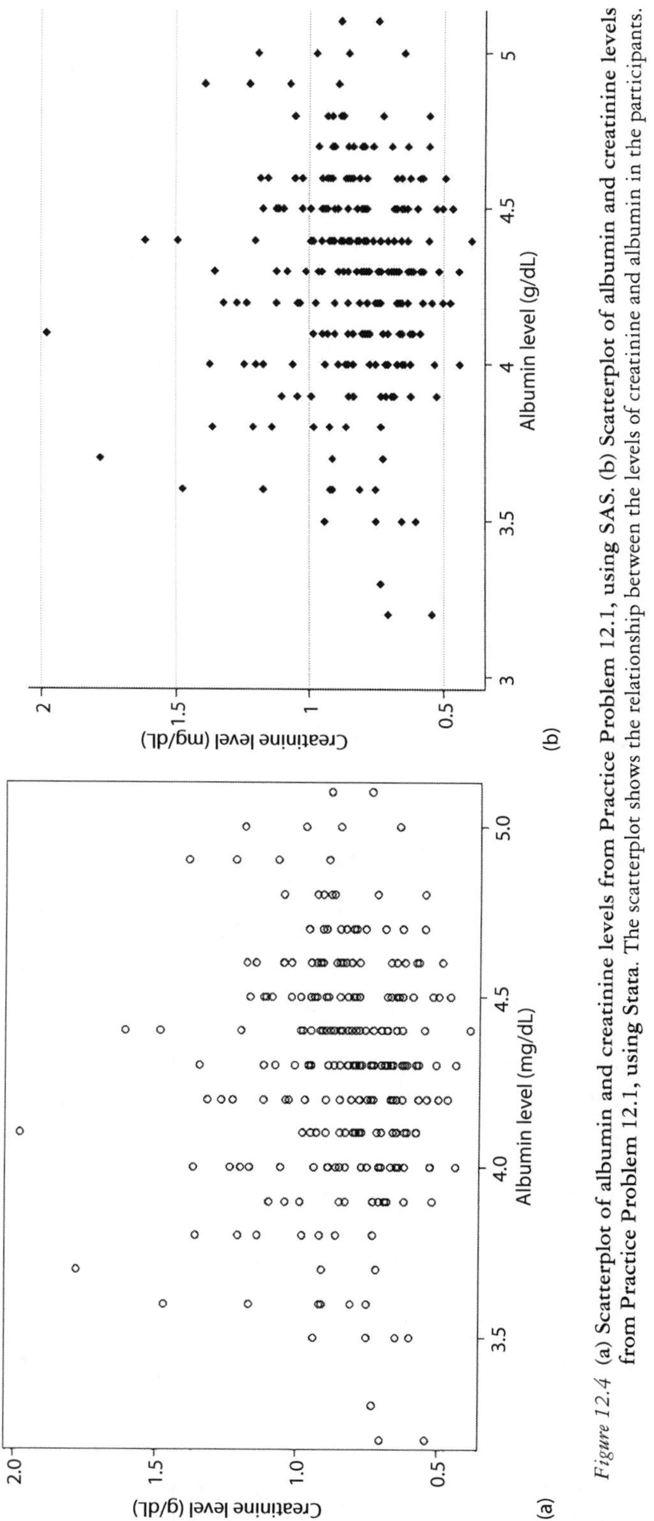

Figure 12.4 **(a) Scatterplot of albumin and creatinine levels from Practice Problem 12.1, using SAS. (b) Scatterplot of albumin and creatinine levels from Practice Problem 12.1, using Stata.** The scatterplot shows the relationship between the levels of creatinine and albumin in the participants.

B What is the Pearson correlation coefficient for these data? Use the following SAS or Stata output.

Pearson Correlation Coefficients, N = 250 Prob > |r| under H0: Rho = 0		
	Albumin	**Creatinine**
albumin	1.00000	0.01067
Albumin Level, g/dL		0.8667
creatinine	0.01067	1.00000
Creatinine Level, mg/dL	0.8667	

```
             | creatinine  albumin
-------------+--------------------
  creatinine |    1.0000
             |
             |
     albumin |    0.0107    1.0000
             |    0.8667
             |
```

C Is there a significant linear relationship between creatinine and albumin levels based on these data? Why or why not?

Spearman rank correlation coefficient (r_s)

The Pearson correlation coefficient is a widely used measure of correlation, but it is sensitive to outliers. This means that it can be heavily influenced by observations that are extremely distant from the other observations in the sample. If the data we are interested in analyzing have outliers, it might be best to use a nonparametric correlation, such as the Spearman rank correlation coefficient (r_s). As a nonparametric measure, the Spearman rank correlation coefficient uses the ranked values of X and Y instead of the actual values of X and Y. Thus, the Spearman rank correlation coefficient is a more robust (i.e., not as sensitive to outliers) estimate of the population correlation than the Pearson correlation coefficient. However, the Spearman rank correlation coefficient is less powerful when the data are normally distributed. The Spearman rank correlation coefficient can also be used when one or more variables are ordinal, whereas the Pearson correlation coefficient is appropriate only when both variables are continuous.

As with the Pearson correlation coefficient, values of the Spearman rank correlation coefficient that are near 0 imply a lack of linear association between X and Y. Values that are close to the extremes of -1 or 1 indicate a high degree of correlation between the variables. The strength of the correlation is interpreted in the same manner as with the Pearson correlation coefficient (see Table 12.1).

The Spearman rank correlation coefficient can be calculated in the same general way as the Pearson correlation coefficient, but by using the ranked values of X and Y (x_{ri}, y_{ri}) instead of x_i and y_i. We rank X and Y independently, giving the rank of 1 to the lowest value of each variable and n to the highest. In the event of a tie, we take the average of the ranks that the observations would have otherwise occupied. For example, if two observations were tied for the fourth rank, they would each be given a rank of 4.5. This is the average of ranks 4 and 5, which are the ranks that the two observations would have occupied.

Equation 12.5 computes the Spearman rank correlation coefficient, where x_{ri} and y_{ri} are the ranks associated with the ith observation (rather than the actual values of x_i and y_i).

$$r_s = \frac{\sum_{i=1}^{n} (x_{ri} - \bar{x}_r)(y_{ri} - \bar{y}_r)}{\sqrt{\left[\sum_{i=1}^{n} (x_{ri} - \bar{x}_r)^2\right]\left[\sum_{i=1}^{n} (y_{ri} - \bar{y}_r)^2\right]}} \tag{12.5}$$

An equivalent method for computing r_s is provided by Equation 12.6, where d_i is the difference between the rank of x_i and y_i, and n is the number of data points in the sample.

$$r_s = 1 - \frac{6\sum_{i=1}^{n} d_i^2}{n(n^2 - 1)} \tag{12.6}$$

As with the Pearson correlation coefficient, we can test the null hypothesis that no correlation exists in the population. Our null hypothesis is that the true population correlation is equal to 0.

$$H_0\text{: } \rho = 0$$

$$H_1\text{: } \rho \neq 0$$

The test statistic (Equation 12.7) to test this null hypothesis, like with the Pearson correlation coefficient test, follows a t-distribution with $n - 2$ degrees of freedom. The test also assumes that the pairs of observations, X and Y, were obtained randomly. However, X and Y do not need to be normally distributed because the Spearman rank correlation coefficient is a nonparametric measure, and this is a nonparametric test. Use this test statistic only if there are at least 10 observations in your dataset.

$$t = r_s\sqrt{\frac{n-2}{1-r_s^2}} \tag{12.7}$$

Using SAS to calculate Spearman rank correlation coefficient

SAS will calculate the Spearman rank correlation coefficient for a set of variables, along with the p-value associated with testing the null hypothesis that the population correlation coefficient is 0. The output generated will be similar in format to the output obtained with the Pearson correlation coefficient. The default correlation in PROC

CORR is Pearson, but we can obtain the $k \times k$ table of the Spearman rank correlation coefficients and p-values by specifying the SPEARMAN option.

```
PROC CORR DATA = dataset SPEARMAN;
    VAR var_1 var_2;
RUN;
```

As before, the output is a $k \times k$ table of the Spearman rank correlation coefficient and, below that, the p-value addressing the null hypothesis that there is no correlation. The values are symmetric along the diagonal. For example, the correlation coefficient between *var_1* and *var_2* is −0.16364, and the p-value is 0.6515. We can conclude that there is a negligible and nonsignificant relationship between *var_1* and *var_2*.

Spearman Correlation Coefficients, N = 10 Prob > |r| under H0: Rho = 0		
	var_1	var_2
var_1	1.00000	-0.16364 0.6515
var_2	-0.16364 0.6515	1.00000

Using Stata to calculate Spearman rank correlation coefficient

Stata will calculate the Spearman rank correlation coefficient for a pair of variables and the p-value associated with testing the null hypothesis that the population correlation coefficient is 0 with the *spearman* command. For a pair of variables, the output presented will be a summary of the number of observations, the estimate of the correlation coefficient, and the p-value.

```
spearman var_1 var_2
```

To obtain the k-by-k table that we obtained when calculating the Pearson correlation coefficient output, we specify the *stats(rho p)* option. With this option specified, the output generated will be similar in format to the output obtained with the Pearson correlation coefficient.

```
spearman var_1 var_2 var_3 var_k, stats(rho p)
```

For a pair of variables, the *spearman* command generates the following output. For example, the correlation coefficient (*Spearman's rho*) between *var_1* and *var_2* is −0.1636, and the p-value (Prob > |t|) is 0.6515. We can conclude that there is a negligible and nonsignificant relationship between *var_1* and *var_2*.

```
Number of obs =         10
Spearman's rho =        -0.1636

Test of Ho: var_1 and var_2 are independent
    Prob > |t| =          0.6515
```

For *k* variables, the *spearman* command generates the following default output. It displays only the correlation coefficients; if you want to also have *p*-values in the output, include the *stats(rho p)* option. The first column of the table shows the relationship between *var_1* and the other variables (including itself), the second column shows the relationship between *var_2* and all of the other variables (including itself), and so on.

```
             |   var_1     var_2     var_3     var_k
-------------+------------------------------------
      var_1  |  1.0000
      var_2  | -0.1636    1.0000
      var_3  |  0.1758   -0.1030    1.0000
      var_k  | -0.2364   -0.4303   -0.0061    1.0000
```

EXAMPLE PROBLEM 12.3

Revisiting Example Problem 12.1, we would like to recalculate our correlation coefficient nonparametrically. First, we will rank each *X* observation and then rank each *Y* observation, with 1 being the rank of the smallest value and 15 being the rank of the largest value. In this dataset, there are no ties.

We, then, will compute the difference between each observation's *X* and *Y* rank (d_i) and square that difference (Table 12.9). We will need the sum of the individual squared differences to compute the Spearman rank correlation coefficient.

We will now compute the Spearman rank correlation coefficient, using Equation 12.6.

Table 12.9 Computing the difference in ranks by hand for Example Problem 12.3

ID	*Weight (X)*	*X Rank* (x_{ri})	*HbA1C (Y)*	*Y Rank* (y_{ri})	d_i	d_i^2
126	269	12	7.3	8	4	16
177	120	2	12.1	15	–13	169
193	224	8	7.5	10	–2	4
207	223	7	9.4	13	–6	36
283	211	6	5.9	2	4	16
308	307	14	5.5	1	13	169
354	296	13	7.2	7	6	36
362	111	1	7.8	12	–11	121
368	162	3	6.9	6	–3	9
703	187	5	7.4	9	–4	16
728	230	9	6.5	3	6	36
810	238	10	6.8	5	5	25
871	252	11	7.6	11	0	0
967	163	4	10.3	14	–10	100
994	341	15	6.6	4	11	121
						$\Sigma = 874$

$$r_s = 1 - \frac{6\sum_{i=1}^{n} d_i^2}{n(n^2-1)} = 1 - \frac{6(874)}{15\left((15)^2-1\right)} = 1 - \frac{5244}{3360} = -0.56$$

The correlation is negative and moderately strong. This coefficient is also similar to our previously calculated Pearson correlation coefficient. We can calculate our test statistic (Equation 12.7) to test our null hypothesis that our two variables are uncorrelated.

$$t = r_s\sqrt{\frac{n-2}{1-r_s^2}} = -0.56\sqrt{\frac{15-2}{1-(-0.56)^2}} = -2.44$$

Due to the symmetrical nature of the t-distribution, the probability of falling below the critical value of –2.44 is equivalent to the probability of being above the critical value of 2.44. Referencing the t table in Appendix Table A.4, with $n - 2 = 13$ degrees of freedom, we find that our test statistic of 2.44 is between 2.160 ($p = 0.025$) and 2.650 ($p = 0.01$). We must double the p-values because they are only for the probability in the upper tail. Thus, we determine p is between 0.05 and 0.02. We, therefore, reject the null hypothesis that there is no correlation ($\rho = 0$) and conclude that weight and HbA1c levels are significantly correlated.

EXAMPLE PROBLEM 12.4

We are interested in the association between diphtheria tetanus toxoid and pertussis (DTP3) immunization coverage and the mortality rate of children younger than 5 years. The dataset *corr_dtp3* comprises data from 194 countries in the GHO data repository that reported on both measures in 2014.[6,7] (See Box 12.5.) Upon examining the data (Figures 12.5 and 12.6), we can see that neither the immunization variable nor the mortality rate variable is normally distributed. Therefore, the Spearman rank correlation coefficient is the appropriate measure to examine the level of association between these two variables.

BOX 12.5 DESCRIPTION OF *corr_dtp3* DATASET

The Global Health Observatory (GHO) is a repository of health-related data from over 194 countries. The *corr_dtp3* dataset contains data on childhood health for 194 countries. Immunization coverage (*dtp3*) is the percentage of children aged 1 year who have had the diphtheria tetanus toxoid and pertussis immunization. The mortality rate (*under5_mortality*) is the number of deaths of children who are under five years old, in the thousands.

Our null hypothesis is that there is no linear relationship between DTP3 immunization and mortality rate of children younger than 5 years. To calculate the Spearman rank correlation coefficient, we will use the code in Table 12.10.

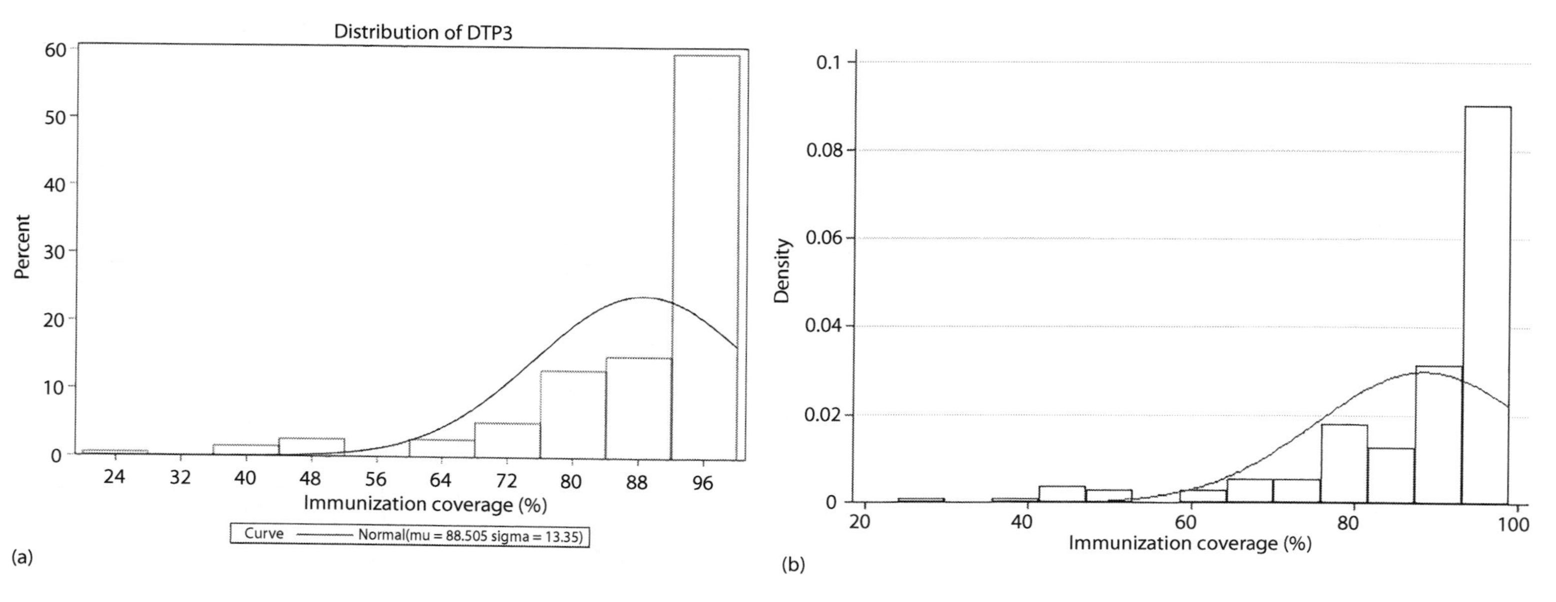

Figure 12.5 **(a) Histogram of distribution of immunization coverage with normal curve overlay from Example Problem 12.4, using SAS. (b) Histogram of distribution of immunization coverage with normal curve overlay from Example Problem 12.4, using Stata.** This histogram shows the distribution of the sample's DTP3 immunization coverage as compared to the expected normal curve. This graph can be used to ascertain whether a parametric or nonparametric test for correlation will be more appropriate.

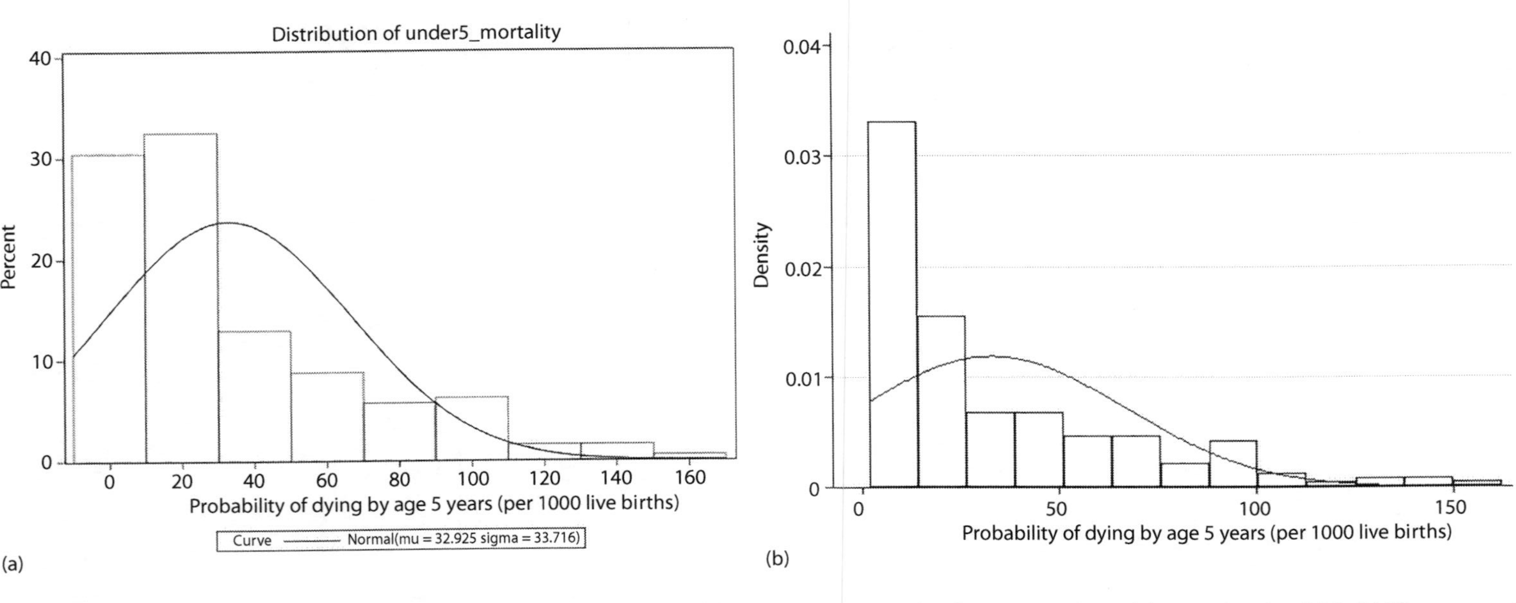

Figure 12.6 **(a) Histogram of distribution of infant mortality rate with normal curve overlay from Example Problem 12.4, using SAS. (b) Histogram of distribution of infant mortality rate with normal curve overlay from Example Problem 12.4, using Stata.** This histogram shows the distribution of the infant mortality rates in the sample as compared to the expected normal curve. This graph can be used to ascertain whether a parametric or nonparametric test for correlation will be more appropriate.

Table 12.10 Code to calculate the Spearman correlation coefficient (Example Problem 12.4)

SAS code	*Stata code*

`PROC CORR DATA = corr_dtp3;`
`VAR dtp3 under5_mortality;`
`RUN;`
	`spearman dtp3 under5_mortality`

Spearman Correlation Coefficients, N = 194 Prob > |r| under H0: Rho = 0		
	DTP3	**Under5_Mortality**
DTP3 Immunization Coverage, %	1.00000	–0.53684 <.0001
Under5_Mortality Probability of Dying by Age 5 Years, per 1000 live births	–0.53684 <.0001	1.00000

```
Number of obs =       194
Spearman's rho =        -0.5368

Test of Ho: dtp3 and under5_mortality are independent
     Prob > |t| =        0.0000
```

From the output, we can see that the Spearman rank correlation coefficient is –0.54. This implies a strong, negative correlation between DTP3 immunization coverage and the probability of dying by 5 years of age. The *p*-value is <0.0001, so we reject our null hypothesis and determine that DTP3 immunization coverage and the mortality rate for those younger than 5 years is negatively (moderate) correlated.

PRACTICE PROBLEM 12.2

For testing the significance of a correlation coefficient, what distribution does the appropriate test statistic follow?

PRACTICE PROBLEM 12.3

Evaluate the following scenarios and determine whether correlation would be a suitable procedure to analyze the data. Why or why not?

A Researchers are interested in investigating the association between a mother's age at conception (measured in years) and her infant's birthweight (measured in ounces).

B We are interested in determining the relationship between maternal mortality rate and race.

C Researchers are interested in investigating the relationship between BMI and patient-reported satisfaction with their health (measured on a five-point Likert scale).

D The health department has compiled state-level data on cigarettes sold (measured in packs) and lung cancer prevalence. They would like to show that increased tobacco sales cause an increase in lung cancer prevalence.

PRACTICE PROBLEM 12.4

Which correlation coefficient is very sensitive to outliers and should be used only if the X and Y variables of interest are normally distributed?

PRACTICE PROBLEM 12.5

We are interested in the correlation between watching TV and drinking soda or pop among students in grades 9 through 12. Data on nutrition, physical activity, and obesity on the state level can be accessed through the Centers for Disease Control and Prevention using estimates obtained from the Youth Risk Behavior Surveillance System.[8] (See Box 12.6.) Use the *soda_pa* dataset for this problem.

BOX 12.6 DESCRIPTION OF *soda_pa* DATASET

Data from the Youth Risk Behavior Surveillance System (YRBSS) (individual level) were aggregated to the state level. The *soda_pa* dataset contains the percentage of students who drank regular soda/pop at least one time per day (*dranksoda*), the percentage of students watching three or more hours of television each school day (*TV_3hours*), and the percentage of students who attended physical education classes daily in an average week (*daily_pe*). Data on soda drinking and TV watching are available from 38 states; data on attending physical education classes are available from 33 states.

A Figure 12.7 are scatterplots of soda drinking versus television watching. On the basis of the scatterplots, what can you say about the relationship between the two variables?

B Do there appear to be any outliers?

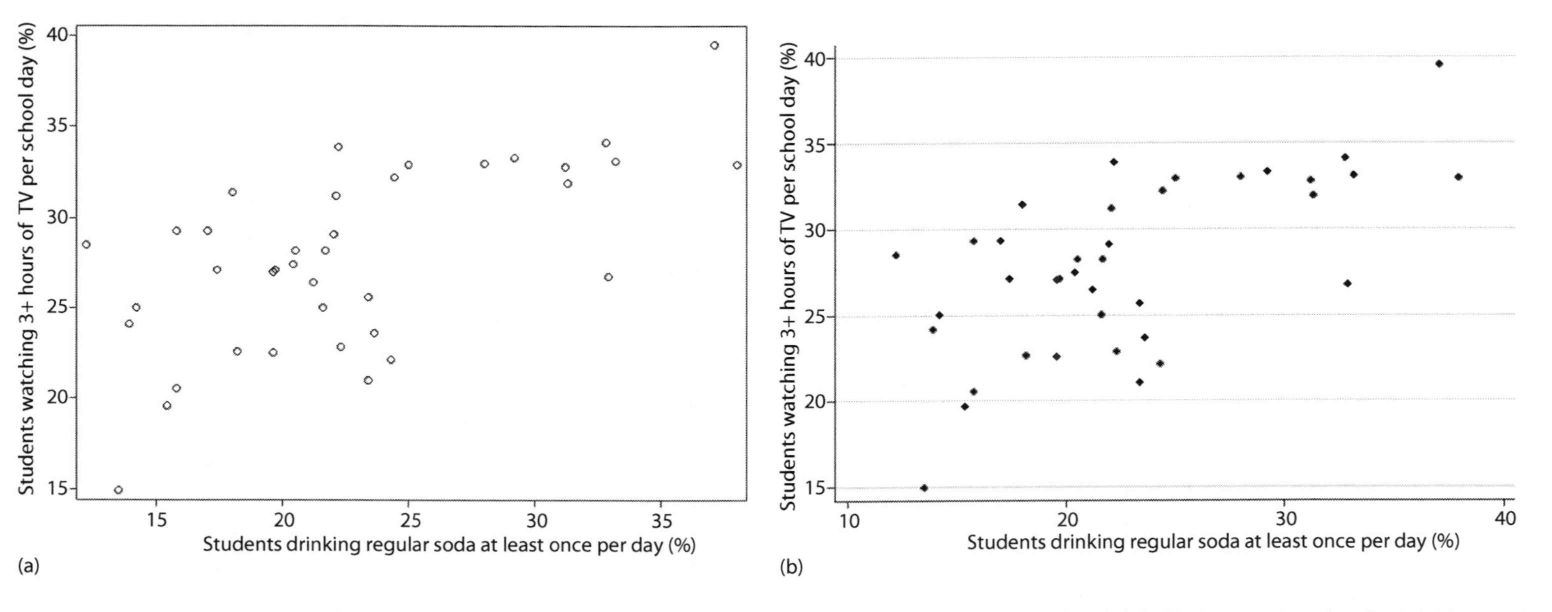

Figure 12.7 **(a) Scatterplot of soda drinking and television watching from Practice Problem 12.5, using SAS. (b) Scatterplot of soda drinking and television watching from Practice Problem 12.5, using Stata.** The scatterplot shows the relationship between the percentage of students drinking soda at least once per day and the percentage of students watching three or more hours of television each school day, at the state level.

C What is the Pearson correlation coefficient for these variables? What does it tell you about the strength of the association? Use SAS and Stata output below.

Pearson Correlation Coefficients Prob > |r| under H0: Rho = 0 Number of Observations	DrankSoda	TV_3hours
DrankSoda	1.00000	0.63396
Students Drinking Regular Soda at		<.0001
Least Once per Day, %	38	38
TV_3hours	0.63396	1.00000
Students Watching 3+ Hours of TV	<.0001	
per School Day, %	38	40

```
             | tv_3ho~s dranks~a
-------------+------------------
   tv_3hours |   1.0000
             |
             |
   dranksoda |   0.6340   1.0000
             |   0.0000
             |
```

D To determine whether there is a significant linear relationship between the two variables, what test should we use? State the null and alternate hypotheses for this test.

E Calculate the test by hand, then check your answer using the output in Practice Problem 12.5—Part (C). What is your conclusion for your test? State your *p*-value in your answer.

F To calculate a more robust measure of association between the two variables, we will calculate the Spearman rank correlation coefficient. If you are using SAS, what option should be specified? If you are using Stata, what command should you use?

G What is the Spearman rank correlation coefficient for these variables (see output below)? What does it tell you about the strength of the association?

Spearman Correlation Coefficients Prob > |r| under H0: Rho = 0 Number of Observations		
	DrankSoda	**TV_3hours**
DrankSoda Students Drinking Regular Soda at Least Once per Day, %	1.00000 38	0.56251 .0002 38
TV_3hours Students Watching 3+ Hours of TV per School Day, %	0.56251 .0002 38	1.00000 40

```
Number of obs =          38
Spearman's rho =          0.5625

Test of Ho: tv_3hours and dranksoda are independent
    Prob > |t| =          0.0002
```

H Using the Spearman rank correlation coefficient, test the null hypothesis that the underlying population correlation is equal to 0. Calculate the test statistic by hand and then check against the software output in Practice Problem 12.5—Part (G).

I How do the Pearson and Spearman correlation coefficients compare?

J Which estimation of correlation do you think is best for these data? Why?

PRACTICE PROBLEM 12.6

Now, using the same dataset (*soda_pa*) as in Practice Problem 12.5, we will investigate the relationship between drinking soda and participation in daily physical education. Data are available for 33 states.

A Figure 12.8 are scatterplots of the two variables. What can you say about the distribution? Are there any outliers?

B What is the Pearson correlation coefficient for these variables (see output below)? What does it tell you about the strength of the association?

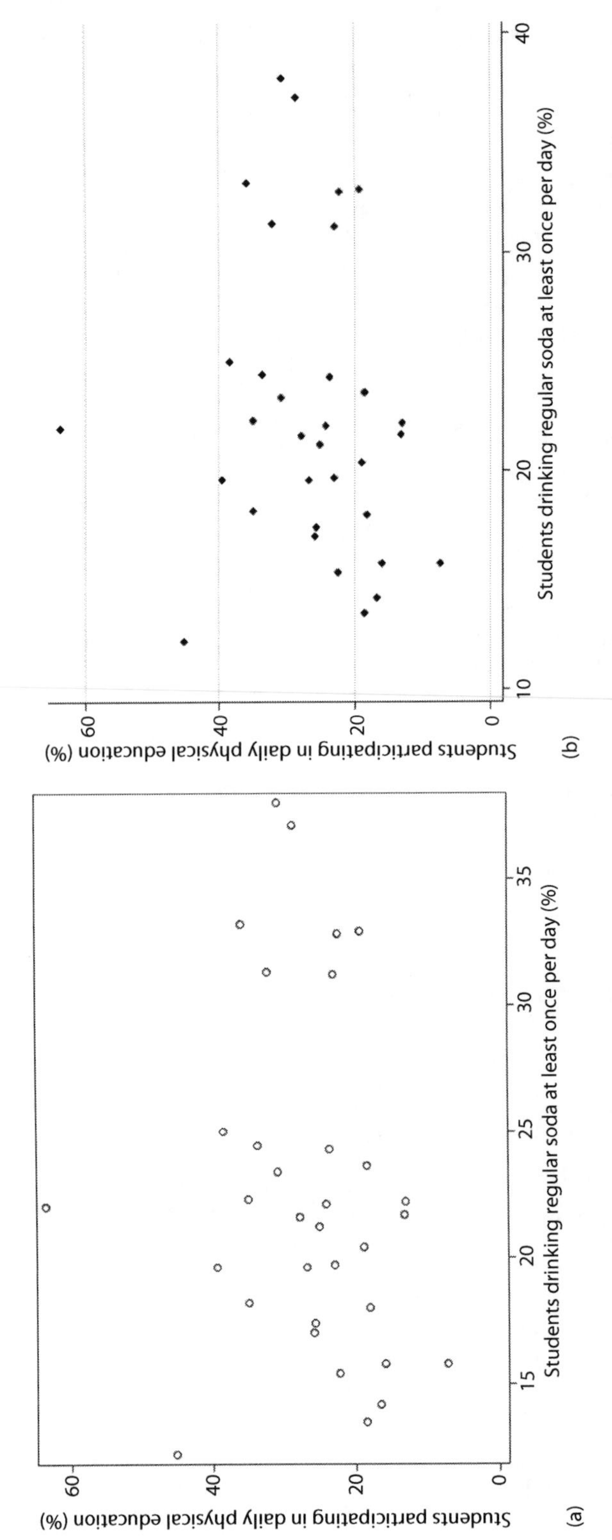

Figure 12.8 **(a) Scatterplot of soda drinking and daily physical education from Practice Problem 12.6, using SAS. (b) Scatterplot of soda drinking and daily physical education from Practice Problem 12.6, using Stata.** The scatterplot shows the relationship between the percentage of students drinking soda at least once per day and the percentage of students who attended physical education classes daily in an average week, at the state level.

Pearson Correlation Coefficients
Prob > |r| under H0: Rho = 0
Number of Observations

	DrankSoda	**TV_3hours**
DrankSoda	1.00000	0.13276
Students Drinking Regular Soda at		.4614
Least Once per Day, %	38	33
Daily_PE	0.13276	1.00000
Students Participating in Daily	.4614	
Physical Education, %	33	37

```
             | daily_pe dranks~a
-------------+------------------
    daily_pe |   1.0000
             |
             |
   dranksoda |   0.1328   1.0000
             |   0.4614
             |
```

C What is the Spearman rank correlation coefficient for these variables (see output below)? What does it tell you about the strength of the association?

Spearman Correlation Coefficients
Prob > |r| under H0: Rho = 0
Number of Observations

	DrankSoda	**TV_3hours**
DrankSoda	1.00000	0.25995
Students Drinking Regular Soda at		.1440
Least Once per Day, %	38	33
Daily_PE	0.25995	1.00000
Students Participating in Daily	.1440	
Physical Education, %	33	37

```
Number of obs =        33
Spearman's rho =          0.2599

Test of Ho: daily_pe and dranksoda are independent
      Prob > |t| =        0.1440
```

D How do the Pearson and Spearman correlation coefficients compare? Which is most appropriate for the data?

E Conduct a test for significance using the most appropriate test for this data. What do you conclude?

References

1. Mukaka MM. Statistics corner: A guide to appropriate use of correlation coefficient in medical research. *Malawi Med J*. 2012;24(3):69–71. doi:10.1016/j.cmpb.2016.01.020.
2. Fan JH, Lyons S, Goodman MS, Blanchard MS, Kaphingst KA. Relationship between health literacy and unintentional and intentional medication nonadherence in medically underserved patients with type 2 diabetes. *Diabetes Educ*. 2016;42(2):199–208. doi:10.1177/0145721715624969.
3. World Health Organization. Global Health Observatory Data Repository: Total fertility rate. http://apps.who.int/gho/data/node.main.HE-1548?lang=en. Updated May 15, 2015. Accessed August 1, 2016.
4. World Health Organization. Global Health Observatory Data Repository: Demand for family planning satisfied. http://apps.who.int/gho/data/view.main.94330. May 15, 2015. Accessed August 1, 2016.
5. National Health and Nutrition Examination Survey. Hyattsville, MD: Centers for Disease Control and Prevention, National Center for Health Statistics. 2014. https://wwwn.cdc.gov/Nchs/Nhanes/Search/nhanes13_14.aspx. Accessed August 1, 2016.
6. World Health Organization. Global Health Observatory Data Repository: Diptheria tetanus toxoid and pertussis (DTP3). http://apps.who.int/gho/data/view.main.80200. Updated July 17, 2015. Accessed August 1, 2016.
7. World Health Organization. Global Health Observatory Data Repository: Number of under-five deaths. http://apps.who.int/gho/data/node.main.ChildMort-1?lang=en. Updated August 27, 2015. Accessed August 1, 2016.
8. Youth Risk Behavior Surveillance System. Atlanta, GA: Centers for Disease Control and Prevention. 2013. www.cdc.gov/yrbs. Updated August 11, 2016. Accessed August 1, 2016.

13 Linear regression

This chapter will focus on investigating the change in a continuous variable in response to a change in one or more predictor variables and will include the following topics:

- Simple linear regression
- Regression concepts
- Methods of least squares
- Linear relationship
- Inference for predicted values
- Evaluation of the model
- Multiple linear regression
- Model evaluation
- Other explanatory variables
- Model selection

Terms

- collinearity
- indicator variable

Simple linear regression

Simple linear regression measures the association between two continuous variables.

- One variable is treated as the response (dependent or outcome) variable, commonly denoted as y.
- The other is the explanatory (independent or predictor) variable, commonly denoted as x.

The concept is similar to correlation; however, regression enables us to investigate how a change in the response variable corresponds to a given change in the explanatory variable. Correlation analysis makes no such distinction. It can only determine whether a linear relationship exists between the two variables of interest, and it determines the strength of that association. The objective of regression is to predict the value of the response variable that is associated with a fixed value of an explanatory variable. Linear regression is used to examine the relationship between a variable (continuous, categorical, or binary) and a continuous outcome, specifically how a change in the explanatory (predictor) variable affects a change in the response (outcome) variable.

Regression concepts

The equation for a line is given by the formula $y = a + bx$.

- The y-intercept is denoted by a and is the value of y when $x = 0$.
- The slope of a line represents the change in y that corresponds to a one-unit change in x and is denoted by b.
  - If the slope is positive, then y increases as x increases.
  - If the slope is negative, then y decreases as x increases.

The mean of all of the values for the response (outcome or dependent) variables is denoted as μ_y (the mean of y). The standard deviation of all of the responses is denoted as σ_y (the standard deviation of y). The mean of the responses given the explanatory variable is $\mu_{y|x}$ (mean of y given x). $\sigma_{y|x}$ = standard deviation of y given x, the standard deviation of the responses given the explanatory variable. The relationship among the standard deviation of y given x, the standard deviation of y, and the Pearson correlation coefficient is known to be the following: $\sigma^2_{y|x} = (1-\rho^2)\sigma^2_y$. By definition, $-1 \leq \rho \leq 1$; therefore, $\sigma_{y|x} \leq \sigma_y$. As such, confidence intervals for the mean value of y given a value of x are smaller (narrower) than the confidence intervals for the mean value of y.

BOX 13.1 LINEAR REGRESSION ASSUMPTIONS

In order to use the linear regression model for analysis, we make assumptions of normality, linearity, homoscedasticity, and independence of the underlying data. Linear regression is an extension of ANOVA, so it will also tolerate minor violations of these assumptions.

- Normality
  - The normality assumption refers to the normal distribution of the outcomes.
  - For a specific predictor value x, which is considered to be measured without error, the distribution of outcome values (y) is normal with mean $\mu_{y|x}$ and standard deviation $\sigma_{y|x}$.
  - We can check this assumption by plotting the data in a histogram.
- Linearity
  - The relationship between the mean of the outcome given the predictor ($\mu_{y|x}$) and the predictor (x) can be described by the straight line: $\mu_{y|x} = \alpha + \beta x$.
  - The linear relationship between the two variables can be assessed visually by plotting a scatter graph (Chapter 1, Lab A, Chapter 12).

- Homoscedasticity
  - Assumption of constant variability across all values of x.
  - Analogous to the assumption of equal variances in the two-sample t-test or the one-way ANOVA.
- Independence
  - Outcomes (y) must be independent observations.
  - Check the distribution of the residuals. They should be randomly distributed.

Method of least squares

The true population regression line is given by Equation 13.1.

$$\mu_{y|x} = \alpha + \beta x \tag{13.1}$$

Because we are interested in finding the best estimate of the population regression line, we estimate the coefficients (α, β) of the population regression line using a single sample of observations.

The least squares regression line is given by Equation 13.2. The hats on the parameters $(\hat{y}, \hat{\alpha}, \hat{\beta})$ denote that they are estimates of the population parameters (y, α, β).

$$\hat{y} = \hat{\alpha} + \hat{\beta}x \tag{13.2}$$

We would like to be able to use the least squares regression line $(\hat{y} = \hat{\alpha} + \hat{\beta}x)$ to make inferences about the population's regression line ($\mu_{y|x} = \alpha + \beta x$). As with any other point estimates, if we used a different sample, we would obtain different estimates $(\hat{\alpha}, \hat{\beta})$.

- $\hat{\alpha}$ is a point estimate of the population intercept α.
- $\hat{\beta}$ is a point estimate of the slope β.

Residuals are the difference between the observed value pair (x_i, y_i) and the least squares regression line (Figure 13.1). They are denoted by the following: $e_i = y_i - \hat{y}_i = y_i - (\hat{\alpha} + \hat{\beta}x_i)$. If $e_i = 0$, this implies that the point (x_i, y_i) lies directly on the fitted line. Since it is rarely true that all points will lie directly on the fitted line, we choose a criterion for fitting a line that minimizes the residuals (makes the residuals as small as possible). We use a mathematical technique called the method of least squares (MLS) for fitting a straight line to a set of points. MLS finds the values of $\hat{\alpha}$ and $\hat{\beta}$ that minimize the sum of the squared residuals. The sum of squared residuals, also called *error sum of squares* or *residual sum of squares*, is given by the following formula:

$$\sum e_i^2 = \sum (y_i - \hat{y}_i)^2 = \sum (y_i - \hat{\alpha} - \hat{\beta}x_i)^2 \tag{13.3}$$

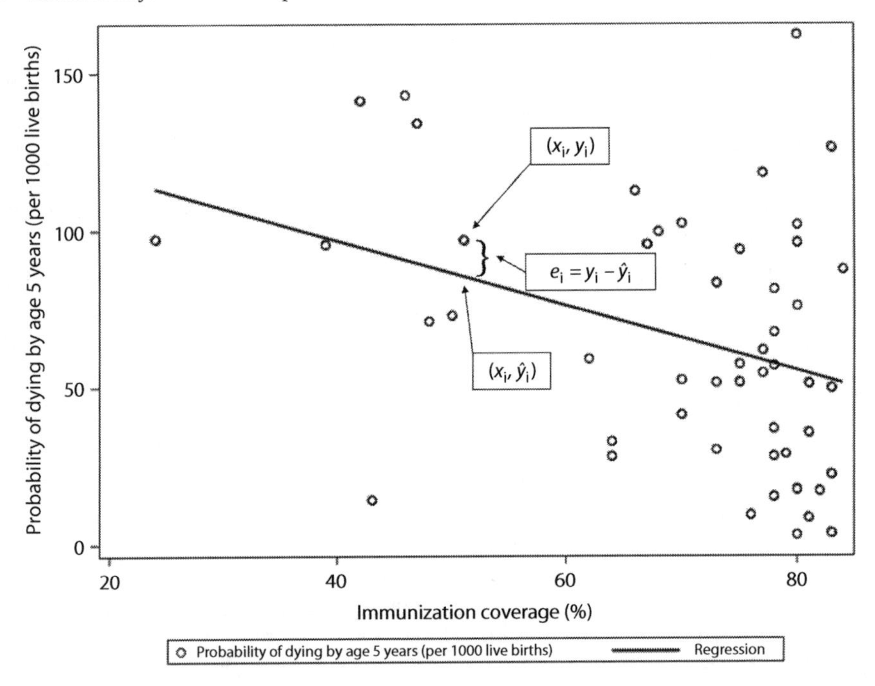

Figure 13.1 **Graphical depiction of observed values, least squares regression line, and residuals.** The open circle points represent the observed values of the data (x is DTP3 coverage among 1-year-olds, y is the probability of dying by age 5 years). The least squares regression line is represented by the solid line. The predicted values ($\hat{y}_i$) for each x_i lie along the least squares regression line. The residuals ($\hat{e}_i$) are the difference between the observed value (y_i) and the predicted value ($\hat{y}_i$).

Linear relationship

The slope is usually the most important coefficient in the linear regression equation. It quantifies the average change in y that corresponds to each one-unit change in x. If $\beta = 0$, then $\mu_{y|x} = \mu_y$. This means that there is no linear relationship between y and x. We use a t-test to investigate whether there is a linear relationship between y and x. The null hypothesis is that the slope is 0.

$$H_0: \beta = 0$$

$$H_1: \beta \neq 0$$

To test the null hypothesis, we calculate a t-statistic, using Equation 13.4. The test statistic follows the t-distribution with n-2 degrees of freedom.

$$t = \frac{\hat{\beta}}{\widehat{se}(\hat{\beta})} \tag{13.4}$$

Where, $\widehat{se}(\hat{\beta}) = \dfrac{S_{y|x}}{\sqrt{\sum_{i=1}^{n}(x_i - \bar{x})^2}}$

and $S_{y|x} = \sqrt{\dfrac{\sum_{i=1}^{n}(y_i - \bar{y})^2}{n-2}}$

The confidence interval for β is given by Equation 13.5.

$$\hat{\beta} \pm t_{n-2}\widehat{se}(\hat{\beta}) \tag{13.5}$$

If we are interested in testing whether the population intercept is equal to a specified value, we use calculations that are analogous to those for the slope. We would use $\hat{\alpha}$ and $\widehat{se}(\hat{\alpha})$ in place of $\hat{\beta}$ and $\widehat{se}(\hat{\beta})$. If the observed data points tend to be far from the intercept, there is very little practical value in making inferences about the intercept. In some instances, a value of $x = 0$ does not make sense. This makes the y-intercept uninterpretable (e.g., if x is the weight of a human). It is not recommended to extrapolate the fitted line beyond the range of observed values of x because the relationship between x and y might be quite different outside of this range.

Inference for predicted values

Predicting a mean outcome value

We can also use the least squares regression line to estimate the mean value of y corresponding to a particular value of x. We can construct a confidence interval for that mean using Equation 13.6.

$$\hat{y} \pm t_{n-2}\widehat{se}(\hat{y}) \tag{13.6}$$

Where $\hat{y}$ is the predicted *mean* value (i.e., fitted value) of normally distributed outcomes and the standard error of $\hat{y}$ is estimated by

$$\widehat{se}(\hat{y}) = S_{y|x}\sqrt{\frac{1}{n} + \frac{(x-\bar{x})^2}{\sum_{i=1}^{n}(x_i - \bar{x})^2}}$$

note the term $(x-\bar{x})^2$ in the expression for the standard error. This quantity assumes a value of 0 when $x = \bar{x}$ and grows large as x moves farther away from the mean. In other words, we are more confident about the mean value of the response when we are closer to the mean value of the explanatory variable.

Predicting an individual outcome value

Instead of predicting the mean value of y for a given value of x, we may prefer to predict an individual value of y for a new member of the population not in the current sample. The predicted individual value is given as $\tilde{y}$ and is identical to the predicted mean $\hat{y}$.

$$\tilde{y} = \hat{\alpha} + \hat{\beta}x = \hat{y} \tag{13.7}$$

However, the standard error of $\tilde{y}$ is not the same as the standard error of $\hat{y}$.

$$\sigma_{\hat{y}} \leq \sigma_{\tilde{y}} \tag{13.8}$$

When computing $\widehat{se}(\hat{y})$, we are interested only in the variability of the estimated mean of the y-values. When considering an individual y, we have an extra source of variability to account for—namely, the dispersion of the y-values themselves around the mean $\hat{y}$.

$$\widehat{se}(\tilde{y}) = \sqrt{s_{y|x}^2 + \widehat{se}(\hat{y})^2} = S_{y|x}\sqrt{1 + \frac{1}{n} + \frac{(x-\bar{x})^2}{\sum_{i=1}^{n}(x_i - \bar{x})^2}} \tag{13.9}$$

The prediction interval (PI) for an individual outcome y is given by Equation 13.10.

$$\tilde{y} \pm t_{n-2}\,\widehat{se}(\tilde{y}) \tag{13.10}$$

The PI for $\tilde{y}$ is wider than the CI for $\hat{y}$. This is due to the extra source of variability.

Evaluation of the model

Now that we have a least squares regression line, we evaluate the model to determine whether it is a good fit that is appropriate for modeling our data. There are several ways to do this, including quantitatively (calculating the coefficient of determination) and visually (examining the residual plots).

- Coefficient of determination (R^2)
  - The percentage of total variability that is explained by the model.
  - It is the square of the Pearson correlation coefficient (see Chapter 12).
  - The range is $0 \leq R^2 \leq 1$.
  - If $R^2 = 1$, all data points in the sample fall directly on the least squares regression line.
  - If $R^2 = 0$, there is no linear relationship between x and y.
  - It can be thought of as the proportion of the variability among the observed values of y that is explained by the linear regression of y on x.

- Residual plots
  - We can create a two-way scatterplot of the residuals (e_i) versus the fitted (predicted) values of the response variable ($\hat{y}_i$) to examine whether a model is a good fit for the data.
  - These plots serve three purposes:
    - Detect outlying observations in the sample.
      - MLS can be very sensitive to outliers, especially if they correspond to relatively large or small values of x.
      - If an outlier is the result of an error in measuring or recording a particular observation (e.g., data entry typo), removal of this point will improve the fit of the regression line.
      - Do not throw away unusual data points that are valid—they might be the most interesting ones in the dataset.
    - Evaluate the assumption of heteroscedasticity.
      - A fan-shaped scatterplot implies that $\sigma_{y|x}$ does not take the same value for all values of x.
      - A fan shape is evidenced by the magnitudes of the residuals either increasing or decreasing as $\hat{y}$ becomes larger.
    - Evaluate the linearity assumption.
      - Do the residuals exhibit a random scatter or follow a distinct trend?
      - A trend suggests that the relationship between x and y might not be linear. A transformation of x, y, or both might be appropriate in this case (see Box 13.2 and Figure 13.2).

BOX 13.2 TRANSFORMATIONS—CORRECTING FOR NONLINEARITY

- Often, a curved linear relationship between two variables can be transformed into a more straightforward linear one.
- If this is possible, we can conduct a linear regression to fit a model to the transformed data.
- When transforming a variable, we are simply measuring it on a different scale.
- Common transformations include $ln(x)$, x^p, or y^p where $p = \ldots -3, -2, -½, ½, 2, 3\ldots$
- The circle of powers graph provides a general guideline for choosing a transformation (see Figure 13.2). If the plotted data resembled the data in Quadrant II, an appropriate transformation would be down in x (raised to a power of $p < 1$) or up in y (raised in power to $p > 1$). The more curvature in the data, the higher (or lower) the value of p will need to be to achieve linearity in the transformation.

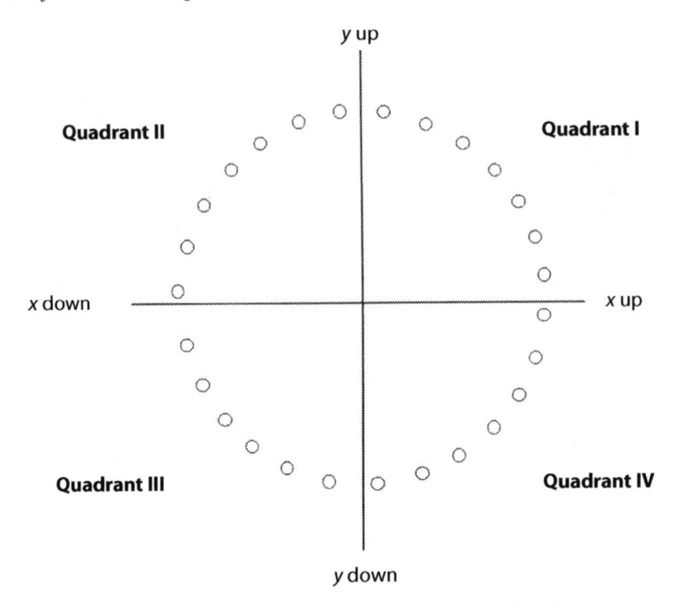

Figure 13.2 **Circle of powers graph.** The graph provides a general guideline for choosing a transformation. If the plotted data resembled the data in Quadrant II, an appropriate transformation would be down in x (raised to a power of $p < 1$) or up in y (raised in power to $p > 1$). The more curvature in the data, the higher (or lower) the value of p will need to be to achieve linearity in the transformation.

BOX 13.3 STRATEGY FOR REGRESSION ANALYSIS

1. Draw a scatterplot of the data.
2. Fit the regression line.
3. Check residuals.
   a. Plot residuals versus predicted values (denoted as $\hat{y}$).
   b. Check for lack of pattern.

EXAMPLE PROBLEM 13.1

Research findings show that breastfed babies have reduced risks of diseases, infections, and death.[1] Evidence also exists that hospital practices can make a difference in breastfeeding rates.[2] We are interested in whether state-level participation in best maternity care practices affects infant mortality rate. Specifically, we want to investigate whether the proportion of hospitals that limit the use of breastfeeding supplements (e.g., formula, glucose water, or water) is related to the state-level infant mortality rate. Going forward, this will be referred to as Example Problem Model 1. Data come from the 2007 Maternity Practices in Infant Nutrition and Care (mPINC) survey,[3] and the infant mortality statistics come from the 2010 period linked birth and infant death dataset.[4] Use the *mpinc_mortality* dataset for the following problems.

BOX 13.4 MATERNITY PRACTICES IN INFANT NUTRITION AND CARE (mPINC) SURVEY

On the mPINC survey, a hospital is indicated as complying with the exclusive breastfeeding benchmark if less than 10% of healthy, full-term, breastfed infants are supplemented with formula, glucose water, or water. The variable *exclusivebf* is the proportion of all hospitals in the state that comply with that standard.

A hospital is indicated as complying with the teaching benchmark if at least 90% of mothers who currently or intend to breastfeed are taught breastfeeding techniques. The variable *teach* is the proportion of all hospitals in the state that comply with that standard.

In the mPINC survey results, subscale scores were calculated for each of the seven domains of interest. The facility discharge care subscale score is a composite of a hospital's assurance of ambulatory breastfeeding support (i.e., physical contact, active reaching out, referrals), and distribution of discharge packs that do not contain infant formula. A dichotomous variable (*discharge*) was created to indicate states with a facility discharge care subscale score greater than or lower than the national average of 43.33 out of 100. A value of 1 indicates that the state has a facility discharge care score that is greater than or equal to the national average. A value of 0 indicates that the state has a facility discharge care score that is less than the national average.

The infant mortality rate is the total number of deaths per 1000 live births (*infant_mortality2010*).

First, we want to visualize the data and the potential relationship between our variables of interest. To do this, we will create a scatterplot of exclusive breastfeeding versus the infant mortality rate per 1000 live births using the code in Table 13.1.

A What can we say about the relationship between exclusive breastfeeding and the infant mortality rate? Does the relationship appear to be linear? Draw a line of best fit on the graph in Figure 13.3.

The relationship between the percentage of hospitals complying with exclusive breastfeeding practices and the infant mortality rate appears to be negative and linear (see Figure 13.4).

Table 13.1 Code for scatterplot (Example Problem 13.1)

Using SAS	*Using Stata*
PROC SGPLOT DATA = mpinc_mortality; SCATTER Y = infant_mortality2010 X = exclusivebf; **RUN;**	**scatter *infant_mortality2010 exclusivebf***

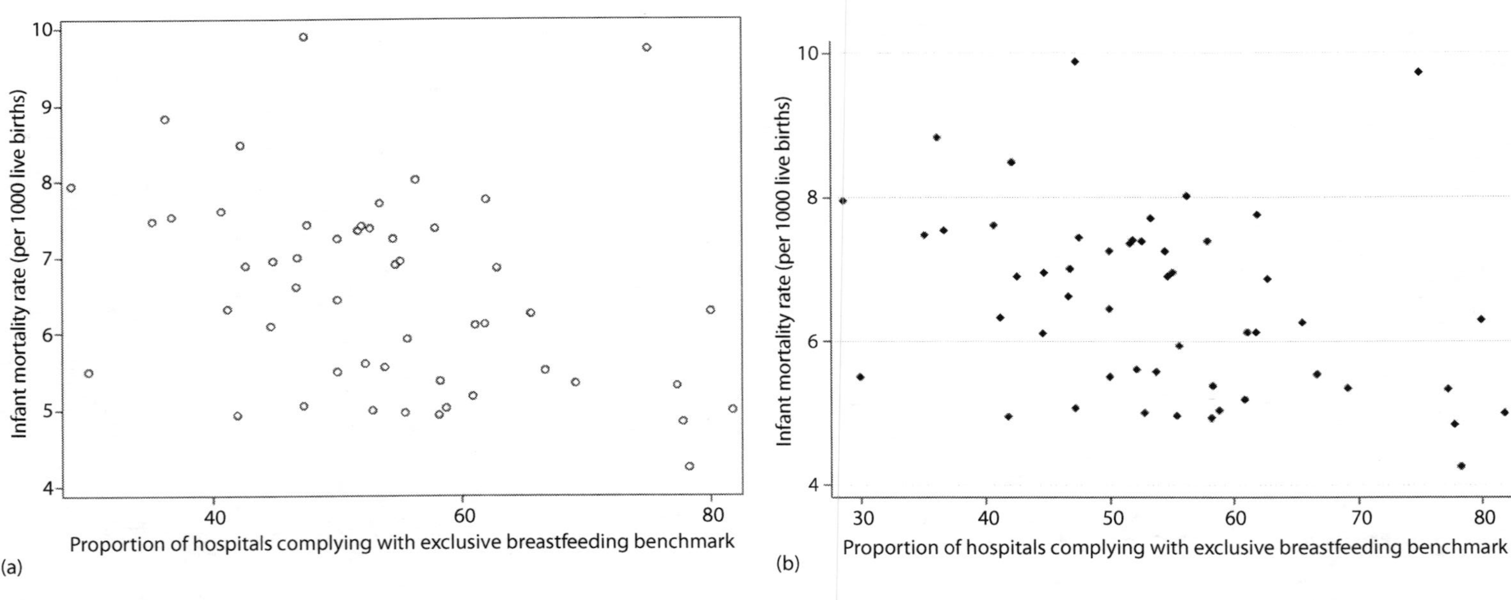

Figure 13.3 **(a) Scatterplot from Example Problem 13.1, using SAS.** [4] **(b) Scatterplot from Example Problem 13.1, using Stata.** The scatterplot shows the relationship between the *x* variable (proportion of hospitals meeting exclusive breastfeeding benchmark) and the *y* variable (infant mortality rate). There is a negative, downward trend. Data for the figure come from mPINC[3] and the linked birth and infant death dataset.[4] From Centers for Disease Control and Prevention, Maternity Practices in Infant Nutrition and Care (mPINC) Survey, http://www.cdc.gov/breastfeeding/data/mpinc/index.htm; Mathews, T. J., and MacDorman, M. F., Natl Vital Stat Reports, 62(8), 1–26, 2013.

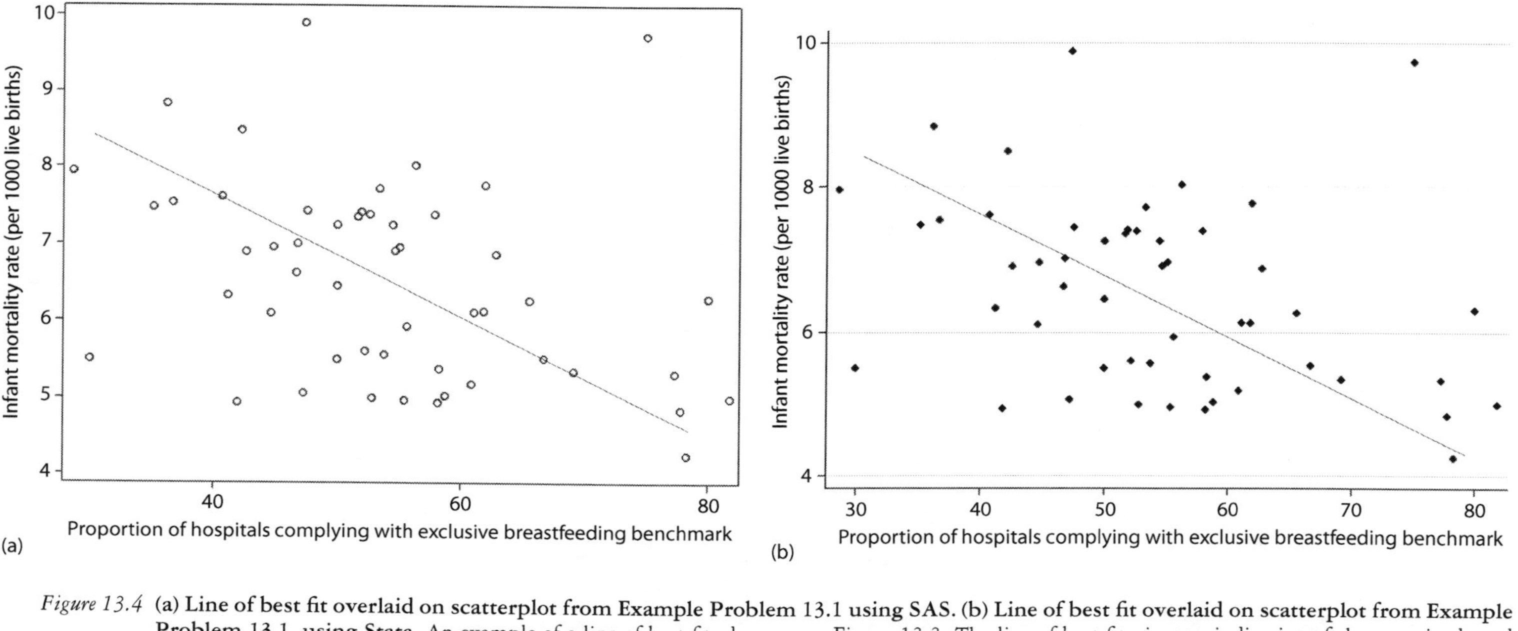

Figure 13.4 **(a) Line of best fit overlaid on scatterplot from Example Problem 13.1 using SAS. (b) Line of best fit overlaid on scatterplot from Example Problem 13.1, using Stata.** An example of a line of best fit, drawn over Figure 13.3. The line of best fit gives an indication of the magnitude and direction of the linear relationship.

Table 13.2 Code for simple linear regression (Example Problem 13.1)

Using SAS	*Using Stata*

In SAS, we use PROC REG. The response variable goes in the MODEL statement, on the left side of the "=" sign. The explanatory variable also goes in the MODEL statement, but after the "=" sign.
 	
PROC REG is a procedure that allows for RUN-group processing (i.e., you can run another model without issuing another PROC REG). To prevent your computer from continuing to run, add a QUIT statement to end PROC REG.
 	
`PROC REG DATA = mpinc_mortality;`
`MODEL infant_mortality2010 =`
`exclusivebf;`
`RUN; QUIT;`
	In Stata, we use the REGRESS command. In this command, the response variable comes first, followed by the explanatory variable.
	
	`regress infant_mortality2010`
	`exclusivebf`

To be more precise, we will use computer software to calculate the least squares regression line (Table 13.2). Our response variable is infant mortality rate (*infant_mortality2010*), and our explanatory variable is exclusive breastfeeding (*exclusivebf*).

B **What is the least squares estimate of the true population intercept ($\hat{\alpha}$)? Interpret this value in words.**

The least squares estimate of the true population intercept is 8.48 infant deaths per 1000 live births. This means that the estimated infant mortality rate is 8.48 when exclusive breastfeeding is 0 (zero percent of hospitals in a state meet the benchmark for exclusive breastfeeding).

Parameter Estimates

Variable	Label	DF	Parameter Estimate	Standard Error	t Value	Pr > |t|
Intercept	Intercept	1	8.48020	0.76212	11.13	<.0001
ExclusiveBF	Proportion of hospitals meeting exclusive breastfeeding benchmark	1	−0.03602	0.01370	−2.63	0.0114

In SAS, this value is found in the Parameter Estimates table. It is denoted as the "parameter estimate" for the intercept ($\hat{\alpha} = 8.48020$).

```
------------------------------------------------------------------------------
infant_~2010 |      Coef.   Std. Err.      t    P>|t|     [95% Conf. Interval]
-------------+----------------------------------------------------------------
 exclusivebf | -.0360227   .0137039   -2.63   0.011    -.0635618   -.0084836
       _cons |  8.480204   .7621157   11.13   0.000     6.948675    10.01173
------------------------------------------------------------------------------
```

In Stata, the estimated value of the intercept is found in the bottom portion of the output. It is denoted as the "coef." for *_cons* ($\hat{\alpha} = 8.480204$).

C **What is the least squares estimate of the true population slope ($\hat{\beta}$)? Interpret this value in words.**

The least squares estimate of the true population slope is −0.036. This means that for every unit increase in exclusive breastfeeding (1%), the infant mortality rate decreases by 0.036.

In the SAS output in the response to Example Problem 13.1—Part (B), this value is also found in the Parameter Estimates table. It is denoted as the "parameter estimate" for *exclusiveBF* ($\hat{\beta} = -0.03602$). It is located below the least squares estimate of the true population intercept ($\hat{\alpha}$).

In the Stata output in the response to Example Problem 13.1—Part (B), this value is also found in the bottom portion of the output box. It is denoted as the "coef." for *exclusivebf* ($\hat{\beta} = -0.0360227$). It is located above the least squares estimate of the true population intercept ($\hat{\alpha}$).

To test whether there is a significant linear relationship between infant mortality rate and the proportion of hospitals meeting the exclusive breastfeeding benchmark, we test to see whether the estimate of the slope is equal to 0.

$$H_0: \beta = 0$$

$$H_1: \beta \neq 0$$

D **Calculate the test statistic by hand, and compare to the SAS or Stata output.**

To calculate the test statistic, we use Equation 13.4.

$$t = \frac{\hat{\beta}}{\hat{se}(\hat{\beta})} = \frac{-0.036}{0.0137} = -2.63$$

Our test statistic follows the t-distribution with $n - 2$ degrees of freedom. In this case, $n = 51$, so we have 49 degrees of freedom.

$$t = -2.63 \sim t_{49}$$

Our test statistic is the same as the t-value in the SAS and Stata output. The test statistic can be found as the "t value" for *exclusivebf* in the SAS output in the response to Example Problem 13.1—Part (B). It can be found as "t" for *exclusivebf* in the Stata output in the response to Example Problem 13.1—Part (B).

After we have calculated our test statistic, we calculate a p-value and draw a conclusion about the linear relationship between the two variables.

E Find the p-value, and compare it to the SAS or Stata output. Draw a conclusion from your test.

From the t-distribution table in Appendix Table A.4, we can see that $0.01 < p < 0.005$. Therefore, we reject the null hypothesis that the slope is equal to 0 and conclude that there is a significant linear relationship. As the proportion of hospitals with exclusive breastfeeding practices increases, the rate of infant mortality decreases.

In SAS, the p-value for the slope is 0.0114. This can be found as the "Pr > |t|" value of *exclusiveBF*. In Stata, the p-value for the slope is 0.011. This can be found as the "P > |t|" value of *exclusivebf*.

The p-values given by both SAS and Stata fall within our calculated range of $0.01 < p < 0.005$.

F Calculate a 95% confidence interval for the slope of the true population regression line. How does it compare to the result of the hypothesis test?

Recall that $t \sim t_{n-2} = t_{51-2} = t_{49}$, which we will estimate by t_{40} (remember to always round down degrees of freedom). A 95% confidence interval for the slope is calculated using Equation 13.5.

$$\hat{\beta} \pm t_{40}\, \hat{se}(\hat{\beta})$$

$$-0.036 \pm 2.021 \times 0.0137$$

$$-0.036 \pm 0.0277$$

$$95\%CI: (-0.064, -0.008)$$

We are 95% confident that the interval (–0.064, –0.008) covers the slope of the true population regression line.

Because the confidence interval does not contain 0, it is consistent with our decision to reject the null hypothesis based on the p-value in Example Problem 13.1—Part E.

Now that we have a fitted regression line, we can recreate the scatterplot (Figure 13.3) and include the fitted regression line. First, we need to calculate the predicted outcome value (infant mortality) for each observation based on the regression equation. See Table 13.3, for sample code.

We then overlay the linear regression line on top of the original scatterplot. See Table 13.4 provides SAS and Stata code and Figure 13.5 shows the resulting graphs.

Table 13.3 Code for calculating predicted values (Example Problem 13.1)

Using SAS	*Using Stata*
In SAS, we request an output dataset within our PROC REG that includes the predicted values. Use the keyword PREDICTED to request the predicted outcome value, and give it an appropriate name, such as *yhat*. **PROC REG** DATA = mpinc_mortality; MODEL infant_mortality2010 = exclusivebf; OUTPUT OUT=pred_data PREDICTED = yhat; **RUN**; **QUIT**;	In Stata, the PREDICT command requests the predicted outcome value. It is stored as a new variable that we give an appropriate name, such as *yhat*. This command must follow our previous REGRESS command (Table 13.2). **predict *yhat***

Table 13.4 Code for scatterplot with regression line (Example Problem 13.1 and Figure 3.5)

Using SAS	*Using Stata*
Make sure to use the dataset that was output from the PROC REG in Table 13.3. Graphs can be overlaid by adding multiple statements to PROC SGPLOT. In this instance, we will have a SCATTER statement (between the observed infant mortality rate and the observed exclusive breastfeeding variable) and a SERIES statement (between the predicted *yhat* and the observed exclusive breastfeeding variable). **PROC SGPLOT** DATA = pred_data; SCATTER Y = infant_mortality2010 X = exclusivebf; SERIES Y = yhat X = exclusivebf; **RUN**; Alternatively, we can use the original dataset and use a REGRESSION statement in PROC SGPLOT to get the overlaid regression line. In this case, the *Y* variable will be our original infant mortality rate variable (*infant_mortality2010*). **PROC SGPLOT** DATA = mpinc_mortality; SCATTER Y = infant_mortality2010 X = exclusivebf; REGRESSION Y = infant_ mortality2010 X = exclusivebf; **RUN**;	Use the TWOWAY command to overlay our SCATTER and LINE graphs. The SCATTER graph is between our observed response variable (*infant mortality rates*) and our observed explanatory variable (*exclusive breastfeeding*). The LINE graph uses the predicted value (*yhat*) as the response variable and the observed explanatory variable (exclusive breastfeeding). **graph twoway (scatter *infant_mortality2010 exclusivebf*) (line *yhat exclusivebf*)**

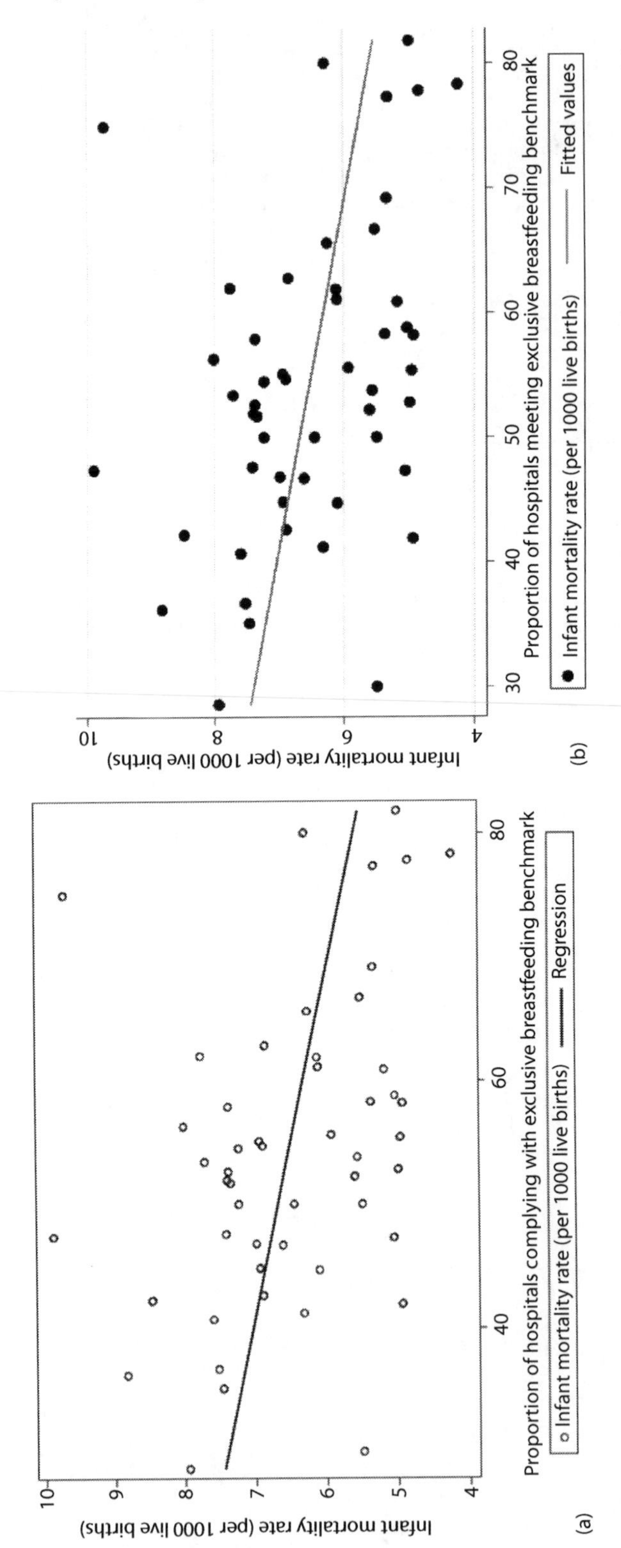

Figure 13.5 (a) **Scatterplot with regression line from Example Problem 13.1, using SAS.** (b) **Scatterplot with regression line from Example Problem 13.1, using Stata.** The least squares regression line is the line that minimizes the residuals of the observed data.

G What is the predicted mean mortality rate ($\hat{y}$) for states where 72% of hospitals meet the exclusive breastfeeding benchmark?

To find the predicted mean mortality rate, we will use Equation 13.2. We plug in 72% as our x value and use the least squares estimates of the true population intercept and slope that we calculated in Parts B and C of Example Problem 13.1.

$$\hat{y} = \hat{\alpha} + \hat{\beta} \times \textit{exclusive breastfeeding}$$

$$\hat{y} = 8.48 - 0.036 \times 72$$

$$\hat{y} = 5.888$$

The mean infant mortality rate is 5.9 deaths per 1000 live births for states where 72% of hospitals meet the exclusive breastfeeding benchmark.

H Suppose that you want to predict the infant mortality rate ($\tilde{y}$) for a state that has 72% of its hospitals in compliance with the exclusive breastfeeding benchmark. What value would you predict?

The prediction for an individual value ($\tilde{y}$) is the same as the prediction for the mean value ($\hat{y}$). As in Example Problem 13.1—Part G, the infant mortality rate would be 5.9 per 1000 live births for a state with 72% of hospitals meeting the breastfeeding benchmark.

$$\tilde{y} = \hat{y} = \hat{\alpha} + \hat{\beta} \times \textit{exclusive breastfeeding} = 5.888$$

The difference between $\hat{y}$ and $\tilde{y}$ becomes apparent when we plot the confidence intervals for both values (Table 13.5; Figure 13.6).

I How do the two types of confidence intervals compare?

The prediction interval is wider than the confidence interval.

Now that we have a model of our data, we want to see how well our least squares regression line fits our data. We do this using the coefficient of determination.

J What is the coefficient of determination, and how does it indicate the adequacy of this model (Example Problem Model 1) in fitting the data?

The coefficient of determination is the percentage of total variability explained by the model. It can be found as "R-Square" in the SAS output box and as "R-squared" in the Stata output box.

$$R^2 = 0.12$$

Table 13.5 Code for scatterplot with confidence and prediction limits (Example Problem 13.1)

Using SAS	*Using Stata*

We can request the upper and lower bounds of the confidence intervals for $\hat{y}$ (CLM) and for $\tilde{y}$ (CLI) to be drawn on the scatterplot. The REG statement of PROC SGPLOT plots the regression line of our Y and X variables. We can, then, request the CLI and CLM options to display the confidence intervals around $\hat{y}$ and $\tilde{y}$. This plot (called a Fit Plot in the SAS output) is also part of the default output in PROC REG.
 	
`PROC SGPLOT DATA = mpinc_mortality;`
`SCATTER Y = infant_mortality2010 X = exclusivebf;`
`REG Y = infant_mortality2010 X = exclusivebf / CLI CLM;`
`RUN;`
 	
Or
 	
`PROC REG DATA = mpinc_mortality;`
`MODEL infant_mortality2010 = exclusivebf;`
`RUN; QUIT;`
	We use the GRAPH TWOWAY command to overlay multiple plots. The LFITCI command allows us to plot the confidence limits for $\hat{y}$. The CIPLOT(RLINE) allows us to designate the confidence limits as lines instead of being shaded. The second LFITCI command specifies the STDF option, which will create the confidence interval around $\tilde{y}$.
	
	`graph twoway (scatter infant_mortality2010 exclusivebf) (lfitci infant_mortality2010 exclusivebf, ciplot(rline)) (lfitci infant_mortality2010 exclusivebf, stdf ciplot(rline))`

Abbreviations: CLI, confidence interval; CLM, confidence limit.

This means that 12% of the variability among the observed values of infant mortality is explained by the linear relationship between infant mortality and proportion of hospitals meeting the exclusive breastfeeding benchmark. The remaining 88% of the variability is not explained by this relationship.

Root MSE	1.21987	**R-Square**	0.1236
Dependent Mean	6.52784	**Adj R-Sq**	0.1057
Coeff Var	18.68713		

```
   Source |       SS           df       MS      Number of obs   =        51
----------+----------------------------------   F(1, 49)        =      6.91
    Model |  10.2822261         1  10.2822261   Prob > F        =    0.0114
 Residual |  72.9156366        49  1.48807422   R-squared       =    0.1236
----------+----------------------------------   Adj R-squared   =    0.1057
    Total |  83.1978627        50  1.66395725   Root MSE        =    1.2199
```

Another way to consider the fit of the model is to produce a plot of the residuals versus the fitted (or predicted) values. SAS displays this plot as the first graph in the Fit Diagnostics panel, which is a default output for output that is being written to an HTML file (ods html;). In Stata, use the command *rvfplot* to obtain the desired plot (Figure 13.7).

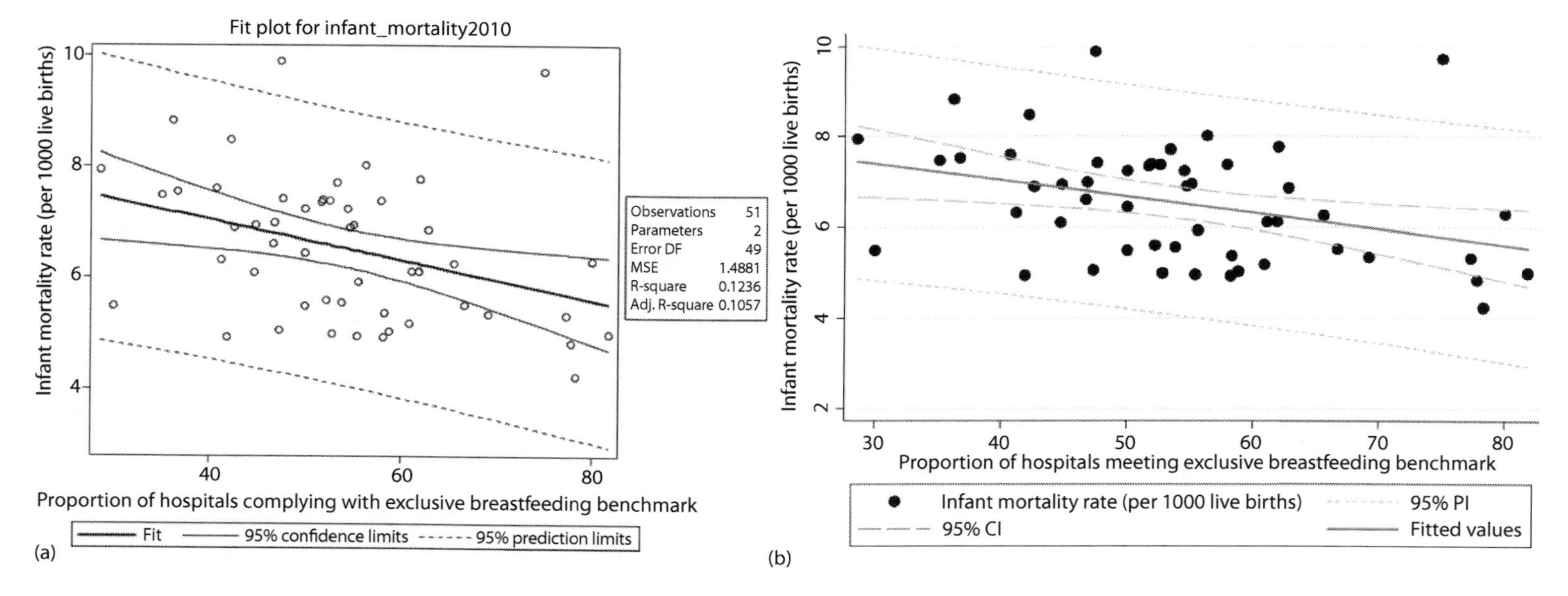

Figure 13.6 (a) **Confidence limits for $\hat{y}$ and $\tilde{y}$ from Example Problem 13.1, using SAS.** The confidence interval corresponds to the mean outcome value ($\hat{y}$) and is represented by the solid, curved lines around the regression line. The prediction interval corresponds to the predicted individual outcome value ($\tilde{y}$). It is represented by the dashed lines. (b) **Confidence limits for $\hat{y}$ and $\tilde{y}$ from Example Problem 13.1, using Stata.** The confidence interval corresponds to the mean outcome value ($\hat{y}$) and is represented by the—curved lines around the fitted values (regression) line. The prediction interval corresponds to the predicted individual outcome value ($\tilde{y}$). It is represented by the short dash lines.

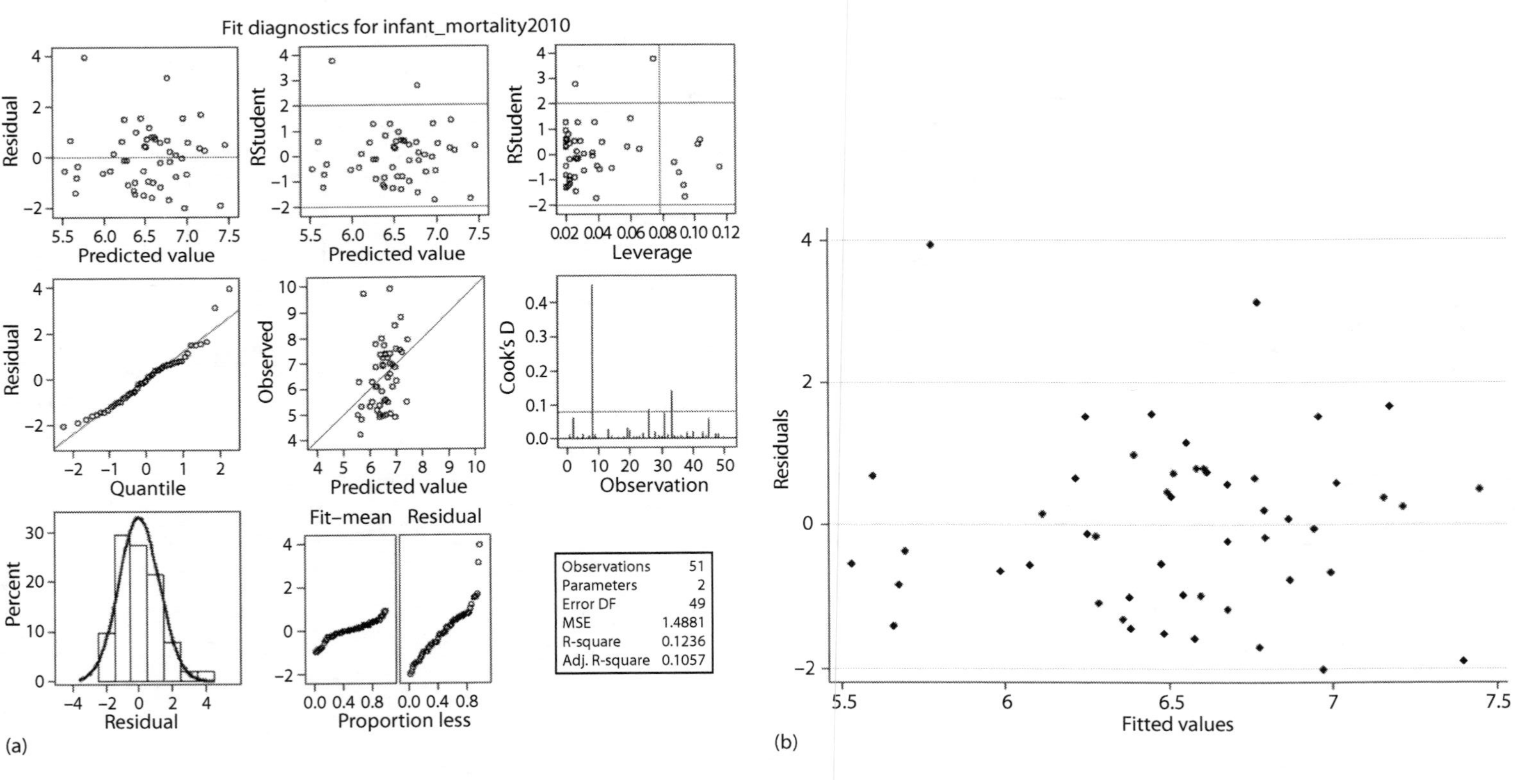

Figure 13.7 **(a) Residual plot for Example 13.1, using SAS.** The residual plot of interest is the top, left graph in the default output of PROC REG. **(b) Residual plot for Example 13.1, using Stata.** This plot shows the distribution of the residuals versus the fitted (or predicted) values. In order to meet the assumptions of homoscedasticity or linearity, the graph should be random scatter, with no obvious pattern.

K What does the plot suggest about whether the assumptions of simple linear regression are met?

There is no obvious pattern. There is no evidence that the assumptions of homoscedasticity or linearity have been violated.

PRACTICE PROBLEM 13.1

Safe and high-quality playgrounds are an important component in the promotion of youth physical activity.[5] Public playgrounds in St. Louis, Missouri were assessed for safety, access, quality, and usability, and summary scores were calculated. These scores were summarized at the neighborhood level. We are interested in the relationship between a neighborhood's overall playground safety score and the percentage of owner-occupied housing in that neighborhood. Going forward, this model will be referred to as Practice Problem Model 1. Use the *pastl_score* dataset to answer the following problems.

BOX 13.5 PLAY ACROSS ST. LOUIS DATA

Each neighborhood was assigned an overall playground safety score (*noscore*) equal to the score of its playground. If there was more than one playground in a neighborhood, the overall playground safety score was made up of the average of the playground scores for that neighborhood. If the neighborhood did not have a playground, the scores from the nearest playground were used. The overall playground safety score was measured as the proportion of safety standards that were met.

The percentage of owner-occupied housing (*perowneroсc*), the percentage of vacant buildings (*pervacant*), and the percentage of the population that is under 18 (*peryouth*) were measured at the neighborhood level as well. These data estimates were taken from the 2010 Census.

The *north* variable is an indicator that describes whether the neighborhood is geographically north (value of 1) or south (value of 0) of Delmar Boulevard.

Note: Estimates in the journal article account for the multilevel nature of the data, which we will not take into account here, as they are beyond the scope of this book. Therefore, the estimate obtained in this problem will be different from what was published.[5]

A Create a scatterplot comparing the overall playground safety score and the percentage of owner-occupied housing. What can you say about the relationship based on this plot?

B What is the least squares estimate of the true population intercept ($\hat{\alpha}$)? Interpret this value in words. Is it meaningful?

C What is the least squares estimate of the true population slope ($\hat{\beta}$)? Interpret this value in words.

D Test to see whether there is a significant linear relationship between percentage of owner-occupied housing and overall neighborhood playground score. Be sure to state the null and alternate hypotheses, the value and distribution of the test statistic, and *p*-value. What do you conclude?

E What is the 95% confidence interval for the population slope? How does this compare to your conclusion from the statistical test in Practice Problem 13.1—Part D?

F What is the predicted mean overall playground score for a neighborhood where 50% of houses are owner occupied?

G Suppose that you want to predict a new overall playground score for a neighborhood with 82% owner-occupied housing. What value would you predict?

H What is the coefficient of determination for this model (Practice Problem Model 1), and what does it say about the model fit?

PRACTICE PROBLEM 13.2

Using the same data from Practice Problem 13.1, we consider whether another neighborhood-level factor, the percentage of vacant buildings, could influence playground scores. This model will be referred to as Practice Problem Model 2. Continue using the *pastl_score* dataset to answer the following problems.

A Create a scatterplot comparing the percentage of vacant buildings and the overall playground safety score. What can you say about the relationship based on this plot?

B What is the least squares estimate of the true population intercept ($\hat{\alpha}$)? Interpret this value in words. Is it meaningful?

C What is the least squares estimate of the true population slope ($\hat{\beta}$)? Interpret this value in words.

D Test to see whether there is a significant linear relationship between percentage of vacant buildings and overall neighborhood playground score. Be sure to state the null and alternative hypotheses, the value and distribution of the test statistic, and *p*-value. What do you conclude?

E What is the 95% confidence interval for the slope of the true population slope? How does this compare to your conclusion from the statistical test in Practice Problem 13.1—Part D (Practice Problem Model 2)?

F What is the predicted mean overall playground score for a neighborhood where 50% of the buildings are vacant?

G Suppose that you want to predict an overall playground score for a new neighborhood with 12% vacant buildings. What value would you predict?

H What is the coefficient of determination for this model (Practice Problem Model 2), and what does it say about the model fit?

Multiple linear regression

Multiple linear regression involves more than one explanatory variable. Again, we are estimating the population regression line using MLS. We can expand the simple linear regression equation (Equation 13.1) to account for multiple explanatory variables:

$$\mu_{y|x} = \alpha + \beta_1 x_1 + \beta_2 x_2 + \ldots + \beta_q x_q$$

The slope β_i is the change in the mean of y that corresponds to a one-unit increase in x_i, given that all other explanatory variables remain constant. For hypothesis testing, the t-test is based on n-q-1 degrees of freedom.

- n is the number of observations.
- q is the number of explanatory variables.

In multiple linear regression, multiple tests are necessary. We are testing whether the slope of each explanatory variable is equal to 0, while holding the rest of the factors (variables) constant. Multiple tests are not independent, so the overall P(Type I error) $> \alpha$, if they are all evaluated at the same α.

Model evaluation

When evaluating the model, the coefficient of determination (R^2) is not useful because R^2 will always increase as the number of explanatory variables increases.

- Using adjusted R^2:
  - Adjusted R^2 increases when the inclusion of a variable improves our ability to predict the response and decreases when it does not.
  - Adjusted R^2 allows for more valid comparisons between models that contain different numbers of explanatory variables.

- Adjusted R^2 is an estimator of the population correlation.
- However, because of the adjustment, it cannot be directly interpreted as the proportion of the variability among the observed values of y that is explained by the linear regression model.

- Residual plots:
    - These are the same as the ones produced for simple linear regression.

EXAMPLE PROBLEM 13.2

Recall that in Example Problem 13.1 we were interested in how hospital-level factors might influence a state's infant mortality rate.[3,4] We concluded that having a high proportion of hospitals adhering to an exclusive breastfeeding standard was related to a lower infant mortality rate.

We now wish to investigate whether the proportion of hospitals that teach breastfeeding techniques affects the infant mortality rate. Given that we have already accounted for the proportion of hospitals that comply with the exclusive breastfeeding benchmark (denoted as x_1), does the inclusion of the proportion of hospitals that teach breastfeeding techniques (denoted as x_2) in the regression model further improve our ability to predict infant mortality? This updated model will be referred to as Example Problem Model 2. Use the *mpinc_mortality* dataset for the following problems.

The population regression model is denoted as the following:

$$\mu_{y|x} = \alpha + \beta_1 x_1 + \beta_2 x_2$$

$$\mu_{y|x} = \alpha + \beta_1 \times \textit{exclusive breastfeeding} + \beta_2 \times \textit{teach techniques}$$

To fit Example Problem Model 2 using code (Table 13.6), we simply add the teaching techniques variable (*teach*) to our model and code from Example Problem 13.1 (Table 13.2).

Parameter Estimates

Variable	Label	DF	Parameter Estimate	Standard Error	t Value	Pr > |t|
Intercept	Intercept	1	8.00811	0.87773	9.12	<.0001
ExclusiveBF	Proportion of hospitals meeting exclusive breastfeeding benchmark	1	–0.05086	0.01940	–2.62	0.0117
Teach	Proportion of hospitals teaching breastfeeding techniques	1	0.02072	0.01921	1.08	0.2861

Table 13.6 Code for multiple linear regression (Example Problem 13.2)

Using SAS	*Using Stata*
PROC REG DATA = mpinc_mortality; MODEL infant_mortality2010 = exclusivebf teach; **RUN**; **QUIT**;	***regress infant_mortality2010 exclusivebf teach***

```
------------------------------------------------------------------------------
infant_~2010 |      Coef.   Std. Err.      t    P>|t|     [95% Conf. Interval]
-------------+----------------------------------------------------------------
 exclusivebf | -.0508596   .0193993    -2.62   0.012    -.0898646   -.0118547
       teach |  .0207213   .0192083     1.08   0.286    -.0178996    .0593422
       _cons |  8.008106   .8777265     9.12   0.000     6.243318    9.772893
------------------------------------------------------------------------------
```

A **What is the equation of the estimated line?**

$$\hat{y} = \hat{\alpha} + \widehat{\beta_1} x_1 + \widehat{\beta_2} x_2$$

$$\widehat{\textit{infant mortality}} = 8.01 - 0.05 \times \textit{exclusive breastfeeding} + 0.02 \times \textit{teach}$$

We now test the null hypotheses that the slopes associated with exclusive breastfeeding and teaching techniques are equal to 0. Because there are two parameters, this requires two separate tests.

Our test statistics follow the t-distribution with n-q-1 degrees of freedom. In this sample, $n = 51$, and $q = 2$, so we have 48 degrees of freedom.

B **What is the conclusion for each of these tests?**

For exclusive breastfeeding, we test the following hypothesis:

$$H_0\colon \beta_1 = 0$$

$$H_1\colon \beta_1 \neq 0$$

To calculate the test statistic, we use Equation 13.4.

$$t = \frac{\hat{\beta}_1}{\hat{se}(\hat{\beta}_1)}$$

$$t = \frac{-0.051}{0.0194}$$

$$t = -2.63 \sim t_{48}$$

From the t-distribution table in Appendix Table A.4, we can see that $0.01 < p < 0.005$. In SAS, the p-value for the slope is 0.0117, and, in Stata, the p-value is 0.012. Therefore, we reject the null hypothesis that the slope is equal to 0 and conclude that there is a significant linear relationship. As the proportion of hospitals with exclusive breastfeeding practices increases, the rate of infant mortality decreases.

We now perform a second hypothesis test. For the teaching techniques benchmark, we test the following hypothesis:

$$H_0: \beta_2 = 0$$

$$H_1: \beta_2 \neq 0$$

$$t = \frac{\hat{\beta}_2}{\widehat{se}(\hat{\beta}_2)}$$

$$t = \frac{0.021}{0.0192}$$

$$t = 1.09 \sim t_{48}$$

From the t-distribution table in Table A.4 of the Appendix, we can see that $p > 0.1$. The p-value for the slope is 0.286 (for both SAS and Stata). Therefore, we fail to reject the null hypothesis that the slope is equal to 0 and conclude that there is not a significant linear relationship.

C **Recall that in Example Problem 13.1 Model 1 (Example Problem Model 1), exclusive breastfeeding alone accounted for 12% of the variability in the model. What percentage of variability do exclusive breastfeeding and teaching techniques together (Example Problem Model 2) explain?**

Root MSE	1.21783	**R-Square**	0.1443
Dependent Mean	6.52784	**Adj R-Sq**	0.1087
Coeff Var	18.65598		

```
    Source |       SS           df       MS      Number of obs   =        51
-----------+----------------------------------   F(2, 48)        =      4.05
     Model |  12.0081905         2  6.00409524   Prob > F        =    0.0237
  Residual |  71.1896723        48  1.48311817   R-squared       =    0.1443
-----------+----------------------------------   Adj R-squared   =    0.1087
     Total |  83.1978627        50  1.66395725   Root MSE        =    1.2178
```

The R^2 for Example Problem Model 2 is 0.1443, according to SAS and Stata. This means that 14.43% of the variability among the observed values of infant mortality is explained by the linear relationship between infant mortality and the proportion of hospitals meeting the benchmarks for exclusive breastfeeding and teaching techniques. The remaining 85.6% is not explained by this relationship.

We can see that the R^2 for Example Problem Model 2 is larger than the R^2 for Example Problem Model 1, but does this have meaning? Is R^2 the most appropriate measure for models with more than one explanatory variable?

No, this is not the most appropriate measure because the R^2 always increases with the addition of more variables. We should use the adjusted R^2 when comparing the models.

D **Find the adjusted R^2 for Example Problem Model 1 (exclusive breastfeeding practices only) and Example Problem Model 2 (exclusive breastfeeding practices and teaching techniques). How does this change in value indicate whether the addition of the teaching techniques variable improves our ability to predict infant mortality rates?**

The adjusted R^2 for Example Problem Model 1 is 0.1057.
The adjusted R^2 for Example Problem Model 2 is 0.1087.

These values can be found below the R-Square value in the SAS output box and below the R-Squared value in the Stata output box. In SAS, it is the "Adj R-Sq" value, and in Stata, it is the "Adj R-Squared" value.

Since the adjusted R^2 for Example Problem Model 2 is larger than the adjusted R^2 for Example Problem Model 1, our ability to predict infant mortality marginally improves (given the small increase) with the addition of the teaching techniques variable.

E **Would you leave teaching techniques in a final model to predict infant mortality rates? Why or why not?**

Because we failed to reject H_0: $\beta_2 = 0$ and because the adjusted R^2 only marginally improved from Example Problem Model 1 to Example Problem Model 2, we would not leave teaching techniques in a final model to predict infant mortality rates.

PRACTICE PROBLEM 13.3

In Practice Problem 13.1, we used the percentage of owner-occupied houses in a neighborhood to predict the overall playground score. We now wish to determine whether the addition of the percentage of youth in a neighborhood improves our ability to predict playground scores. This model will be referred to as Practice Problem Model 3. Use the *pastl_score* dataset to answer the following problems.

A What is the equation of the estimated line?

B At the $\alpha = 0.05$ significance level, test the null hypothesis that the slope associated with the percentage of owner-occupied housing and the percentage of youth is equal to 0. Note: These are two separate tests.

C Recall that in Practice Problem 13.1—Part (H) (Practice Problem Model 1) we calculated the amount of variability in the model that was attributed to the explanatory variable for percentage of owner-occupied housing. What percentage of variability do percentage of owner-occupied housing and percentage of youth together (Practice Problem Model 3) explain?

D What would you use to compare this model to Practice Problem Model 1? Compare the values for both models.

E Would you leave percentage of youth in a final model to predict neighborhood playground scores? Why or why not?

Other explanatory variables

Indicator variables

So far, our predictor variables have been continuous, but regression analysis can be generalized to incorporate discrete or nominal explanatory variables as well. One example is the indicator variable.

Indicator Variable (Dummy Variable): A dichotomous (0,1) variable with values that do not have any quantitative meaning.

A regression model with one continuous explanatory variable and one dichotomous explanatory variable can be thought of as two different models.

- Each model corresponds to a different level of the two possible values for the dichotomous variable.
- The intercepts of each model's regression line will be different, but both models' regression lines will have the same slope.

Categorical variables

The concept of dichotomous variables can be extended to include categorical variables. For each categorical variable with m levels, create $m - 1$ indicator variables, and enter them all into the model.

- Each level will be represented by the set of indicator variables.
- The *m*th level will be represented when all the $m - 1$ indicators are set to 0. This representation is the reference level for the categorical variable.

BOX 13.6 TRANSFORMING A CATEGORICAL VARIABLE INTO INDICATOR VARIABLES

If we have a categorical variable with five levels indicating race ethnicity (non-Hispanic White, non-Hispanic Black, Asian, Hispanic, and other), we would create four indicator variables (non-Hispanic Black, Asian, Hispanic, and other). This would leave non-Hispanic White as our reference level. Table 13.7 displays the transformation from a five-level categorical variable to a series of four indicator variables. Notice that non-Hispanic Whites receive a value of 0 for each of the indicators. Those who are non-Hispanic Black receive a value of 1 for the non-Hispanic Black indicator and a 0 for the Asian, Hispanic, and other indicators. All four indicator variables will be entered into the model as predictors.

Interaction terms

In some situations, one explanatory variable has a different effect on the predicted response *y*, depending on the value of a second explanatory variable; this is referred to as moderation or effect modification. To model this relationship, we create an interaction term.

Interaction Term: A variable generated by multiplying together the values of two variables x_i and x_j to create a third variable, x_ix_j.

Do this in a DATA step in SAS, or use the *generate* command in Stata to create the new variable. When entering an interaction term (x_ix_j) into the model, the main effects (x_i and x_j) must remain in the model.

Table 13.7 Transformation of a categorical variable into indicator variables

Categorical variable	*Indicator variable*			
	Non-Hispanic Black	*Asian*	*Hispanic*	*Other*
Non-Hispanic White	0	0	0	0
Non-Hispanic Black	1	0	0	0
Asian	0	1	0	0
Hispanic	0	0	1	0
Other	0	0	0	1

EXAMPLE PROBLEM 13.3

Recall the model that we established in Example Problem 13.2, using the *mpinc_mortality* dataset.[3,4] We concluded that having a high proportion of hospitals adhering to an exclusive breastfeeding standard was related to a lower infant mortality rate but that the addition of the proportion of hospitals that teach breastfeeding techniques did not improve the model. Another hospital factor that might influence infant mortality rates is the overall facility discharge score and whether that score is above the national average (denoted as x_3). This model will be referred to as Example Problem Model 3.

To fit Example Problem Model 3 using code (Table 13.8), we add the *discharge* variable to our model that only contains the *exclusive breastfeeding* variable (Example Problem Model 1).

Parameter Estimates

Variable	Label	DF	Parameter Estimate	Standard Error	t Value	Pr > |t|
Intercept	Intercept	1	8.25254	0.69826	11.82	<.0001
ExclusiveBF	Proportion of hospitals meeting exclusive breastfeeding benchmark	1	–0.02486	0.01294	–1.92	0.0607
Discharge	Above national facility discharge care score average	1	–1.13215	0.34221	–3.31	0.0018

```
------------------------------------------------------------------------------
infant_~2010 |      Coef.   Std. Err.      t    P>|t|     [95% Conf. Interval]
-------------+----------------------------------------------------------------
exclusivebf | -.0248591   .0129422     -1.92   0.061     -.0508811     .0011629
  discharge | -1.132148   .3422121     -3.31   0.002     -1.820212    -.4440843
      _cons |   8.25254   .6982564     11.82   0.000      6.848601     9.656478
------------------------------------------------------------------------------
```

A **What is the equation of the estimated line?**

$$\hat{y} = \hat{\alpha} - \widehat{\beta_1} x_1 + \widehat{\beta_3} x_3$$

$$\widehat{\textit{infant mortality}} = 8.25 - 0.02 \times \textit{exclusive breastfeeding} - 1.13 \times \textit{discharge}$$

Table 13.8 Code for multiple linear regression with indicator variable (Example Problem 13.3)

Using SAS	*Using Stata*
PROC REG DATA = mpinc_mortality; MODEL infant_mortality2010 = exclusivebf discharge; **RUN; QUIT;**	**regress *infant_mortality2010 exclusivebf discharge***

B Interpret the estimated coefficients for exclusive breastfeeding and for the facility discharge score in words.

Within each level of discharge, the mean infant mortality rate decreases by 0.02 for each percentage point increase in the proportion of hospitals meeting the exclusive breastfeeding benchmark.

States with a facility discharge score that is lower than the national average have a mean infant mortality rate that is 1.13 infant deaths per 1000 live births higher than for states with a score greater or equal to the national average, when the proportion of hospitals meeting the exclusive breastfeeding benchmark is the same.

We now test the null hypothesis that the slope associated with facility discharge care is equal to 0.

Our test statistic follows the t-distribution with n-q-1 degrees of freedom. In this case, $n = 51$ and $q = 2$, so we have 48 degrees of freedom.

C What is the conclusion for this test?

For facility discharge care, we test the following hypothesis:

$$H_0: \beta_3 = 0$$

$$H_1: \beta_3 \neq 0$$

Using the test statistic,

$$t = \frac{\hat{\beta}_3}{\hat{se}(\hat{\beta}_3)}$$

$$t = \frac{-1.132}{0.3422}$$

$$t = -3.31 \sim t_{48}$$

Using statistical software (SAS or Stata), we see that the test statistic is −3.31. In SAS, the p-value for the slope is 0.0018. In Stata, the p-value for the slope is 0.002. Therefore, we reject the null hypothesis that the slope is equal to 0 and conclude that there is a significant linear relationship. We conclude that states with a facility discharge score that is lower than the national average have a higher mean infant mortality rate than states that are at or above the national average.

D How has Example Problem Model 1 (Example Problem 13.1) changed by adding the indicator for facility discharge score?

In order to compare the two models, we use the adjusted R^2 value.

Root MSE	1.11221	R-Square	0.2863
Dependent Mean	6.52784	Adj R-Sq	0.2566
Coeff Var	17.03794		

```
     Source |       SS           df       MS      Number of obs   =        51
-----------+----------------------------------   F(2, 48)        =      9.63
      Model |  23.8213086         2  11.9106543   Prob > F        =    0.0003
   Residual |  59.3765541        48  1.23701154   R-squared       =    0.2863
-----------+----------------------------------   Adj R-squared   =    0.2566
      Total |  83.1978627        50  1.66395725   Root MSE        =    1.1122
```

The adjusted R^2 for Example Problem Model 1 is 0.1057.

The adjusted R^2 for this model (Example Problem Model 3) is 0.2566.

Since the adjusted R^2 for Example Problem Model 3 is larger than the adjusted R^2 for Example Problem Model 1, we conclude that our ability to predict infant mortality rates improves with the addition of the dichotomous variable for the facility discharge score.

Since our results indicate a significant relationship between infant mortality rates and the facility discharge score dichotomous variable, the model can be thought of as two regression lines (one for states with a facility discharge score below the national average and one for states at or above the national average).

When $x_3 = 1$ (at or above the national average),

$$\hat{y} = 8.25 - 0.02 \times \textit{exclusive breastfeeding} - 1.13 \times (1)$$

$$\hat{y} = 7.12 - 0.02 \times \textit{exclusive breastfeeding}$$

When $x_3 = 0$ (below the national average),

$$\hat{y} = 8.25 - 0.02 \times \textit{exclusive breastfeeding} - 1.13 \times (0)$$

$$\hat{y} = 8.25 - 0.02 \times \textit{exclusive breastfeeding}$$

If we sketch this relationship, it will look like Figure 13.8.

We could add another variable to the model to determine whether an increase in proportion of hospitals meeting the exclusive breastfeeding benchmark has a different effect in states that have a facility discharge score that is lower than the national average versus states that have a facility discharge score higher or equal to the national average. This added variable would be an interaction between the *exclusive breastfeeding* variable and the facility discharge score indicator.

If the interaction variable significantly adds to the model, that means that the effect of exclusive breastfeeding on infant mortality rates would be different

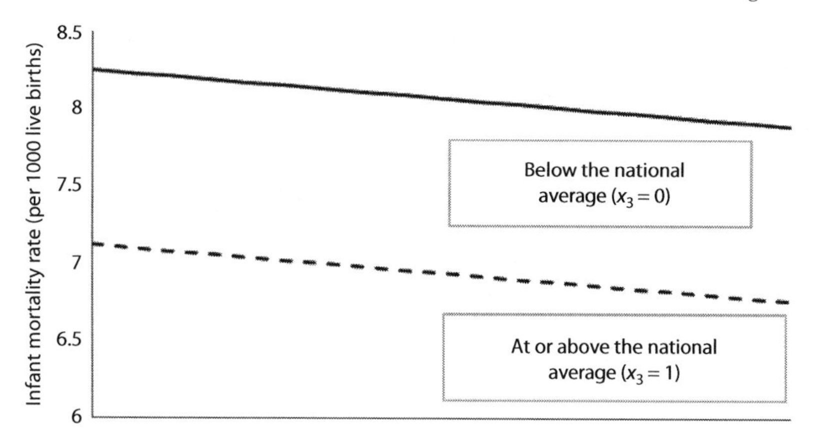

Figure 13.8 **Indicator variables and their effect on the regression model for Example Problem 13.3.** The top line can be thought of as the regression line of the model when facility discharge scores are below the national average, and the bottom line is a representation of the regression line of the model when facility discharge scores are at or above the national average.

in states that have facility discharge scores that are lower than the national average versus states with scores higher or equal to the national average.

Upon adding the interaction term to the model, the regression equation will look like the following:

$$\hat{y} = \hat{\alpha} + \widehat{\beta_1} x_1 + \widehat{\beta_3} x_3 + \widehat{\beta_4}(x_1 \times x_3)$$

$$\hat{y} = \hat{\alpha} + \widehat{\beta_1} \textit{exclusivebf} + \widehat{\beta_3} \textit{discharge} + \widehat{\beta_4}(\textit{exclusivebf} \times \textit{discharge})$$

If discharge = 1, then the following is true:

$$\hat{y} = \hat{\alpha} + \widehat{\beta_1} \textit{exclusivebf} + \widehat{\beta_3}(1) + \widehat{\beta_4 \textit{exclusivebf}} \times (1)$$

$$\hat{y} = (\hat{\alpha} + \widehat{\beta_3}) + (\widehat{\beta_1} + \widehat{\beta_4}) \textit{exclusivebf}$$

If discharge = 0, then the following is true:

$$\hat{y} = \hat{\alpha} + \widehat{\beta_1} \textit{exclusivebf} + \widehat{\beta_3}(0) + \widehat{\beta_4} \textit{exclusivebf} \times (0)$$

$$\hat{y} = \hat{\alpha} + \widehat{\beta_1} \textit{exclusivebf}$$

The interaction term makes the slope and the intercept different in the two regression equations.

If we sketch this relationship, it will look like Figure 13.9. Also see Table 13.9 for code to create on interaction term.

Add the interaction term to Example Problem Model 3 (see Table 13.10). The resulting model (with the added interaction term) will be referred to as Example Problem Model 4.

Parameter Estimates

Variable	Label	DF	Parameter Estimate	Standard Error	t Value	Pr > |t|
Intercept	Intercept	1	7.51435	1.18273	6.35	<.0001
ExclusiveBF	Proportion of hospitals meeting exclusive breastfeeding benchmark	1	–0.01064	0.02249	–0.47	0.6384
Discharge	Above national facility discharge care score average	1	0.02542	1.53261	0.02	0.9868
ebf_discharge		1	–0.02136	0.02756	–0.78	0.4422

```
------------------------------------------------------------------------------
infant_m~2010 |      Coef.   Std. Err.      t    P>|t|     [95% Conf. Interval]
--------------+---------------------------------------------------------------
  exclusivebf |  -.0106358   .0224878    -0.47   0.638    -.0558754    .0346037
    discharge |   .0254216   1.532611     0.02   0.987    -3.057793    3.108636
ebf_discharge |  -.0213563   .0275556    -0.78   0.442    -.0767911    .0340784
        _cons |   7.514353   1.182728     6.35   0.000     5.135011    9.893695
------------------------------------------------------------------------------
```

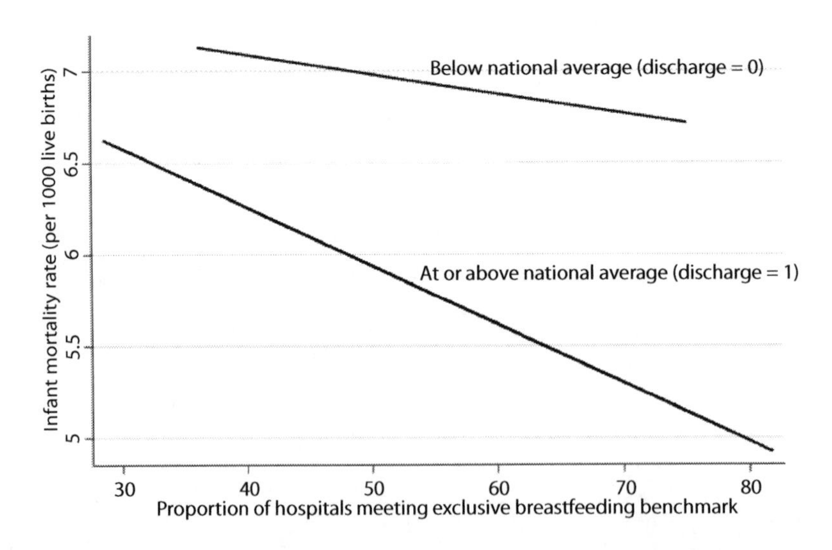

Figure 13.9 **Regression model for Example Problem 13.3 with moderation (interaction).** The top line can be thought of as the regression line of the model when facility discharge scores are below the national average, and the bottom line is a representation of the regression line of the model when facility discharge scores are at or above the national average.

Table 13.9 Code for calculating an interaction term (Example Problem 13.3)

Using SAS	*Using Stata*

To create an interaction term, use a DATA step.
 	
`DATA mpinc_mortality_1;`
`SET mpinc_mortality;`
`ebf_discharge = exclusivebf *`
`discharge;`
`RUN;`
	To create an interaction term, use the *generate* command. The new variable is added to your working dataset.
	
	`generate ebf_discharge =`
	`exclusivebf*discharge`

Table 13.10 Code for regression with an interaction term (Example Problem 13.3)

Using SAS	*Using Stata*

Remember to run your PROC REG on the new dataset that you created.
 	
`PROC REG DATA =`
`mpinc_mortality_1;`
`MODEL infant_mortality2010 =`
`exclusivebf discharge`
`ebf_discharge;`
`RUN; QUIT;`
	`regress infant_mortality2010`
	`exclusivebf discharge ebf_discharge`

To determine whether the interaction term improves our ability to predict infant mortality rates, we need to test the null hypothesis that the slope of the interaction term is 0 and examine the change in the value of the adjusted R^2.

E **Test to see whether there is a significant linear relationship between the interaction term and the overall neighborhood playground score in Example Problem Model 4. Be sure to state the null and alternate hypotheses, the value and distribution of the test statistic, and *p*-value. What do you conclude?**

$$H_0: \beta_4 = 0$$

$$H_1: \beta_4 \neq 0$$

$$t = \frac{\widehat{\beta_4}}{\widehat{se}(\widehat{\beta_4})}$$

$$t = \frac{-0.021}{0.0276}$$

$$t = -0.76 \sim t_{48}$$

Using statistical software (SAS or Stata), we get $t = -0.78$ and $p = 0.442$. Therefore, we fail to reject the null hypothesis that the slope is equal to 0 and conclude that there is not a significant linear relationship.

F **What is the adjusted R^2 value, and how does it compare to the adjusted R^2 found for Example Problem Model 3 in Example Problem 13.3—Part D?**

The adjusted R^2 for Example Problem Model 3 is 0.2566.
The adjusted R^2 for this model (Example Problem Model 4) is 0.2503.
Because the adjusted R^2 for this model is less than the adjusted R^2 for Example Problem Model 3, we can conclude that adding the interaction does not increase our ability to predict infant mortality rates. On this basis—and our failure to reject the null hypothesis in Example Problem 13.3—Part E—we would decide to exclude the interaction term from the final model.

Model selection

When you have many variables of interest, how do you choose the final model?

- You should have some prior idea about what is important, based on some subject area knowledge.
- You could construct all possible models.
  - This is thorough but time consuming.
  - Perform a regression analysis for each possible combination of variables.
- You could perform stepwise model selection.

Automatic Model Selection: An automatic approach to finding a subset of explanatory variables that produces the best fit regression line.

The three types of selection discussed in this book are forward selection, backward elimination, and stepwise selection. It is possible to end up with different final models from each of the stepwise approaches.

- Forward selection
  - Start with no explanatory variables in the model, and introduce variables one at a time.
  - The model is evaluated after the introduction of each variable.
  - The process continues until some specified statistical criterion is achieved.
- Backward elimination
  - Begin with all explanatory variables in the model, and drop variables one at a time.
  - The model is evaluated after each variable has been dropped.
  - The process continues until some specified statistical criterion is achieved.
- Stepwise selection
  - This method uses both forward selection and backward elimination techniques.
  - Start with no explanatory variables in the model, and introduce variables into the model, one at a time.

- All previous variables in the model are checked at each step to ensure that they maintain their statistical significance.
- A variable entered in one step might be dropped out in a later step.

BOX 13.7 USING SAS FOR AUTOMATIC MODEL SELECTION

In SAS, use the SELECTION=option in the MODEL statement of PROC REG to specify which type of automatic model selection the program should use to determine a final model. For forward selection, use SELECTION=FORWARD. For backward elimination, use SELECTION=BACKWARD. Finally, for stepwise selection, use SELECTION=STEPWISE.

You can also adjust the inclusion and exclusion criteria, but this is optional. For the inclusion criterion, use the SLENTRY=value option to adjust the significance level for entry into the model. The default is 0.5 for forward selection and 0.15 for stepwise selection. For the exclusion criterion, use the SLSTAY=value for the significance level to stay in the model. The default is 0.1 for backward elimination and 0.15 for stepwise selection. The order of the variables that are specified in the model statement is the order that they will be entered into the model, if forward selection is specified.

The output of PROC REG using automatic model selection is an abbreviated version of the PROC REG output that we discussed previously. For each step in the process, SAS provides an ANOVA and a parameter estimates table for the resulting model. The final table provides a summary of what happened at each step (which single variable was added or removed). See Table 13.11 for the code to run each of these methods.

Once you are satisfied with your final model, it is a good idea to run it again (including only the variables in the final model) without the automatic selection method specified. SAS deletes observations list-wise at each step, and, if a more restrictive variable does not end up in the final model, it is possible that observations were deleted that could be included in the final model.

BOX 13.8 USING STATA FOR AUTOMATIC MODEL SELECTION

To run automatic model selection in Stata, use the *stepwise* command with the appropriate option before your *regress* command. The pr(*value*) option allows you to specify the significance level for removal from the model. For example, if you specified pr(0.05), variables that had a *p*-value of greater than 0.05 would be kicked out of the model. The pe(*value*) option allows you to specify the significance level for addition into the model. You must specify at least one pr(*value*) or pe(*value*), as this indicates to Stata which automatic model selection method to use. See Table 13.11 for the code to run each of these methods.

In Stata, the output is the same as a regular *regress* command, with the exception of a statement at the beginning summarizing the variables that were added and dropped.

Table 13.11 Example code to run automatic model selection on three explanatory variables

Automatic model selection method	*Software code*

Backward elimination	SAS Code:
	`PROC REG DATA = dataset;`
	`MODEL outcome = var1 var2 var3 / selection=backward;`
	`RUN; QUIT;`
	
	Stata Code:
	`stepwise, pr(value): regress outcome var1 var2 var3`

Forward selection	SAS Code:
	`PROC REG DATA = dataset;`
	`MODEL outcome = var1 var2 var3 / selection=forward;`
	`RUN; QUIT;`
	
	Stata Code:
	`stepwise, pe(value): regress outcome var1 var2 var3`

Stepwise selection	SAS Code:
	`PROC REG DATA = dataset;`
	`MODEL outcome = var1 var2 var3 / selection=stepwise;`
	`RUN; QUIT;`
	
	Stata Code:
	`stepwise, pr(value) pe(value) forward: regress outcome var1 var2 var3`

Collinearity

Regardless of the strategy used when selecting a model, we should always check for collinearity.

Collinearity: A condition that occurs when two or more of the explanatory variables are correlated to the extent that they convey essentially the same information about the observed variability in the outcome y.

- One symptom of collinearity is the instability of the estimated coefficients and their standard errors.
- Standard errors often become very large, implying that there is a great deal of sampling variability in the estimated coefficients.
- The variance inflation factor (VIF) quantifies the degree of severity of collinearity in the model.

PRACTICE PROBLEM 13.4

Upon examining the neighborhoods further in the *pastl_score* dataset,[5] we notice that the neighborhoods with high percentages of vacant buildings are clustered in the north of the city, north of Delmar Boulevard. We are interested in whether an interaction between the geographic location of the neighborhood (north or south of Delmar Boulevard) affects the neighborhood playground score.

A What is the regression equation for a model that includes the percentage of vacant buildings and the indicator for north or south of Delmar Boulevard (Practice Problem Model 4)?

B Interpret the estimated coefficients for the slopes in words.

C Test to see whether there is a significant linear relationship between the indicator (*north*) and the overall neighborhood playground score in Practice Problem Model 4. Be sure to state the null and alternate hypotheses, the value and distribution of the test statistic, and p-value. What do you conclude?

D How has Practice Problem Model 2 from (Practice Problem 13.2) changed by adding the indicator?

E Create an interaction term between the percentage of vacant buildings and the indicator for north or south of Delmar Boulevard. What is the regression equation for this model (Practice Problem Model 5)?

F Test to see whether there is a significant linear relationship between the interaction term and the overall neighborhood playground score in Practice Problem Model 5. Be sure to state the null and alternate hypotheses, the value and distribution of the test statistic, and p-value. What do you conclude?

G What is the adjusted R^2 value for Practice Problem Model 5, and how does it compare to the adjusted R^2 value found for the model in Practice Problem 13.2 (Practice Problem Model 2)?

PRACTICE PROBLEM 13.5

A What is the equation for the *true* population regression line for simple linear regression?

B What is the equation for the *true* population regression line for multiple linear regression?

PRACTICE PROBLEM 13.6

Compare and contrast when you use the R^2 value versus when you use the adjusted R^2 value.

References

1. Centers for Disease Control and Prevention. Hospital actions affect breastfeeding. *Vital Signs*. http://www.cdc.gov/vitalsigns/breastfeeding2015/index.html. Updated October 6, 2015. Accessed September 16, 2016.
2. Baby-Friendly USA. The ten steps to successful breastfeeding. http://www.babyfriendlyusa.org/about-us/baby-friendly-hospital-initiative/the-ten-steps/. Accessed September 16, 2016.
3. Centers for Disease Control and Prevention. Maternity Practices in Infant Nutrition and Care (mPINC) Survey. http://www.cdc.gov/breastfeeding/data/mpinc/index.htm. Updated November 4, 2016. Accessed December 10, 2016.
4. Mathews TJ, MacDorman MF. Infant mortality statistics from the 2010 period linked birth/infant death data set. *Natl Vital Stat Reports*. 2013;62(8):1–26. http://www.cdc.gov/nchs/data/nvsr/nvsr62/nvsr62_08.pdf. Accessed December 10, 2016.
5. Arroyo-Johnson C, Woodward K, Milam L, Ackermann N, Goodman MS, Hipp JA. Still separate, still unequal: Social determinants of playground safety and proximity. *J Urban Heal*. 2016;93(4):627–638. doi:10.1007/s11524-016-0063-8.

14 Logistic regression

This chapter will focus on logistic regression analysis and will include the following topics:

- Interpretation of coefficients
- Hypothesis tests and confidence intervals for estimated regression coefficients
- Model evaluation

Term

- c statistic

Introduction

There are many situations in which the response of interest is dichotomous rather than continuous. Most commonly, the binary variable is a yes/no variable indicating an event or condition. If we use linear regression in a case in which the outcome is dichotomous, we can have predicted values that are less than 0 or greater than 1 even though the outcome can take only values 0 or 1. Thus, we need a different model for dichotomous/binary data than we used for linear regression with a continuous outcome. In these cases in which the response variable Y is dichotomous, we use logistic regression.

Many of the concepts in logistic regression are the same as in linear regression, a topic that was introduced in Chapter 13. Following is a list of the shared concepts:

- Indicator variables
- Interactions
- Model selection techniques

However, some concepts are different from the linear regression model:

- Residuals
- Model evaluation
- Interpretation of coefficients

In linear regression, it is helpful to look at two-way scatterplots to get a sense of the correlation between the predictor and the outcome. However, when the outcome is dichotomous, all points on the scatterplot will be on the two lines corresponding to the two levels of the outcome. Thus, two-way scatterplots in a logistic regression case do not give us much useful information about the relationship between the predictor and the outcome. (See Figure 14.1.)

The mean of a dichotomous random variable Y, designated by p, is the proportion of times that Y takes the value 1. In symbols, mean of $Y = P(Y = 1) = p$. Just as we estimated the mean value of the response when Y was continuous, we would like to be able to estimate the probability p (its mean) associated with a dichotomous response.

If an event occurs with probability p, the odds in favor of the event are $\frac{p}{1-p}:1$. Modeling the probability with a logistic function is equivalent to fitting a linear regression model in which the continuous response Y has been replaced by the logarithm of the odds of success for a dichotomous random variable. Instead of assuming that the relationship between p and X is linear, we assume that the relationship between $\ln\left(\frac{p}{1-p}\right)$ and X is linear. Thus, in logistic regression, we are modeling the log odds of an event.

$$\ln\left(\frac{p}{1-p}\right) = \alpha + \beta_1 x_1 + \ldots + \beta_q x_q \tag{14.1}$$

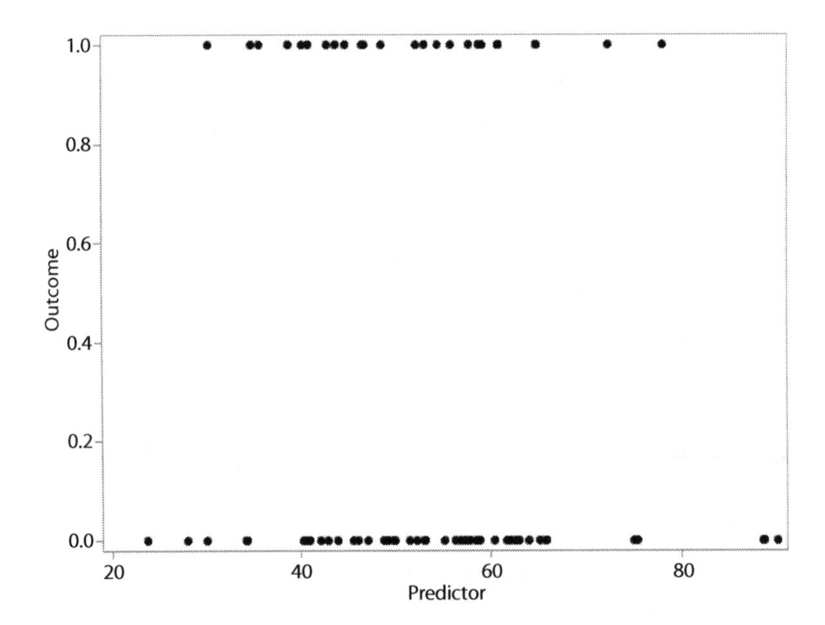

Figure 14.1 **Two-way scatterplot with dichotomous outcome.** When the outcome variable is dichotomous, it is difficult to assess the association between the explanatory variable and the outcome using a two-way scatterplot.

We cannot apply the method of least squares, which assumes that the response is continuous and normally distributed. Instead, we use maximum likelihood estimation (MLE). MLE uses the information in a sample to find the parameter estimates that are most likely to have produced the observed data. We can start with the basic logistic regression equation and solve for $\hat{p}$.

$$\begin{aligned}
\ln\left(\frac{\hat{p}}{1-\hat{p}}\right) &= \hat{\alpha}+\hat{\beta}_1x_1+\ldots+\hat{\beta}_qx_q \\
\frac{\hat{p}}{1-\hat{p}} &= e^{\hat{\alpha}+\hat{\beta}_1x_1+\ldots+\hat{\beta}_qx_q} \\
\hat{p} &= e^{\hat{\alpha}+\hat{\beta}_1x_1+\ldots+\hat{\beta}_qx_q}(1-\hat{p}) \\
\hat{p} &= e^{\hat{\alpha}+\hat{\beta}_1x_1+\ldots+\hat{\beta}_qx_q} - e^{\hat{\alpha}+\hat{\beta}_1x_1+\ldots+\hat{\beta}_qx_q}\hat{p} \\
\left(1+e^{\hat{\alpha}+\hat{\beta}_1x_1+\ldots+\hat{\beta}_qx_q}\right)\hat{p} &= e^{\hat{\alpha}+\hat{\beta}_1x_1+\ldots+\hat{\beta}_qx_q} \\
\hat{p} &= \frac{e^{\hat{\alpha}+\hat{\beta}_1x_1+\ldots+\hat{\beta}_qx_q}}{1+e^{\hat{\alpha}+\hat{\beta}_1x_1+\ldots+\hat{\beta}_qx_q}}
\end{aligned} \tag{14.2}$$

The expression for $\hat{p}$ is called a logistic function. Some of the properties of a logistic function are:

- It cannot yield a value that is either negative or greater than 1. This is beneficial because it restricts the estimated value of p to the required range.
- It is S-shaped, with a steeper slope in the middle and a shallower slope as the predicted probability approaches 0 or 1. (See Figure 14.2.)

In addition to graphing the data, we can create a table of probabilities to see the relationship between the explanatory variable and the predicted probability of the outcome. Table 14.1 shows how the association between the outcome and explanatory variable can be assessed by examining a table of the values of the explanatory variable, x_1, and the corresponding predicted probability of the outcome, $\hat{p}$. In the table, we can see that as x_1 increases, so does $\hat{p}$.[1]

If an event occurs with probability $p=\frac{e^{\alpha+\beta X_i}}{1+e^{\alpha+\beta X_i}}$, the odds in favor of the event are

$$\begin{aligned}
\frac{p}{1-p} = \frac{\frac{e^{\alpha+\beta X_i}}{1+e^{\alpha+\beta X_i}}}{1-\frac{e^{\alpha+\beta X_i}}{1+e^{\alpha+\beta X_i}}} &= \frac{\frac{e^{\alpha+\beta X_i}}{1+e^{\alpha+\beta X_i}}}{\frac{1}{1+e^{\alpha+\beta X_i}}} \\
&= e^{\alpha+\beta X_i}
\end{aligned} \tag{14.3}$$

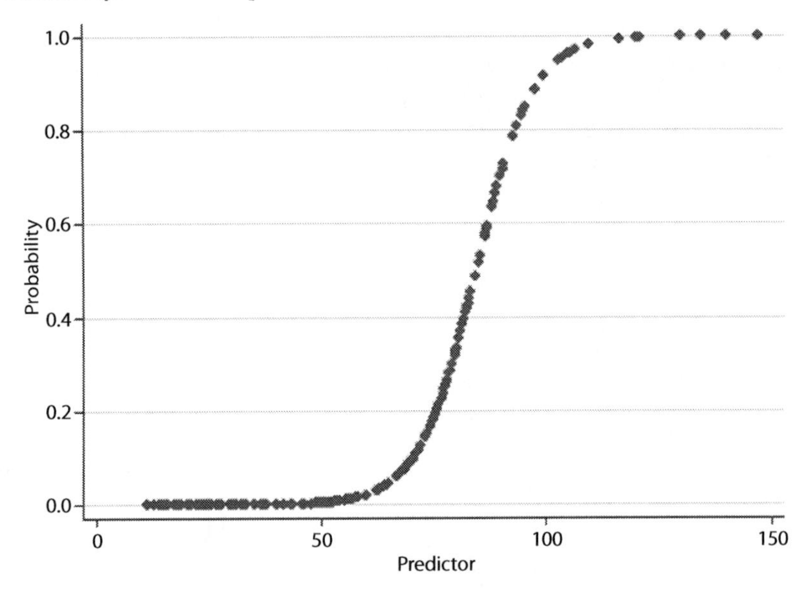

Figure 14.2 **Logistic distribution function.** The relationship between the predicted probability of the outcome and the values of the explanatory variable is an S-shaped function. The slope of the logistic function is shallow when the predicted probability is near 0 or 1 and is steeper in the middle. Data for the figure come from National Health and Nutrition Examination Survey, Centers for Disease Control and Prevention, National Center for Health Statistics, Hyattsville, MD, 2014, https://wwwn.cdc.gov/Nchs/Nhanes/Search /nhanes13{_}14.aspx.

Table 14.1 Relationship between explanatory variable and predicted probability of the outcome

x_1	$\hat{p}$
13.1	0.00001
32.6	0.00030
43.5	0.00165
53.8	0.00817
58.1	0.01586
63.2	0.03451
74.9	0.18178
80.7	0.35466
86.6	0.58000
97.6	0.88499
129.9	0.99916

If we take the natural logarithm, then we eliminate the exponentiation and have a function for the log odds dependent only on the values of α, β, and the explanatory variables x_i.

$$\ln\left(\frac{p}{1-p}\right) = \ln\left(e^{\alpha+\beta X_i}\right) = \alpha + \beta X_i \tag{14.4}$$

Interpretation of coefficients

The logistic regression model can be generalized to include discrete or nominal explanatory variables in addition to continuous ones. The estimated regression coefficient $\hat{\beta}$ is the change in the log odds of the outcome corresponding to a one-unit increase in x. When we have a dichotomous variable, the interpretation is slightly different since there are only two levels of x. Thus, the log odds change by $\hat{\beta}$ when increasing from x_i = 0 to x_i = 1, which means $\hat{\beta}$ is the difference in the log odds between the two levels of the binary predictor. Table 14.2 shows that the type of explanatory variable influences the interpretation of the estimated log odds and estimated odds ratio $(\widehat{\text{OR}})$.

We can also transform the estimated regression coefficient $\hat{\beta}$ into an $\widehat{\text{OR}}$ by calculating the antilogarithm of the regression coefficient.

$$\widehat{\text{OR}} = e^{\hat{\beta}} \tag{14.5}$$

The result is the $\widehat{\text{OR}}$ or relative odds comparing a one-unit increase in the explanatory variable. Sometimes, it is preferable to report an odds ratio corresponding to more than one unit of change in the predictor variable. For example, the odds ratio corresponding to a five-pound increase in weight might be more meaningful than the odds ratio corresponding to a one-pound increase in weight. In this case, $\widehat{\text{OR}} = e^{c\hat{\beta}}$, where c is the number of units of the explanatory variable. For the weight example, the OR corresponding to a five-pound increase in weight is

$$\widehat{\text{OR}} = e^{5\times\hat{\beta}}.$$

For dichotomous explanatory variables, the antilogarithm of $\hat{\beta}_i$, $e^{\hat{\beta}_i}$, is the estimated odds ratio for the response y comparing the two possible levels of x_i. The same results could be obtained by arranging the sample data in a 2 × 2 contingency table. The $\widehat{\text{OR}}$

Table 14.2 Interpretations for estimated coefficients

Type of predictor	*Interpretation of* $\hat{\beta}$	*Interpretation of* $e^{\hat{\beta}}$
Continuous	For each one-unit increase in x, the log odds of y changes by $\hat{\beta}$.	$e^{\hat{\beta}} = \widehat{\text{OR}}$ is the relative odds of y comparing a one-unit increase in x.
Dichotomous	The log odds of y changes by $\hat{\beta}$ when increasing from x_i = 0 to x_i = 1 ($\hat{\beta}$ is the difference in the log odds of y between the two levels of x).	$e^{\hat{\beta}} = \widehat{\text{OR}}$ is the estimated odds ratio for y comparing the two possible levels of x_i.

is estimated by computing the cross-product of the entries in the contingency table $\left(\frac{ad}{bc}\right)$ that was introduced in Chapter 10 and is identical to that obtained from the logistic regression model.

In order to estimate the odds of the event given predictor values, plug in the appropriate values of $\hat{\alpha}$, x_i, and $\hat{\beta}_i$ into Equation 14.3. To determine the predicted probability of the event given values of x_i, we plug in $\hat{\alpha}$, x_i, and $\hat{\beta}_i$ into Equation 14.2.

Hypothesis tests and confidence intervals for estimated regression coefficients

The hypothesis test for the estimated regression coefficient tests the null hypothesis that there is no relationship between the predictor and the outcome, H_0: $\beta = 0$, against the alternative H_1: $\beta \neq 0$. The null and alternative hypotheses can also be written in terms of the OR: H_0: OR $= 1$ versus H_1: OR $\neq 1$.

Test statistic $Z = \frac{\hat{\beta}}{\hat{se}(\hat{\beta})}$ follows a standard normal distribution. A confidence interval for the OR can be calculated from the model by computing a confidence interval for the coefficient $\hat{\beta}$ and taking the antilogarithm of its upper and lower limits. Table 14.3 provides a summary of hypothesis testing and confidence intervals for logistic regression. In a hypothesis test for the coefficient, we wish to test whether $\beta = 0$. In a hypothesis test for the odds ratio the null value is 1.

Model evaluation

In linear regression, the R^2 and adjusted R^2 indicate the proportion of variation in the outcome explained by the predictor variables. Unfortunately, we do not have an analogous measure for logistic regression. However, the c statistic can be used to assess model fit.

c Statistic: The area under the ROC curve that indicates how well the model predicts who will have the outcome and who will not. The c statistic ranges from 0.5 (poor discrimination) to 1 (perfect discrimination).

As a guideline, a c statistic ≥ 0.70 is considered acceptable.

Table 14.3 Hypothesis tests and confidence intervals for estimated regression coefficients

Component	*Formula*
Hypotheses	H_0: $\beta = 0$ vs. H_1: $\beta \neq 0$ (alternatively, H_0: OR $= 1$ vs. H_1: OR $\neq 1$)
Test statistic	$Z = \frac{\hat{\beta}}{\hat{se}(\hat{\beta})}$
Distribution of test statistic under H_0	Standard normal
Odds ratio (OR)	$\widehat{OR} = e^{\hat{\beta}}$
Confidence interval for OR	$\left(e^{lower\ CI\ for\ \hat{\beta}}, e^{lower\ CI\ for\ \hat{\beta}}\right)$

Logistic regression in SAS

We run logistic regressions in SAS using PROC LOGISTIC. The MODEL statement specifies the dichotomous outcome on the left side of the equals sign. When the binary outcome has levels 0 and 1, the SAS default is to calculate the probability that the outcome = 0. However, typically, binary variables are set up so that outcome = 1 indicates "yes" to the event, and it is the level that we want to model. When we insert the EVENT option, SAS models the probability that the outcome equals that level. Thus, specifying EVENT = "1" means that the probability that the outcome = 1 is modeled rather than outcome = 0.

We list predictor variables to the right of the equals sign. For continuous, binary, or ordinal predictor variables, we do not need a CLASS statement. However, if we have a categorical predictor variable and want SAS to produce dummy variables for the various levels, we use a CLASS statement. The CLASS statement includes the name of the categorical variable and an indication of the reference level.

The output will show estimates comparing all levels of the categorical variable to the level specified in the REF = option. The default parameterization method in PROC LOGISTIC is effect coding rather than reference coding. To change this, specify the PARAM = REF option in the CLASS statement. When we use reference coding, we can interpret $e^{\hat{\beta}}$ as summarized in Table 14.2.

```
PROC LOGISTIC DATA = dataset_name;
      CLASS pred_cat (REF = "1") / PARAM = REF;
      MODEL outcome (EVENT = "1") = pred_cont pred_bin pred_cat;
RUN;
```

The LOGISTIC Procedure

Model Information	
Data Set	WORK.DATASET_NAME
Response Variable	outcome
Number of Response Levels	2
Model	binary logit
Optimization Technique	Fisher's scoring

Number of Observations Read	75
Number of Observations Used	75

Response Profile

Ordered Value	Outcome	Total Frequency
1	0	46
2	1	29

Probability modeled is outcome = 1.

Class Level Information			
Class	Value	Design	Variables
pred_cat	1	0	0
	2	1	0
	3	0	1

Model Convergence Status

Convergence criterion (GCONV=1E-8) satisfied.

Model Fit Statistics		
Criterion	Intercept Only	Intercept and Covariates
AIC	102.085	95.672
SC	104.403	107.260
-2 Log L	100.085	85.672

Testing Global Null Hypothesis: BETA = 0			
Test	Chi-Square	DF	Pr > ChiSq
Likelihood Ratio	14.4127	4	0.0061
Score	13.0680	4	0.0109
Wald	10.8986	4	0.0277

Type 3 Analysis of Effects			
Effect	DF	Wald Chi-Square	Pr > ChiSq
pred_cont	1	1.2285	0.2677
pred_bin	1	6.2501	0.0124
pred_cat	2	7.4064	0.0246

Analysis of Maximum Likelihood Estimates						
Parameter		DF	Estimate	Standard Error	Wald Chi-Square	Pr > ChiSq
Intercept		1	–1.1595	1.1410	1.0327	0.3095
pred_cont		1	–0.0226	0.0204	1.2285	0.2677
pred_bin		1	1.4101	0.5640	6.2501	0.0124
pred_cat	2	1	1.7579	0.7837	5.0314	0.0249
pred_cat	3	1	1.8992	0.7190	6.9764	0.0083

Odds Ratio Estimates			
Effect	Point Estimate	95% Wald Confidence Limits	
pred_cont	0.978	0.939	1.017
pred_bin	4.096	1.356	12.373
pred_cat 2 vs 1	5.800	1.248	26.947
pred_cat 3 vs 1	6.680	1.632	27.343

Association of Predicted Probabilities and Observed Responses			
Percent Concordant	75.4	Somers' D	0.508
Percent Discordant	24.6	Gamma	0.508
Percent Tied	0.0	Tau-a	0.244
Pairs	1334	c	0.754

Many output tables are produced by default. The "Response Profile" box gives the number of observations in each level of the outcome. The "Type 3 Analysis of Effects" table shows tests for each predictor, including a chunk test for categorical variables. The test statistic follows a chi-squared distribution, and the *p*-value appears under the "Pr > ChiSq" column.

The parameter estimates from the model are found in the "Analysis of Maximum Likelihood Estimates" output box. The "Estimate" column shows the value of $\hat{\beta}$ for each variable. The standard error column shows the standard error of the parameter estimate. The value of the test statistic and the *p*-value for the hypothesis test for each predictor (H_0: $\beta = 0$) appear in the "Wald Chi-Square" and "Pr > ChiSq" columns, respectively. Notice that the test statistic calculated by SAS follows a chi-squared distribution, rather than a *Z*-distribution as in Table 14.3.

The "Odds Ratio Estimates" box shows the $\widehat{OR}$ in the "Point Estimate" column and the confidence interval for the $\widehat{OR}$ in the "95% Wald Confidence Limits" column. When there is a categorical predictor in a CLASS statement, there is a separate line in the "Analysis of Maximum Likelihood Estimates" and "Odds Ratio Estimates" tables for each level that is compared to the reference level. The name of the level is shown after the variable name. The final output box, "Association of Predicted Probabilities and Observed Responses," shows the value of the c statistic in the bottom right cell.

Logistic regression in Stata

The *logistic* command in Stata runs a logistic regression. We first specify the outcome variable, followed by one or more predictor variables. For categorical predictors, we use i. before the variable name to tell Stata to use dummy variables for the various levels.

```
logistic outcome pred_cont pred_bin i.pred_cat
```

```
Logistic regression                          Number of obs     =         75
                                             LR chi2(4)        =      14.41
                                             Prob > chi2       =     0.0061
Log likelihood = -42.836153                  Pseudo R2         =     0.1440
------------------------------------------------------------------------------
     outcome | Odds Ratio   Std. Err.      z    P>|z|     [95% Conf. Interval]
-------------+----------------------------------------------------------------
   pred_cont |   .9776963    .019897    -1.11   0.268     .9394663    1.017482
    pred_bin |   4.096224   2.310354     2.50   0.012      1.35609    12.37311
             |
    pred_cat |
          2  |   5.800111   4.545464     2.24   0.025     1.248423    26.94702
          3  |   6.680461   4.803496     2.64   0.008     1.632155    27.34333
             |
       _cons |   .3136386   .3578648    -1.02   0.310      .033512    2.935343
------------------------------------------------------------------------------
```

The global test for the regression, including the test statistic, degrees of freedom, and *p*-value, appears in the upper right corner of the output. The OR for each predictor is shown in the "Odds Ratio" column. The 95% confidence interval for the OR appears in the "[95% Conf. Interval]" column. The value of the test statistic and the *p*-value for the hypothesis test for each predictor (H_0: $\beta = 0$) are shown in the "z" and "Pr>|z|" columns, respectively.

If there is a factor variable as a predictor, the levels being compared to the reference level are listed in the left-most column under the name of the categorical variable. In the example shown, we are comparing levels 2 and 3 of *pred_cat* with level 1. To get the estimated coefficients $\hat{\beta}_i$, we can run the *logit* command directly after the *logistic* command. This will run the regression and produce the estimated regression coefficients rather than the OR.

```
logit
```

```
Logistic regression                          Number of obs     =         75
                                             LR chi2(4)        =      14.41
                                             Prob > chi2       =     0.0061
Log likelihood = -42.836153                  Pseudo R2         =     0.1440
------------------------------------------------------------------------------
     outcome |      Coef.   Std. Err.      z    P>|z|     [95% Conf. Interval]
-------------+----------------------------------------------------------------
   pred_cont |  -.0225562   .0203509    -1.11   0.268    -.0624433    .0173309
    pred_bin |   1.410065   .5640205     2.50   0.012     .3046056    2.515525
             |
```

```
pred_cat |
       2 |   1.757877   .7836857     2.24   0.025     .2218814   3.293873
       3 |   1.899187   .7190366     2.64   0.008     .4899011   3.308473
         |
   _cons |  -1.159514    1.14101    -1.02   0.310    -3.395852   1.076824
------------------------------------------------------------------------------
```

The "Coef." column shows the value of the estimated regression coefficients. The standard error of $\hat{\beta}_i$ appears in the "Std. Err." Column. The test statistic and p-value for the test corresponding to the null hypothesis $\beta = 0$ appear in the "z" and "Pr|z|" columns. A 95% confidence interval is produced by default in the "[95% Conf. Interval]" column. Note: To request the estimated coefficients rather than $\widehat{OR}$, we could also add the *coef* option to the end of the logistic command, separated by a comma, as shown in the following code:

```
logistic outcome pred_cont pred_bin i.pred_cat, coef
```

In order to get the c-statistic in Stata, we use the *lroc* command after a *logistic* or *logit* command:

```
lroc, nograph
```

EXAMPLE PROBLEM 14.1

Suppose that we are interested in identifying factors that influence the probability that an adult will develop diabetes. In our data, *diabetes* is a dichotomous random variable that takes the value of 1 if the condition is present and 0 if it is not. We use a sample of 400 adults to estimate the probability, p, of diabetes.[1] To begin, we would like to determine whether BMI affects p. The data are in the dataset *ch14_diabetes*.

A Why is logistic regression an appropriate method for investigating the association between probability of diabetes and BMI?

Diabetes is a dichotomous outcome, so logistic regression is the appropriate analysis method. In this case, $y = 0$ indicates no diabetes; $y = 1$ indicates diabetes.

B Write the logistic regression model.

$$\ln\left(\frac{p}{1-p}\right) = \ln(\text{odds of diabetes}) = \alpha + \beta \times \text{body mass index}$$

C Fit this model using SAS or Stata.

We use PROC LOGISTIC in SAS to run the logistic regression model. In the MODEL statement, we specify *diabetes* as the outcome and *bmi* as the predictor. We want to model the probability that an adult has diabetes, so we add (EVENT = "1") in the model line to the left of the equals sign. We do not need a CLASS statement since *bmi* is a continuous variable.

```
PROC LOGISTIC DATA = ch14_diabetes;
      MODEL diabetes (EVENT = "1") = bmi;
RUN;
```

The LOGISTIC Procedure

Model Information		
Data Set	WORK.CH14_DIABETES	
Response Variable	Diabetes	Diabetes
Number of Response Levels	2	
Model	binary logit	
Optimization Technique	Fisher's scoring	

Number of Observations Read	400
Number of Observations Used	400

Response Profile		
Ordered Value	Diabetes	Total Frequency
1	0	352
2	1	48

Probability modeled is diabetes=1.

BOX 14.1 DESCRIPTION OF *ch_diabetes* DATASET

The National Health and Nutrition Examination Survey (NHANES) asked respondents, "Other than during pregnancy, have you ever been told by a doctor or a health professional that you have diabetes or sugar diabetes?" Respondents could answer "Yes," "No," "Borderline," "Don't know," or could refuse to answer the question. Those who indicated "Yes" are coded as *diabetes* = 1, whereas those who reported "No" are represented by *diabetes* = 0. Respondents who selected a level other than "Yes" or "No" were excluded from the sample. The survey also asked, "Including living and deceased, were any of your close biological that is, blood relatives including father, mother, sisters or brothers, ever told by a health professional that they had diabetes?" Response options included "Yes," "No," "Don't know," or refusal to answer. The variable *family_risk* takes a value of 1 for those who answered affirmatively and 0 for those who answered negatively. Respondents who refused to answer or didn't know were excluded from the sample. Finally, measured weight and height were used to calculate BMI, which is recorded in the continuous variable *bmi*. The sample in the dataset *ch14_diabetes* is further limited to those respondents more than 18 years old with nonmissing BMI.

Model Convergence Status
Convergence criterion (GCONV=1E-8) satisfied.

Model Fit Statistics		
Criterion	Intercept Only	Intercept and Covariates
AIC	295.540	271.291
SC	299.531	279.273
–2 Log L	293.540	267.291

Testing Global Null Hypothesis: BETA=0			
Test	Chi-Square	DF	Pr > ChiSq
Likelihood Ratio	26.2495	1	<.0001
Score	30.5642	1	<.0001
Wald	25.7293	1	<.0001

Analysis of Maximum Likelihood Estimates					
Parameter	DF	Estimate	Standard Error	Wald Chi-Square	Pr > ChiSq
Intercept	1	–5.0596	0.6583	59.0651	<.0001
bmi	1	0.1003	0.0198	25.7293	<.0001

Odds Ratio Estimates			
Effect	Point Estimate	95% Wald Confidence Limits	
bmi	1.105	1.063	1.149

Association of Predicted Probabilities and Observed Responses			
Percent Concordant	71.7	Somers' D	0.436
Percent Discordant	28.0	Gamma	0.438
Percent Tied	0.3	Tau-a	0.092
Pairs	16896	c	0.718

The *logistic* command in Stata runs a logistic regression. We first specify the outcome, *diabetes*, followed by the predictor variable, *bmi*. We are interested in the estimated coefficient $\hat{\beta}$ as well as the $\widehat{OR}$, so we can run the *logit* command after the logistic command.

```
logistic diabetes bmi

logistic diabetes bmi

Logistic regression                             Number of obs     =        400
                                                LR chi2(1)        =      26.25
                                                Prob > chi2       =     0.0000
Log likelihood = -133.64526                     Pseudo R2         =     0.0894

------------------------------------------------------------------------------
    diabetes | Odds Ratio   Std. Err.      z    P>|z|     [95% Conf. Interval]
-------------+----------------------------------------------------------------
         bmi |   1.105471   .0218523     5.07   0.000      1.06346    1.149141
       _cons |   .0063462   .0041781    -7.69   0.000     .0017463    .0230631
------------------------------------------------------------------------------

logit

Logistic regression                             Number of obs     =        400
                                                LR chi2(1)        =      26.25
                                                Prob > chi2       =     0.0000
Log likelihood = -133.64526                     Pseudo R2         =     0.0894

------------------------------------------------------------------------------
    diabetes |      Coef.   Std. Err.      z    P>|z|     [95% Conf. Interval]
-------------+----------------------------------------------------------------
         bmi |   .1002714   .0197674     5.07   0.000     .0615281    .1390147
       _cons |    -5.0599   .6583682    -7.69   0.000    -6.350278   -3.769522
------------------------------------------------------------------------------
```

D Write the equation for the estimated log-odds of diabetes for an adult with a BMI of x_i.

$$\ln\left(\frac{\hat{p}}{1-\hat{p}}\right) = -5.06 + 0.10 \times x_i$$

E Interpret the coefficient of BMI in this model using the fitted values and the appropriate units of measurement.

For each one-unit increase in BMI, the log odds of having diabetes increases by 0.10, on average.

F At the $\alpha = 0.05$ significance level, test the null hypotheses that the coefficient associated with BMI is equal to 0, using the output from the statistical software. What do you conclude?

We wish to test H_0: $\beta_{bmi} = 0$ versus H_1: $\beta_{bmi} \neq 0$.

$$Z = \frac{\hat{\beta}}{\widehat{se}(\hat{\beta})} = \frac{0.10}{0.02} = 5.00$$

The p-value is $P(|Z| > 5.00) < 0.0001$, which means that we reject the null hypothesis. We have evidence that the probability of having diabetes differs depending on an adult's BMI.

G **What is the $\widehat{\text{OR}}$ for diabetes associated with a one-unit increase in BMI?**

$$\widehat{OR} = e^{\hat{\beta}} = e^{0.10} = 1.11$$

H **What is the $\widehat{\text{OR}}$ for diabetes associated with a five-unit increase in BMI?**

$$\widehat{OR} = e^{5 \times \hat{\beta}} = e^{5 \times 0.10} = e^{0.50} = 1.65$$

I **Given an adult from this population whose BMI is 28, what is the predicted probability (i.e., predicted from the model in Example Problem 14.1—Part (C)) that this adult will have diabetes?**

$$\hat{p} = \frac{e^{\hat{\alpha} + \hat{\beta}_1 x_1 + \ldots + \hat{\beta}_q x_q}}{1 + e^{\hat{\alpha} + \hat{\beta}_1 x_1 + \ldots + \hat{\beta}_q x_q}} = \frac{e^{-5.06 + 0.10 \times 28}}{1 + e^{-5.06 + 0.10 \times 28}} = \frac{0.10}{1.10} = 0.09$$

An adult with a BMI of 28 has a 9% probability of having diabetes.

EXAMPLE PROBLEM 14.2

We are interested in investigating—using logistic regression—the association between employment status and whether someone has ever been tested for HIV. The data are contained in the dataset *ch14_hiv_test*.[2]

A **Using the variable *hiv_test* as the outcome, which indicates ever been tested for HIV, fit a logistic regression model with employment status as the single explanatory variable.**

PROC LOGISTIC runs a logistic regression in SAS. We specify *hiv_test* as the outcome in the MODEL statement and indicate that the event of interest is having an HIV test by adding the EVENT = "1" option. *Employed* is the predictor variable, which is listed to the right of the equals sign in the MODEL statement.

```
PROC LOGISTIC DATA = ch14_hiv_test;
              MODEL hiv_test (EVENT = "1") = employed;
RUN;
```

The LOGISTIC Procedure

Model Information		
Dataset	WORK.CH14_HIV_TEST	
Response Variable	hiv_test	Ever Had Been Tested for HIV
Number of Response Levels	2	
Model	binary logit	
Optimization Technique	Fisher's scoring	

Number of Observations Read	250
Number of Observations Used	250

Response Profile		
Ordered Value	hiv_test	Total Frequency
1	0	182
2	1	68

Probability Modeled Is hiv_test=1.

Model Convergence Status
Convergence criterion (GCONV=1E-8) satisfied.

BOX 14.2 DESCRIPTION OF *ch14_test* DATASET

The Behavioral Risk Factor Surveillance System (BRFSS) asked respondents, "Have you ever been tested for HIV? Do not count tests you may have had as part of a blood donation. Include testing fluid from your mouth." Respondents could answer "Yes," "No," "Don't know," or could refuse to answer the question. Those who indicated "Yes" are coded as *hiv_test* = 1, whereas those who reported "No" are represented by *hiv_test* = 0. Respondents who selected a level other than "Yes" or "No" were excluded from the sample. The survey also asked about employment status. Respondents who answered that they were employed for wages or were self-employed were coded as *employed* = 1. Respondents were considered not employed (*employed* = 0) if they reported being out of work for one year or more, out of work for less than one year, a homemaker, a student, retired, or unable to work. Respondents who refused to answer the question were excluded from the sample.

Model Fit Statistics		
Criterion	Intercept Only	Intercept and Covariates
AIC	294.619	296.202
SC	298.140	303.245
–2 Log L	292.619	292.202

Testing Global Null Hypothesis: BETA=0			
Test	Chi-Square	DF	Pr > ChiSq
Likelihood Ratio	0.4173	1	0.5183
Score	0.4171	1	0.5184
Wald	0.4166	1	0.5186

Analysis of Maximum Likelihood Estimates					
Parameter	DF	Estimate	Standard Error	Wald Chi-Square	Pr > ChiSq
Intercept	1	–1.0776	0.2047	27.7197	<.0001
employed	1	0.1837	0.2847	0.4166	0.5186

Odds Ratio Estimates			
Effect	Point Estimate	95% Wald Confidence Limits	
employed	1.202	0.688	2.099

Association of Predicted Probabilities and Observed Responses			
Percent Concordant	27.3	Somers' D	0.046
Percent Discordant	22.8	Gamma	0.092
Percent Tied	49.9	Tau-a	0.018
Pairs	12376	c	0.523

We will use the *logistic* command to run the logistic regression in Stata. The outcome variable *hiv_test* is listed first after the *logistic* command, followed by the predictor variable *employed*. Including the *coef* option requests the estimated regression coefficients rather than the $\widehat{OR}$, and, then, we can run the command again without the *coef* option to get the $\widehat{OR}$.

logistic *hiv_test employed*, coef

```
Logistic regression                             Number of obs     =        250
                                                LR chi2(1)        =       0.42
                                                Prob > chi2       =     0.5183
Log likelihood = -146.10085                     Pseudo R2         =     0.0014

------------------------------------------------------------------------------
    hiv_test |      Coef.   Std. Err.      z    P>|z|     [95% Conf. Interval]
-------------+----------------------------------------------------------------
    employed |    .183741   .2846572     0.65   0.519    -.3741768    .7416588
       _cons |  -1.077559   .2046663    -5.26   0.000    -1.478697   -.6764203
------------------------------------------------------------------------------
```

logistic *hiv_test employed*

```
Logistic regression                             Number of obs     =        250
                                                LR chi2(1)        =       0.42
                                                Prob > chi2       =     0.5183
Log likelihood = -146.10085                     Pseudo R2         =     0.0014

------------------------------------------------------------------------------
    hiv_test | Odds Ratio   Std. Err.      z    P>|z|     [95% Conf. Interval]
-------------+----------------------------------------------------------------
    employed |   1.201705   .3420738     0.65   0.519     .6878553    2.099415
       _cons |   .3404255   .0696736    -5.26   0.000     .2279344    .5084338
------------------------------------------------------------------------------
```

B **Interpret the estimated coefficient of employment status.**

The log odds of ever having an HIV test are higher by 0.18, on average, for those who are employed versus those who are not employed.

C **What are the estimated odds of ever being tested for HIV for individuals who are employed relative to those who are not?**

The output in Example Problem 14.2—Part (A) gives $\widehat{OR} = 1.20$. Those who are employed have 1.20 times the odds of ever having been tested for HIV compared with those who are not employed.

D **What is the 95% confidence interval for the population OR?**

The 95% confidence interval for the odds ratio is (0.69, 2.10). We are 95% confident that the OR comparing those who are employed to those who are unemployed lies in the interval (0.69, 2.10).

E **Does this interval contain the value 1? What does this tell us?**

The 95% confidence interval for the OR contains the null value of 1. Thus, we would fail to reject the null hypothesis that there is no association between ever having an HIV test and employment status (H_0: OR = 1) at the 0.05 level of significance.

PRACTICE PROBLEM 14.1

Let's return to the dataset used in Example Problem 14.1. We, now, attempt to determine whether having a close relative with diabetes (from here on referred to as "family risk") influences the probability that an adult has diabetes. To do this, we fit a logistic regression as before, but this time including the predictor *family_risk* instead (let's denote it as $x_2 = 1$, indicating a close relative has diabetes; $x_2 = 0$ indicates no close relatives with diabetes).

A Run the regression in a statistical program.

B At the $\alpha = 0.05$ significance level, test the null hypothesis that the coefficient associated with family risk is equal to 0, using the output from SAS or Stata. What do we conclude?

C Use the estimated regression coefficient to calculate the estimated relative odds of having diabetes for those with a family risk of diabetes versus those without a family risk of diabetes. Interpret the OR in words.

D How does the reported OR for family risk from the program output compare with what we calculated in Practice Problem 14.1—Part (C)?

E Now, suppose that instead of receiving the entire dataset, we receive a 2 × 2 table (Table 14.4). What would be the estimate of the OR relating the odds of diabetes for those with a family risk versus those without a family risk? The 2 × 2 table in Table 14.4 shows counts for 400 subjects and information on their diabetes status and family risk of diabetes.

F How does this value compare to the OR estimated using logistic regression?

Table 14.4 Data for Practice Problem 14.1

		Diabetes		
		Yes	*No*	*Total*
Family risk	Yes	37	116	153
	No	11	236	247
	Total	48	352	400

EXAMPLE PROBLEM 14.3

Many Americans have activity limitations due to health problems, and we are interested in the factors that influence the presence of these limitations. In particular, we would like to investigate the association between activity limitations and race, BMI, and sex using a sample of 600 subjects.[2] The data are in the dataset *ch14_limitations*.

BOX 14.3 DESCRIPTION OF *ch14_limitations* DATASETS

The Behavioral Risk Factor Surveillance System (BRFSS) asked, "Are you limited in any way in any activities because of physical, mental, or emotional problems?" Respondents could answer "Yes," "No," "Don't know," or could refuse to answer the question. Those who indicated "Yes" are coded as *limitation* = 1, whereas those who reported "No" are coded as *limitation* = 0. Respondents who selected a level other than "Yes" or "No" were excluded from the sample. Measured weight and height were used to calculate BMI, which is recorded in the continuous variable called *bmi*. The variable *female* takes a value of 1 for female respondents, and the value 0 is for male respondents. The survey asked, "What is the highest grade or year of school you completed?" Responses for this question were categorized into a three-level variable, excluding those who did not report their education level. The levels of the variable *education* are "No College," "Some College," and "Graduated College." Finally, the variable *race* categorizes respondents on the basis of their self-reported racial category and information on Hispanic origin. The three categories of the variable *race* are "White," "Black," and "Other." Note that the "White" and "Black" categories only include non-Hispanic respondents; Hispanic respondents are in the "Other" category. The sample in the dataset *ch14_limitations* is limited to subjects who have nonmissing values for the *limitations*, *bmi*, *education*, and *race* variables.

A Fit a logistic regression with the presence of an activity limitation as the response and with race, BMI, and sex as explanatory variables. For race, make "White" the reference group.

In SAS, we specify the variable *limitation* as the outcome and *race*, *bmi*, and *female* as the predictors. Because *race* is a categorical variable, we must include a CLASS statement, which also specifies "White" as the reference group in the REF = option.

```
PROC LOGISTIC DATA = ch14_limitations;
             CLASS race (REF = "White") / PARAM = REF;
             MODEL limitation (EVENT = "1") = race bmi female;
RUN;
```

The LOGISTIC Procedure

Model Information		
Dataset	WORK.CH14_LIMITATIONS	
Response Variable	Limitation	Activity Limitation
Number of Response Levels	2	
Model	binary logit	
Optimization Technique	Fisher's scoring	

Number of Observations Read	600
Number of Observations Used	600

Response Profile		
Ordered Value	Limitation	Total Frequency
1	0	448
2	1	152

Probability modeled is limitation = 1.

Class Level Information			
Class	Value	Design Variables	
race	Black	1	0
	Other	0	1
	White	0	0

Model Convergence Status
Convergence criterion (GCONV=1E-8) satisfied.

Model Fit Statistics		
Criterion	Intercept Only	Intercept and Covariates
AIC	681.161	668.450
SC	685.558	690.435
–2 Log L	679.161	658.450

Testing Global Null Hypothesis: BETA = 0			
Test	Chi-Square	DF	Pr > ChiSq
Likelihood Ratio	20.7112	4	0.0004
Score	21.3790	4	0.0003
Wald	20.1051	4	0.0005

Type 3 Analysis of Effects			
Effect	DF	Wald Chi-Square	Pr > ChiSq
race	2	0.1834	0.9124
bmi	1	14.6933	0.0001
female	1	6.5940	0.0102

Analysis of Maximum Likelihood Estimates						
Parameter		DF	Estimate	Standard Error	Wald Chi-Square	Pr > ChiSq
Intercept		1	-3.0312	0.4712	41.3891	<.0001
race	Black	1	0.1420	0.3325	0.1823	0.6694
race	Other	1	0.00445	0.3114	0.0002	0.9886
bmi		1	0.0569	0.0149	14.6933	0.0001
female		1	0.5147	0.2004	6.5940	0.0102

Odds Ratio Estimates			
Effect	Point Estimate	95% Wald Confidence Limits	
race Black vs White	1.153	0.601	2.212
race Other vs White	1.004	0.546	1.849
bmi	1.059	1.028	1.090
female	1.673	1.130	2.478

Association of Predicted Probabilities and Observed Responses			
Percent Concordant	60.3	Somers' D	0.207
Percent Discordant	39.6	Gamma	0.207
Percent Tied	0.1	Tau-a	0.078
Pairs	68096	C	0.603

In Stata, we use the *logistic* command to run the regression. However, we must first transform the variable *race* into a format that Stata can understand. In the dataset, *race* has three levels: "White," "Black," and "Other." We need to use the *egen* command with the label option to make a new variable called *race_cat* that takes values 1, 2, and 3 but retains the names (called *labels*) of the levels. The *race_cat* variable now has levels 1 = Black, 2 = other race, and 3 = White.

```
egen race_cat = group(race), label
```

Once we have the new categorical variable, we can run the logistic regression. We, first, specify the outcome variable, *limitation*, followed by the explanatory variables *race_cat*, *bmi*, and *female*. Because *race_cat* is categorical, we use the i. function to make it into a factor variable in the regression. We would also like the reference level of *race_cat* to be "White," so we specify ib3. before *race_cat*, indicating that the reference level is the third level of the variable. We will subsequently run the logit command to get the estimated regression coefficients.

```
logistic limitation ib3.race_cat bmi female

Logistic regression                             Number of obs     =        600
                                                LR chi2(4)        =      20.71
                                                Prob > chi2       =     0.0004
Log likelihood = -329.22497                     Pseudo R2         =     0.0305

------------------------------------------------------------------------------
  limitation | Odds Ratio   Std. Err.      z    P>|z|     [95% Conf. Interval]
-------------+----------------------------------------------------------------
    race_cat |
      Black  |   1.152568   .3832716     0.43   0.669     .6006344    2.211682
      Other  |   1.004457   .3127767     0.01   0.989      .545603    1.849209
             |
         bmi |   1.058595   .0157256     3.83   0.000     1.028218     1.08987
      female |   1.673172   .3353815     2.57   0.010     1.129588     2.47834
       _cons |   .0482563   .0227368    -6.43   0.000     .0191644    .1215102
------------------------------------------------------------------------------

logit

Logistic regression                             Number of obs     =        600
                                                LR chi2(4)        =      20.71
                                                Prob > chi2       =     0.0004
Log likelihood = -329.22497                     Pseudo R2         =     0.0305

------------------------------------------------------------------------------
  limitation |      Coef.   Std. Err.      z    P>|z|     [95% Conf. Interval]
-------------+----------------------------------------------------------------
    race_cat |
      Black  |   .1419921   .3325372     0.43   0.669    -.5097689    .7937531
      Other  |   .0044472   .3113888     0.01   0.989    -.6058636     .614758
             |
         bmi |   .0569427   .0148552     3.83   0.000      .027827    .0860583
      female |   .5147211   .2004465     2.57   0.010     .1218531     .907589
       _cons |   -3.03123   .4711683    -6.43   0.000    -3.954703   -2.107757
------------------------------------------------------------------------------
```

B Interpret the estimated coefficients for race, adjusted for sex and BMI.

Holding all the other variables in the model constant, the log odds of having an activity limitation are higher by 0.14, on average, for blacks versus whites. Holding all the other variables in the model constant, the log odds of having an activity limitation are higher by 0.004, on average, for people of other races versus whites.

C What is the adjusted OR comparing black individuals to white individuals? What about comparing people of other races to whites?

$\widehat{OR}_{b\ vs.\ w} = 1.15$. Blacks have 1.15 times the odds of having an activity limitation due to a health problem compared to whites, adjusting (controlling) for BMI and sex.

$\widehat{OR}_{o\ vs.\ w} = 1.00$. People of other races have 1.00 times the odds of having an activity limitation due to a health problem compared to whites, adjusting (controlling) for BMI and sex.

D Now let's look at sex. What is the estimated relative odds for an activity limitation comparing females and males, adjusting for race and BMI?

Females have 1.67 times the odds of an activity limitation compared with males, adjusting for race and BMI.

E What is the 95% confidence interval for the OR for sex that adjusts for race and BMI? Does the interval contain the null value of 1? What does this tell us?

The 95% confidence interval for the OR is (1.13, 2.48). We are 95% confident that the adjusted OR comparing females and males lies in the interval (1.13, 2.48). This interval does not contain the null value of 1, which leads us to reject the null hypothesis. We have statistically significant evidence of an association between presence of an activity limitation and sex, controlling for race and BMI.

F We are curious to see whether the relationship between presence of an activity limitation and BMI differs for females and males. Run the regression again, this time including an interaction term between BMI and sex. Interpret the output for the interaction term.

To add the interaction term in SAS, we put a vertical pipe ("|") between the variables *bmi* and *female*.

```
PROC LOGISTIC DATA = ch14_limitations;
       CLASS race (REF = "White") / PARAM = REF;
       MODEL limitation (EVENT = "1") = race bmi|female;
RUN;
```

Selected output boxes follow.

The LOGISTIC Procedure

Testing Global Null Hypothesis: BETA = 0			
Test	Chi-Square	DF	Pr > ChiSq
Likelihood Ratio	20.8307	5	0.0009
Score	21.8500	5	0.0006
Wald	20.3266	5	0.0011

Type 3 Analysis of Effects			
Effect	DF	Wald Chi-Square	Pr > ChiSq
race	2	0.1488	0.9283
bmi	1	3.8979	0.0483
female	1	0.0442	0.8334
bmi*female	1	0.1194	0.7297

Analysis of Maximum Likelihood Estimates						
Parameter		DF	Estimate	Standard Error	Wald Chi-Square	Pr > ChiSq
Intercept		1	–2.8200	0.7693	13.4369	0.0002
race	Black	1	0.1283	0.3351	0.1467	0.7017
race	Other	1	–0.00056	0.3119	0.0000	0.9986
bmi		1	0.0499	0.0253	3.8979	0.0483
female		1	0.1975	0.9388	0.0442	0.8334
bmi*female		1	0.0109	0.0314	0.1194	0.7297

Odds Ratio Estimates			
Effect	Point Estimate	95% Wald Confidence Limits	
race Black vs White	1.137	0.589	2.193
race Other vs White	0.999	0.542	1.842

In Stata, we use two pound signs ("##") between the variables *bmi* and *female* to create an interaction in the model. We also add c. to the beginning of the *bmi* variable to indicate that it should be treated as a continuous variable in the interaction.

```
logistic limitation ib3.race_cat c.bmi##female, coef

Logistic regression                             Number of obs     =        600
                                                LR chi2(5)        =      20.83
                                                Prob > chi2       =     0.0009
Log likelihood = -329.16525                     Pseudo R2         =     0.0307

------------------------------------------------------------------------------
  limitation |      Coef.   Std. Err.      z    P>|z|     [95% Conf. Interval]
-------------+----------------------------------------------------------------
    race_cat |
       Black |   .1283473   .3351365     0.38   0.702    -.5285082    .7852029
       Other |  -.0005618    .311918    -0.00   0.999    -.6119098    .6107862
             |
         bmi |   .0498725   .0252607     1.97   0.048     .0003624    .0993826
    1.female |   .1974524   .9387537     0.21   0.833    -1.642471    2.037376
             |
female#c.bmi |
           1 |   .0108576   .0314211     0.35   0.730    -.0507265    .0724418
             |
       _cons |  -2.819972   .7692984    -3.67   0.000    -4.327769   -1.312174
------------------------------------------------------------------------------
```

Note that when we model an interaction between two variables, the main effects of these variables are also included in the regression model. From the output, the estimated regression coefficient for the *bmi* × *female* interaction is $\hat{\beta}_{int} = 0.01$. The interaction term is not significant at the $\alpha = 0.05$ level of significance, as the *p*-value is 0.7297 (SAS) or 0.730 (Stata).

PRACTICE PROBLEM 14.2

We will continue with the dataset introduced in Example Problem 14.3 regarding activity limitations due to health problems, *ch14_limitations*. We want to see whether there is an association between education level and presence of an activity limitation. We also want to adjust for BMI in the model.

A Run the logistic regression with *education* and *bmi* as the explanatory variables and *limitations* as the outcome. Make "Graduated College" the reference level for the education variable.

B What is the estimated OR comparing those with no college education with those who graduated from college? Interpret the value in words.

C What are the estimated odds of an activity limitation for those who have some college education relative to those who graduated from college? Interpret the value in words.

D What is the 95% confidence interval for the OR comparing those with some college education with those who graduated from college? What information can we obtain from the interval?

E Interpret the regression coefficient for BMI.

F What are the relative odds of an activity limitation corresponding to a five-unit change in BMI?

G What is the predicted probability of having an activity limitation for someone who has no college education and a BMI of 34?

References

1. National Health and Nutrition Examination Survey. Hyattsville, MD: Centers for Disease Control and Prevention, National Center for Health Statistics. 2014. https://wwwn.cdc.gov/Nchs/Nhanes/Search/nhanes13{_}14.aspx. Accessed February 23, 2016.
2. Behavioral Risk Factor Surveillance System. Atlanta, GA: Centers for Disease Control and Prevention. 2014. http://www.cdc.gov/brfss/annual_data/annual_2014.html. Updated September 11, 2015. Accessed February 23, 2016.

15 Survival analysis

This chapter will focus on a basic introduction to survival analysis and will include the following topics:

- Log-rank test
- Survival curve
- Survival table
- The life-table method
- The product-limit method
- Using statistical software for survival analysis

Terms

- censoring
- failure
- life-table method
- product-limit method

Introduction

Survival analysis is used when we want to study a time to an event. The variable of interest is the time, T, to an event; this time is sometimes referred to as the survival time or failure time. Examples include time to death, time to diagnosis of diabetes, time from start of therapy to remission of a cancer, and time from HIV diagnosis to onset of AIDS.

Although measurements of survival times are continuous, their distributions are rarely normal. Analysis of this type of data generally focuses on estimating the probability that an individual will survive for a given length of time. A common circumstance in working with survival data is that some people in the sample are not observed up to their time of "failure."

Failure: The occurrence of the event in question (e.g., death, diagnosis of diabetes, remission of cancer, onset of AIDS).

Censoring: The incomplete observation of a time to "failure."

An observation is censored if the event time is not observed. This may happen for many reasons. For example, a patient may drop out of a study before her cancer goes into remission. The presence of censoring distinguishes the analysis of survival data from other types of analysis. A distribution of survival times can be characterized by a survival function represented by $S(t)$. The graph of $S(t)$ versus t is called a survival curve. Figure 15.1 shows an example of a survival curve.

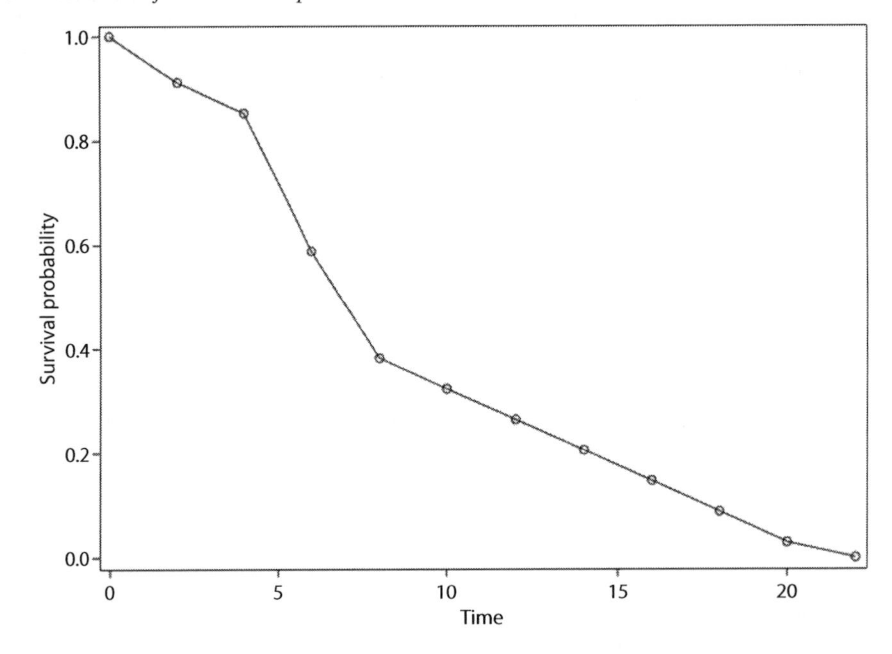

Figure 15.1 **Example of a life-table survival curve.** On the *y*-axis is the survival probability, and on the *x*-axis is time.

The goal is to estimate the distribution of the survival times or, equivalently, the survival function $S(t)$. $S(t)=P(T>t)=$ proportion of individuals who have not experienced the event by time *t*. There are two methods to estimate $S(t)$: The life-table method and the product-limit method.

Life-Table Method: The classical method of estimating a survival curve. In the life table, the following elements are included:

- The time interval is represented as $[t, t+n]$.
- Survival times are grouped within intervals of fixed length.
- The proportion of individuals alive at time *t* who "fail" prior to $t + n$ (also called the *hazard function*) is represented as ${}_nq_t$.
- The number of individuals still alive at time *t* is represented as l_t.
- If l_0 is the number of individuals alive at time 0 and l_t is the number of these individuals still alive at time *t*, the proportion of individuals who have not yet "failed" at time *t* can be calculated as

$$S(t) = \frac{l_t}{l_0} \tag{15.1}$$

- The proportion of individuals who do not fail during a given interval is represented by $1 - {}_nq_t$.
- For the time intervals in the life table not containing an event, the estimated hazard function is 0, and the estimated proportion of individuals who do not "fail" is equal to 1.

- From the life table, we can use the proportion of individuals who do not "fail" in each interval to estimate the survival function using the multiplicative rule of probability.

$$\hat{S}(t) = \hat{S}(t-1) \times (1 - {}_{n}t_{q}) \tag{15.2}$$

- The estimated survival function $\hat{S}(t)$ changes only during the time intervals in which at least one "event" occurs.
- For smaller datasets, there can be many intervals without a single event. In these instances, it might not make sense to present the survival function this way.

Product-Limit Method (also called the Kaplan–Meier method): A nonparametric technique that uses the exact survival time for each individual in a sample instead of grouping the times into intervals.

- $\hat{S}(t)$ is assumed to remain the same over the time period between events. It changes precisely when someone "fails." Using the multiplicative rule of probability, the proportions of individuals who do not fail can be used to estimate the survival function just as in the life-table method.
- The estimated survival function will look different for different samples. It is an estimate of the true population survival function.
- This method can be adjusted to account for partial information about survival times that is available from censored observations.
  - A censored observation is denoted by a plus (+) sign.
  - $\hat{S}(t)$ does not change from its previous value if the observation at time t is censored.
  - The censored observation is not used to calculate the probability of failure at any subsequent time point.
- For the product-limit survival table, the following conditions are true:
  - Time equals the exact times at which events occur.
  - The proportion of patients alive just prior to time t who, then, fail at time t is represented by q_t.
  - The proportion of individuals who do not fail at t is represented by $1 - q_t$.

Comparing two survival functions

- Instead of simply characterizing survival times for a single group of subjects, we often want to compare the distributions of survival times for two different populations.
- Our goal is to determine whether survival differs systematically between the groups.
- If there are no censored observations in either group, we can use the Wilcoxon rank-sum test (Chapter 9) to compare the median survival times.
- If censored observations exist, one method that can be used is a nonparametric technique known as the log-rank test.
  - We want to test the null hypothesis: H_0: $S_1(t) = S_2(t)$.
  - To do this, we start by plotting survival curves for both groups on the same graph.
  - Does one curve consistently lie above the other? Or do the curves overlap?
  - Next, we conduct the log-rank test.
  - Is the difference between the two curves greater than might be observed by chance alone?
  - Care must be taken not to ignore important confounding variables when present as they may mask the true effect.

EXAMPLE PROBLEM 15.1

Suppose that we are interested in the age at which people are diagnosed with asthma. A random sample of 25 participants in the 2014 NHANES survey[1] is presented in Table 15.1.

We begin our analysis by summarizing the asthma diagnosis time data using the classic life-table method which is shown in Table 15.2. Using the previous information we were given on participants' age at diagnosis of asthma (see Table 15.1), we create a

Table 15.1 Age at diagnosis of asthma for 25 randomly selected participants with asthma from the 2014 NHANES survey[a]

Participant[b]	*Age*[c]
75583	1
76766	1
77031	1
79583	1
80385	1
81154	1
75802	2
80540	2
81572	3
80806	4
76799	5
78909	5
80178	5
80938	5
81402	6
79506	9
75872	12
82199	12
77805	17
83278	19
79669	20
79386	22
79902	30
75523	50
75070	72

Source: National Health and Nutrition Examination Survey, Centers for Disease Control and Prevention, National Center for Health Statistics, Hyattsville, MD, 2014, https://wwwn.cdc.gov/Nchs/Nhanes/Search/nhanes13_14.aspx.

[a] The data can be used to estimate the survival functions. The data are presented in three segments for the sake of efficiency.

[b] An identification number represents each participant.

[c] Each number represents the age at which the participant was diagnosed as having asthma.

BOX 15.1 DESCRIPTION OF DATA ON THE AGE AT DIAGNOSIS OF ASTHMA[1]

The dataset (*age_asthma_15_1b*) for Example Problem 15.1 and Example Problem 15.2 come from the 2014 National Health and Nutrition Examination Survey (NHANES). The data presented in Table 15.1 consist of a random sample of 25 participants who had received a diagnosis of asthma and had nonmissing data. Table 15.4 includes the data in Table 15.1 combined with a random sample of 10 participants who had not received a diagnosis of asthma and who had nonmissing data—these data are also in the dataset *age_asthma_15_1b*. The main variable that we are considering in these examples—age at diagnosis of asthma—comes from the NHANES question "How old {were you/was SP} when {you were/s/he was} first told {you/he/she} had asthma (az-ma)?" The response options were ages 1 to 79 years, and values of 80 years or more were all coded as 80 years. The respondent could also refuse to answer or respond that he or she did not know—participants in these two response categories (and other categories with missing responses) were excluded from this sample. Further along in this chapter, we will also use the variables *asthma* and *gender*. Asthma, used as the censoring variable, comes from the NHANES question "The following questions are about different medical conditions. Has a doctor or other health professional ever told {you/SP} that {you have/s/he/SP has} asthma (az-ma)?" The responses were yes, no, refused, or don't know. Refused, don't know, and other missing responses were excluded from this sample. Gender responses come from the NHANES question "Gender of the participant." Responses were "male" or "female," and there were no missing responses for this question.

survival table using the life-table method (see Table 15.2). We can see in Table 15.2 that as the time (age) interval increases, the survival function decreases.

Review the contents of each column. The first column specifies the time interval in years (t to $t + n$); the second column specifies the number of individuals who have not been diagnosed as having asthma at that time period (l_t).

A For the time intervals in the life table not containing a failure (diagnosis of asthma), the estimated proportion of individuals diagnosed with asthma is equal to what number?

Zero

B What does the life table indicate as the probability that a patient will be diagnosed with asthma after age 5 years? After age 30 years?

$\hat{S}(5) = P(t > 5) = 0.60$

$\hat{S}(30) = P(t > 30) = 0.12$

Table 15.2 Life-table method of estimating S(*t*) for age at diagnosis of asthma

t to $t + n$[a]	${}_nq_t$[b]	l_t[c]	$1 - {}_nq_t$[d]	*Estimate of S(t)*[e]
1–5	0.40	25	0.60	1.00
5–10	0.40	15	0.60	0.60
10–15	0.22	9	0.78	0.36
15–20	0.29	7	0.71	0.28
20–25	0.40	5	0.60	0.20
25–30	0.00	3	1.00	0.12
30–35	0.33	3	0.67	0.12
35–40	0.00	2	1.00	0.08
40–45	0.00	2	1.00	0.08
45–50	0.00	2	1.00	0.08
50–55	0.50	2	0.50	0.08
55–60	0.00	1	1.00	0.04
60+	1.00	1	0.00	0.04

[a] The time frame in years.
[b] The proportion of individuals alive at time t who "fail" prior to $t + n$.
[c] The number of individuals still alive at time t.
[d] The proportion of individuals who do not "fail" during the given interval.
[e] The estimate of the survival function.

Since we are dealing with a relatively small group of participants, we might prefer to estimate the survival function using the product-limit method. The product-limit method of estimating $S(t)$ is a nonparametric technique that uses the exact recurrence time for each individual instead of grouping the times into intervals. In this case, the participants who were diagnosed with asthma at age 1 year would not be grouped with the participants who were diagnosed with asthma at the age of 2 years.

Table 15.3 displays the product-limit estimate of $S(t)$ for the sample of 25 participants. Review the contents of each column. We can see that as the time (age) interval increases, the survival function decreases.

C What does the product-limit estimate indicate as the probability that a participant will be diagnosed with asthma after age 5 years? After age 30 years?

$$\hat{S}(5) = P(t > 5) = 0.44$$

$$\hat{S}(30) = P(t > 30) = 0.08$$

D How do the values in Example Problem 15.1—Part (C) compare with what was predicted using the life-table method in Example Problem 15.1—Part (B)?

The values in Example Problem 15.1—Part (C) are somewhat lower than the values predicted using the life-table method.

The product-limit method for estimating a survival curve can be modified to take into account the partial information about age at diagnosis of asthma that is

Table 15.3 Product-limit method of estimating S(*t*) diagnosis of asthma

Time[a]	q_t[b]	$1 - q_t$[c]	*Estimate of* $S(t)$[d]
0	0.00	1.00	1.00
1	0.26	0.74	0.76
2	0.11	0.89	0.68
3	0.06	0.94	0.64
4	0.06	0.94	0.60
5	0.27	0.73	0.44
6	0.09	0.91	0.40
9	0.10	0.90	0.36
12	0.22	0.78	0.28
17	0.14	0.86	0.24
19	0.17	0.83	0.20
20	0.20	0.80	0.16
22	0.25	0.75	0.12
30	0.33	0.67	0.08
50	0.50	0.50	0.04
72	1.00	0.00	0.00

[a] Time (i.e., age) in years.
[b] The proportion of patients alive just prior to time *t* who have "failed" at that time.
[c] The proportion of individuals who do not "fail" at *t*.
[d] The estimate of the survival function.

available from censored observations. Censored survival times for an additional 10 participants who were never diagnosed with asthma are reported in Table 15.4. They are considered censored observations in this example because they never experienced a "failure," meaning that they were never diagnosed as having asthma.

The calculation for the product-limit estimate of the survival function is shown in Table 15.5. Using the previous information that we were given on participants' age at diagnosis of asthma in Table 15.4, including the additional censored observations, we can create a survival table using the product-limit method. We can see that as the time (age) increases, the survival function decreases.

E What does Table 15.5 indicate as the probability that a participant will be diagnosed as having asthma after age 5 years? After age 30 years?

$\hat{S}(5) = P(t > 5) = 0.59$

$\hat{S}(30) = P(t > 30) = 0.26$

F Is this estimate of survival function at age 5 years different from the previous estimate? Why would you expect this?

Yes, the estimate that contains the censored observations is higher than the one without. We would expect this to change because there are censored observations that occur before age 5 years.

Table 15.4 Age of randomly selected NHANES 2014 participants (10 without reported asthma and 25 with reported asthma)[a]

Participant[b]	*Age*[c]
75583	1
76766	1
77031	1
79583	1
80385	1
81154	1
75802	2
80540	2
76085	2+
80914	2+
81572	3
80806	4
76799	5
78909	5
80178	5
80938	5
81402	6
79506	9
77412	9+
75872	12
82199	12
74658	12+
79792	13+
77805	17
83278	19
79669	20
79386	22
79100	28+
79902	30
79217	33+
75523	50
76877	52+
82963	60+
80379	67+
75070	72

Source: National Health and Nutrition Examination Survey, Centers for Disease Control and Prevention, National Center for Health Statistics, Hyattsville, MD, 2014, https://wwwn.cdc.gov/Nchs/Nhanes/Search/nhanes13_14.aspx.

[a] The data are presented in three segments for the sake of efficiency. Also, the 25 participants with asthma were reported in Table 15.1.

[b] An identification number represents each participant.

[c] Each number represents the age at which the participant was diagnosed as having asthma. Participants without asthma are denoted by a plus (+) sign.

Table 15.5 Product-limit method of estimating S(*t*) diagnosis of asthma, with censoring[a]

Time[b]	q_t[c]	$1 - q_t$[d]	$S(t)$[e]
0	0.00	1.00	1.00
1	0.17	0.83	0.83
2	0.07	0.93	0.77
3	0.04	0.96	0.74
4	0.04	0.96	0.71
5	0.17	0.83	0.59
6	0.05	0.95	0.56
9	0.06	0.94	0.52
12	0.13	0.88	0.46
13	0.00	1.00	0.46
17	0.08	0.92	0.42
19	0.09	0.91	0.38
20	0.10	0.90	0.34
22	0.11	0.89	0.31
28	0.00	1.00	0.31
30	0.14	0.86	0.26
33	0.00	1.00	0.26
50	0.20	0.80	0.21
52	0.00	1.00	0.21
60	0.00	1.00	0.21
67	0.00	1.00	0.21
72	1.00	0.00	0.00

a The estimates here are slightly different from the estimates calculated in Table 15.3 because of the additional censored observations that were included.

b Time (i.e., age) in years.

c The proportion of patients alive just prior to time *t* who have "failed" at that time.

d The proportion of individuals who do not "fail" at *t*.

e The estimate of the survival function.

G Is it also different at age 30 years? Did you expect this?

Yes, the estimate that contains the censored observations is higher than the one without. We would expect this to change because there are censored observations that occur before age 30 years.

H We can also create a table similar to Table 15.5 using SAS or Stata. Create tables for the survivor functions using both the product-limit method and the life-table method using SAS or Stata. The data presented in this problem are saved in the dataset *asthma_age_15b*.

Instructions for Example Problem 15.1—Part H

Generating Survival Tables in SAS and Stata

SAS

In order to create survivor function tables in SAS, we will use PROC LIFETEST. This procedure will allow us to compute tables, along with several other items we will learn about later in this chapter, for both the life table and product-limit methods.

After making sure that we have our dataset *asthma_age_15b* saved in our mylib library, we will use PROC LIFETEST:

```
PROC LIFETEST
DATA=mylib.asthma_age_15b;
     TIME age_time*asthma(0);
RUN;
```

The default method for PROC LIFETEST is the product-limit method. To get the life-table method, we would simply add METHOD=life to the PROC LIFETEST line:

```
PROC LIFETEST
DATA=mylib.asthma_age_15b
METHOD=life INTERVALS=0 to 60
by 5;;
     TIME age_time*asthma(0);
RUN;
```

To get the life-table method table similar to what we presented in Table 15.2, we can use the INVERVALS option. We want to see a table from 0 to 60 with interval lengths of 5 (see SAS code above).

The SAS output created after running PROC LIFETEST, using the product-limit method, is shown after this table. The survival function estimate is presented in the Survival column. The life-table method output is shown after the product-limit method output.

Stata

In order to create survivor function tables in Stata, we can use the *sts list* command. This will create a survival function table using the product-limit method. In order to use this command, we first have to declare our data as survival data by using the *stset* command:

```
stset age_time, failure(asthma)
```

After the *stset* command, we type our time variable, *age_time* in this example, then let Stata know our failure (censor) variable, *asthma* in this example. Since asthma is already coded as 1 = asthma/failure, 0 = no asthma/censored, Stata knows that 0 is the censored observation. If asthma was coded differently, we would have to let Stata know the censored observation value. Next, to create the product-limit table, we use the *sts list* command:

```
sts list
```

If we wanted to get the survival function table using the life-table method, we could use the *ltable* command:

```
ltable age_time asthma,
intervals(5)
```

The *intervals*(5) option tells Stata that we would like our intervals at a length of 5.
The Stata output created after running the *sts list* command, using the product-limit method, is shown after this table, following the SAS output. The life-table method output is shown after the product-limit method output.

SAS Product-Limit Output:

The LIFETEST Procedure

Product-Limit Survival Estimates

age_time		Survival	Failure	Survival Standard Error	Number Failed	Number Left
0.0000		1.0000	0	0	0	35
1.0000		.	.	.	1	34
1.0000		.	.	.	2	33
1.0000		.	.	.	3	32
1.0000		.	.	.	4	31
1.0000		.	.	.	5	30
1.0000		0.8286	0.1714	0.0637	6	29
2.0000		.	.	.	7	28
2.0000		0.7714	0.2286	0.0710	8	27
2.0000	*	.	.	.	8	26
2.0000	*	.	.	.	8	25
3.0000		0.7406	0.2594	0.0745	9	24
4.0000		0.7097	0.2903	0.0776	10	23
5.0000		.	.	.	11	22
5.0000		.	.	.	12	21
5.0000		.	.	.	13	20
5.0000		0.5863	0.4137	0.0852	14	19
6.0000		0.5554	0.4446	0.0861	15	18
9.0000		0.5246	0.4754	0.0867	16	17
9.0000	*	.	.	.	16	16
12.0000		.	.	.	17	15
12.0000		0.4590	0.5410	0.0874	18	14
12.0000	*	.	.	.	18	13
13.0000	*	.	.	.	18	12
17.0000		0.4208	0.5793	0.0880	19	11
19.0000		0.3825	0.6175	0.0880	20	10
20.0000		0.3442	0.6558	0.0871	21	9
22.0000		0.3060	0.6940	0.0854	22	8
28.0000	*	.	.	.	22	7
30.0000		0.2623	0.7377	0.0836	23	6
33.0000	*	.	.	.	23	5
50.0000		0.2098	0.7902	0.0817	24	4
52.0000	*	.	.	.	24	3
60.0000	*	.	.	.	24	2
67.0000	*	.	.	.	24	1
72.0000		0	1.0000	.	25	0

Note: The marked (asterisk) survival times are censored observations.

SAS Life-Table Method Output:

Life Table Survival Estimates

Interval (Lower,	Upper)	Number Failed	Number Censored	Effective Sample Size	Conditional Probability of Failure	Conditional Probability Standard Error	Survival	Failure
0	5	10	2	34.0	0.2941	0.0781	1.0000	0
5	10	6	1	22.5	0.2667	0.0932	0.7059	0.2941
10	15	2	2	15.0	0.1333	0.0878	0.5176	0.4824
15	20	2	0	12.0	0.1667	0.1076	0.4486	0.5514
20	25	2	0	10.0	0.2000	0.1265	0.3739	0.6261
25	30	0	1	7.5	0	0	0.2991	0.7009
30	35	1	1	6.5	0.1538	0.1415	0.2991	0.7009
35	40	0	0	5.0	0	0	0.2531	0.7469
40	45	0	0	5.0	0	0	0.2531	0.7469
45	50	0	0	5.0	0	0	0.2531	0.7469
50	55	1	1	4.5	0.2222	0.1960	0.2531	0.7469
55	60	0	0	3.0	0	0	0.1968	0.8032
60	.	1	2	2.0	0.5000	0.3536	0.1968	0.8032

Life-Table Survival Estimates						
Survival Standard Error	Median Residual Lifetime	Median Standard Error	Evaluated at the Midpoint of the Interval			
			PDF	PDF Standard Error	Hazard	Hazard Standard Error
0	11.2784	6.2120	0.0588	0.0156	0.068966	0.021482
0.0781	16.3986	4.9756	0.0376	0.0138	0.061538	0.024824
0.0873	24.3750	7.2618	0.0138	0.00938	0.028571	0.020151
0.0882	37.5568	5.7571	0.0150	0.0101	0.036364	0.025607
0.0879	.	.	0.0150	0.0101	0.044444	0.031232
0.0848	.	.	0	.	0	.
0.0848	.	.	0.00920	0.00886	0.033333	0.033217
0.0833	.	.	0	.	0	.
0.0833	.	.	0	.	0	.
0.0833	.	.	0	.	0	.
0.0833	.	.	0.0112	0.0106	0.05	0.049608
0.0816	.	.	0	.	0	.
0.0816	.	.	.	.	.	.

Stata Product-Limit Method Output:

```
      failure _d:  asthma
analysis time _t:  age_time
```

Time	Beg. Total	Fail	Net Lost	Survivor Function	Std. Error	[95% Conf.	Int.]
1	35	6	0	0.8286	0.0637	0.6577	0.9191
2	29	2	2	0.7714	0.0710	0.5946	0.8785
3	25	1	0	0.7406	0.0745	0.5603	0.8558
4	24	1	0	0.7097	0.0776	0.5271	0.8323
5	23	4	0	0.5863	0.0852	0.4025	0.7310
6	19	1	0	0.5554	0.0861	0.3732	0.7041
9	18	1	1	0.5246	0.0867	0.3445	0.6767
12	16	2	1	0.4590	0.0874	0.2845	0.6173
13	13	0	1	0.4590	0.0874	0.2845	0.6173
17	12	1	0	0.4207	0.0880	0.2490	0.5833
19	11	1	0	0.3825	0.0880	0.2152	0.5481
20	10	1	0	0.3442	0.0871	0.1831	0.5118
22	9	1	0	0.3060	0.0854	0.1527	0.4742
28	8	0	1	0.3060	0.0854	0.1527	0.4742
30	7	1	0	0.2623	0.0836	0.1183	0.4322
33	6	0	1	0.2623	0.0836	0.1183	0.4322
50	5	1	0	0.2098	0.0817	0.0784	0.3838
52	4	0	1	0.2098	0.0817	0.0784	0.3838
60	3	0	1	0.2098	0.0817	0.0784	0.3838
67	2	0	1	0.2098	0.0817	0.0784	0.3838
72	1	1	0	0.0000	.	.	.

Stata Life-Table Method Output:

Interval		Beg. Total	Deaths	Lost	Survival	Std. Error	[95% Conf. Int.]	
0	5	35	10	2	0.7059	0.0781	0.5224	0.8296
5	10	23	6	1	0.5176	0.0873	0.3370	0.6712
10	15	16	2	2	0.4486	0.0882	0.2735	0.6092
15	20	12	2	0	0.3739	0.0879	0.2076	0.5402
20	25	10	2	0	0.2991	0.0848	0.1477	0.4668
25	30	8	0	1	0.2991	0.0848	0.1477	0.4668
30	35	7	1	1	0.2531	0.0833	0.1111	0.4235
50	55	5	1	1	0.1968	0.0816	0.0686	0.3731
60	65	3	0	1	0.1968	0.0816	0.0686	0.3731
65	70	2	0	1	0.1968	0.0816	0.0686	0.3731
70	75	1	1	0	0.0000	.	.	.

EXAMPLE PROBLEM 15.2

Rather than work with survival times drawn from a single population, we often want to compare the distributions of times for two different groups. For example, we might wish to compare the age of diagnosis of asthma for participants who are male versus those who are female. For this problem, we will continue using the dataset *asthma_age_15b*.

A Using statistical software, plot the survival curves of both males and females using the product-limit estimates.

B Look at the plotted results. Does either curve drop down to the horizontal axis?

Instructions for Example Problem 15.2—Part (A)

Plotting Survival Curves in SAS and Stata

SAS	*Stata*
In order to plot a survival curve in SAS, we will use PROC LIFETEST. This procedure will allow us to compute survival curves, along with tables, for both the life-table and product-limit methods. After making sure that we have our dataset *asthma_age_15b* saved in our mylib library, we will use PROC LIFETEST:	In order to plot a survival curve in Stata, we can use the *sts graph* command. First, we have to make sure that our data are declared as survival data, which should already be the case if you followed the process presented in Example Problem 15.1.

PROC LIFETEST
DATA=mylib.asthma_age_15b;
    TIME age_time*asthma(0);
    STRATA gender;
RUN;
	Next, to create the graph, we use the *sts graph* command, with a by(gender) option:
	
	sts graph, by(*gender*)

Along with other tables, including the survivor function estimates discussed in Example Problem 15.1—Part (H), we obtain the survival curve presented in Figure 15.2. The graph shows the survival curves for both males and females. If we wanted to plot a survival curve using the life-table method, we could just add the METHOD=life option to our PROC LIFETEST statement.	We will obtain the survival curve presented in Figure 15.3. The graph shows the survival curves for both males and females. If we wanted to plot a survival curve using the life-table method, we could use the *ltable* command with a *graph* option: `ltable age_time asthma, graph by(gender)`

The curve for the females drops to the horizontal axis; however, the curve for the males does not.

C What does this indicate about each of the estimated survival probabilities?

This indicates that the estimated survival probability for females reaches 0, whereas the male survival probability does not reach 0.

D Why did this occur in this case for the male group?

This occurred in the male group because the last observation is censored.

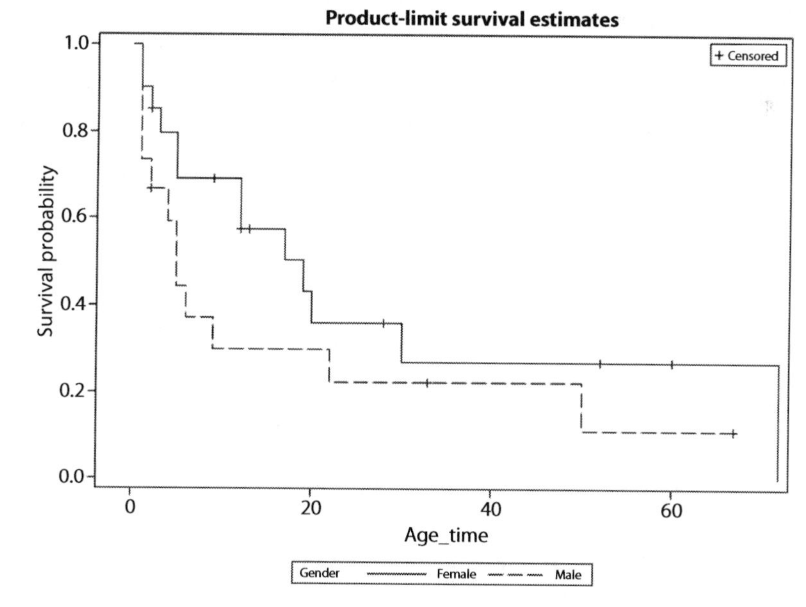

Figure 15.2 **SAS product-limit survival curve of age at diagnosis of asthma by sex.** The SAS-made product-limit survival curve (also known as Kaplan–Meier curve) of age at diagnosis of asthma, stratified by sex is presented in the figure. The solid black line represents females, and the dashed black line represents males. Both curves trend downward as age increases; however, the male curve appears to decrease slightly faster than the female curve.

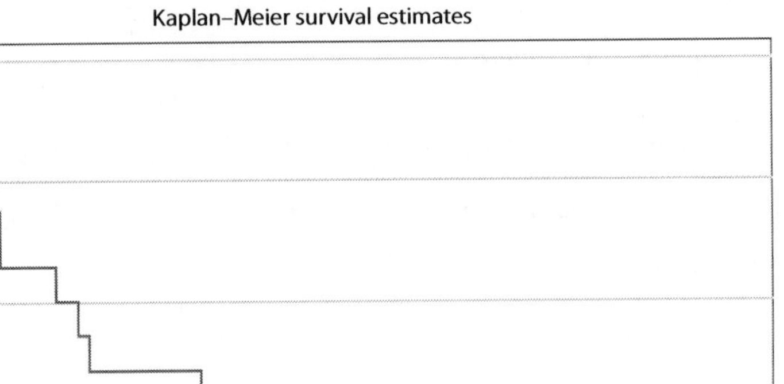

Figure 15.3 **Stata product-limit survival curve of age at diagnosis of asthma by gender.** The black line represents females and the light gray line represents males.

E Based on the plotted survival curves alone, which group of participants appears to fare better?

On the basis of the curve, females appear to fare better because the curve is higher at almost all time points, except for at the very end, so there is a higher probability of not being diagnosed with asthma.

We can conduct a log-rank test to determine whether the apparent difference is statistically significant.

F What is the appropriate null and alternative hypothesis?

The null hypothesis for the log-rank test would be

$H_0\colon S_M(t) = S_F(t)$ $\qquad$ $H_1\colon S_M(t) \neq S_F(t)$

where $S_M(t)$ is the survival function of the females and $S_F(t)$ is the survival function of the males.

G Conduct the test at the $\alpha=0.05$ level. What do you conclude?

In order to conduct a log-rank test, we can use statistical software.

Instructions for Example Problem 15.2—Part G

How to Conduct a Log-Rank Test in SAS and Stata

SAS

To obtain the log-rank test in SAS, we can use the same code that we ran in Example Problem 15.2—Part (A):

```
PROC LIFETEST
DATA=mylib.asthma_age_15b;
     TIME age_time*asthma(0);
     STRATA gender;
RUN;
```

Within the output, we will see the box "Test for Equality over Strata" like below:

Test of Equality over Strata

Test	Chi-Square	DF	Pr > Chi-Square
Log-Rank	1.8429	1	0.1746
Wilcoxon	2.6115	1	0.1061
–2Log(LR)	1.5616	1	0.2114

The first line gives us the log-rank test. Here, we see that the p-value is greater than 0.05; thus, we would fail to reject the null hypothesis and conclude that there is no evidence to suggest that the distribution of age at diagnosis of asthma is different in males and females.

Stata

To obtain the log-rank test in Stata, we can use the *sts test* command:

```
sts test gender
```

We specify that we want to test by gender and obtain the resulting output:

```
Log-rank test for equality of
survivor functions

       |   Events            Events
gender |   observed          expected
-------+-------------------------
Female |         13             16.08
Male   |         12              8.92
-------+-------------------------
Total  |         25             25.00
             chi2(1) =          1.84
             Pr>chi2 =        0.1746
```

We see the p-value is 0.1746, which is greater than 0.05. Thus, we would fail to reject the null hypothesis and would conclude that there is no evidence to suggest that the distribution of age at diagnosis of asthma is different in males and females.

PRACTICE PROBLEM 15.1

Suppose that we are interested in age at first heart attack. Listed here are the ages in years when a participant had a heart attack: 35, 46, 23, 71, 41, 64, 50, 70. The group is composed of eight randomly selected NHANES[1] participants with nonmissing data. None of the observations are censored in the list of the ages in years when a participant had a heart attack.

A What is the median survival time for these patients?

B For fixed intervals of length 10 years, use the life-table method to estimate the survival function S(t).

BOX 15.2 DESCRIPTION OF DATA FOR PRACTICE PROBLEM 15.1[1]

The data presented in Practice Problem 15.1 come from a random sample of 2014 NHANES participants that had a valid response option for the age at first heart attack. The question asked in the 2014 NHANES survey was "How old {were you/was SP} when {you were/s/he was} first told {you/s/he} had a heart attack (also called myocardial infarction)?" The age responses ranged from 16 to 79 years, and ages 80 and older were all coded as 80 years. The respondent could also refuse to answer or respond that he or she did not know—participants in these two response categories (and other categories with missing responses) were excluded from this sample.

C Construct a survival curve based on the life-table estimate of S(*t*).

D Use the product-limit method to estimate the survival function.

E Construct a survival curve based on the product-limit estimate.

PRACTICE PROBLEM 15.2

In 2012, an additional survey was conducted as part of the NHANES survey that targeted youths. That survey was called the NHANES National Youth Fitness Survey (NNYFS).[2] In the dataset *nnyfs_plank* is a stratified random sample of 60 participants in the NNYFS survey who completed both a plank hold test and a cardiovascular fitness test. There are five variables included in this sample dataset. The variable ID

BOX 15.3 DESCRIPTION OF DATA FOR PRACTICE PROBLEM 15.2[2]

In the dataset *nnyfs_plank* is a stratified random sample of 60 participants in the NNYFS survey who completed both a plank hold test and a cardiovascular fitness test. The variable *ID* comes from the NNYFS variable *seqn*, which is the ID number given to each participant. The variable *bmi* comes from the NNYFS variable BMI category for children/adolescents that classifies the youths as underweight, normal weight, overweight, or obese. The first two categories were combined to create the underweight/normal weight category, and the latter two categories were combined to create the overweight/obese category. The variable *cardiofit* comes from the NNYFS variable cardiovascular fitness level and was left as coded by NNYFS. The variables *plank* and *plank_time* come from the NNYFS variable for the number of the seconds that plank position is held. If participants did not have missing values for these variables, the variable *plank* was coded as 1. *Plank_time* contains values that appeared in the NNYFS variable for the number of seconds that plank position was held.

is an identification number for each participant. The variable *bmi* is a two-category (dichotomous) variable, where 0 = underweight or normal weight and 1 = overweight or obese, as classified by the NNYFS survey administrators. The variable *cardiofit* is a three-category variable, where 1 = healthy fitness zone, 2 = needs improvement—some risk, and 3 = needs improvement—high risk. According to the NNYFS,[2] this variable is based on gender- and age-specific cutoff points of an estimated VO_2max. The variable plank contains a 1 for youths who completed the plank hold test and a 0 for the youths who did not. In this sample, all youths completed the plank hold test, so they all have a value of 1. The final variable in the dataset *plank_time* is the number of seconds that the youth held the plank position.

A Use the product-limit method to estimate the survival function in each BMI group.

B Construct survival curves based on the product-limit estimate.

C On the basis of the survival curve, does it appear that the youths in one group have a longer plank hold time than those in the other group?

D Test the hypothesis that the distributions of plank hold times are identical in the two BMI groups.

E For the overweight or obese children, test the null hypothesis that the distributions of plank hold times are identical for youths in each cardio fitness category. What do you conclude?

References

1. National Health and Nutrition Examination Survey. Hyattsville, MD: Centers for Disease Control and Prevention, National Center for Health Statistics. 2014. https://wwwn.cdc.gov/Nchs/Nhanes/Search/nhanes13_14.aspx. Accessed February 23, 2016.
2. National Health and Nutrition Examination Survey, NNYFS 2012. Centers for Disease Control and Prevention, National Center for Health Statistics. https://wwwn.cdc.gov/Nchs/Nhanes/Search/Nnyfs12.aspx. Published 2012. Accessed January 11, 2016.

Lab E: Data analysis project

A random sample of 1,000 births from the 2010 birth cohort-linked birth and infant death dataset is provided in the *labe_births_2010* dataset.[1] Use the sample to answer the following questions. The questions are just a guide, and it is important to conduct descriptive analyses to explore the dataset, write the null and alternative hypotheses, interpret confidence intervals, and draw conclusions. Include all assumptions, justifications, interpretations, and explanations in the answers.

Part one

First, we will look at the variables of interest and then recode missing values. (Note: Table E.1 shows the variables that we will use in this lab. A description of each variable and the values of each variable are shown.)

A Run basic descriptive statistics for the variables *gest_age*, *birth_wt*, *del_method*, *mothers_age*, *wt_gain*, and *preg_htn*.

B Using Table E.1, recode the unknown values of each variable so that they are understood to be missing by SAS or Stata.

C Now, run the descriptive statistics again. Are all of the unknown variables excluded from the analysis?

Part two

Suppose that we are interested in finding whether babies born prematurely had the same mean birthweight as the general population. We already know that the true mean birthweight of the population of babies born in the United States in 2010 is 3261 grams. Create a subsample of premature babies (gestational age < 36 weeks).

A How many premature babies are there in the sample?

B What are the sample mean and sample standard deviation of birthweight among premature babies?

C Use the sample to construct a 95% confidence interval for the true mean birthweight of premature babies. Interpret the confidence interval. Does the interval contain the

Table E.1 Variables for Lab E

Variable	*Description*	*Level*
gest_age	Gestational age in weeks	22–47 = Weeks of gestation 99 = Unknown
birth_wt	Birthweight in grams	227–8165 9999 = Unknown
del_method	Delivery method	1 = Vaginal 2 = C-section 9 = Unknown
mothers_age	Mother's age in years	12 = 10 to 12 years 13 = 13 years 14 = 14 years ... 49 = 49 years 50 = 50 to 54 years
wt_gain	Weight gain during pregnancy in pounds	0–97 = Weight gain in pounds 98 = ≥ 98 Pounds 99 = Unknown
preg_htn	Pregnancy-associated hypertension	1 = Yes 2 = No 9 = Unknown

true mean birthweight of the general population? What do you conclude about the mean birthweight of the population of babies born at less than 36 weeks gestational age compared with the general population?

D Using the random sample, test the null hypothesis that premature babies had a mean birthweight of 3261 grams, the mean birthweight of the general population. Use a two-sided test at the $\alpha = 0.05$ level of significance. What type of test do we perform? What is the test statistic? What distribution does the test statistic follow? What is the p-value? What do we conclude?

E Do the conclusions drawn from the confidence interval and hypothesis test agree? Would we expect that they would?

F Because we have data on all babies born in the United States in 2010, we know that the true mean birthweight for the population of premature babies is 2283 grams. Did we make a correct conclusion with the hypothesis test based on the sample of babies? If not, what type of error did we make?

Part three

Investigate whether the mean birthweight of male babies was the same as that of female babies in the 2010 U.S. cohort. Since we do not know what the true mean birthweight is in either population, we will perform a hypothesis test using the sample. Use a two-sided test at the $\alpha = 0.05$ level of significance.

A What are the two populations that we are comparing?

B What are the null and alternative hypotheses?

C What is the probability that we will reject the null hypothesis if, in fact, the null hypothesis is true?

D What are the sample mean and sample standard deviation for each group? How many boys and how many girls are in the sample? Recall that *female* = 1 for females and *female* = 0 for males.

E Does it appear as if the assumption of equal variances is valid?

F Using the random sample, test the null hypothesis that male babies and female babies had the same mean birthweight. What type of test do we perform? What is the value of the test statistic? What distribution does the test statistic follow? What is the p-value? What do we conclude?

G What is the 95% confidence interval for the true difference in mean birthweight between males and females? Does the confidence interval contain 0? Would we expect it to? Why or why not?

Part four

Next, we will use several statistical methods to investigate whether there is an association between vaginal birth and gestational age in the population of babies born in the United States in 2010. Specifically, do babies born after 40 weeks gestational age have the same proportion of vaginal births as babies born at 40 weeks gestational age or less? For each test, use the sample of babies. Please, note that multiple tests are valid for this analysis; in fact, some are algebraically identical.

To answer these questions, we will work with two variables, *gest_age* and *del_method*. Refer to Table E.1 for the variable names as well as the range of observed values and the values for unknown measurements.

In order to compare the proportion of vaginal births for babies born at a gestational age $\leq$ 40 weeks, the variable *gest_age* needs to be dichotomized, and *del_method* will be used to create a new indicator. Create a new variable called *gest_lte40*, which will recode *gest_age* into a binary variable as shown in Table E.2. Likewise, recode *del_method* into a new variable called *vag_birth*. (Note: Table E.2 shows a description and values for two new indicator variables that we will use in the analysis.)

Using the sample, test the null hypothesis that the proportion of vaginal births for babies born at a gestational age $\leq$ 40 weeks is the same as the proportion for babies born at a gestational age > 40 weeks. Use a two-sample test of proportions at the 0.05 level of significance.

Table E.2 New indicator variables

Variable	*Description*	*Level*
gest_lte40	Gestational age ≤ 40 indicator	1 = Yes (gest_age ≤ 40) 0 = No (gest_age > 40) . = Unknown (gest_age = .)
vag_birth	Vaginal delivery indicator	1 = Yes (del_method = 1) 0 = No (del_method = 2) . = Unknown (del_method = .)

A Write the code to create the new variables *gest_lte40* and *vag_birth*.

B State the null and alternative hypotheses.

C For each group of babies, what is the point estimate of the population proportion of vaginal births?

D What is the point estimate for the true difference in proportion of vaginal births between the two groups?

E What is the 95% confidence interval for the difference in proportions?

F Draw a conclusion about the null hypothesis based on the confidence interval.

G What are the value and distribution of the test statistic?

H What is the *p*-value?

I Draw a conclusion about the null hypothesis based on the results of the hypothesis test.

Part five

Test the same null hypothesis as in Part Four, this time using a chi-square test.

A Display the sample data as a 2 × 2 contingency table.

B Why is McNemar's test not an appropriate method for analyzing these data?

C Perform the hypothesis test using an appropriate statistic.

D What are the value and distribution of the test statistic?

E What is the *p*-value?

F Draw a conclusion about your null hypothesis based on the results of the hypothesis test.

G How does the chi-square test statistic compare with the test statistic from the two-sample test of proportions?

H How does the *p*-value of the chi-squared test compare with that of the two-sample test of proportions?

I Under what situation is the chi-square test not a valid way to test for an association between two dichotomous variables?

Part six

Test the same hypothesis as in part four, this time using odds ratios to analyze these data.

A What are your null and alternative hypotheses in terms of the odds ratio?

B What are the estimated odds of vaginal birth for babies born at a gestational age ≤ 40 weeks in the sample? Note: This can be calculated by hand using a 2×2 table or through a logistic regression.

C What are the estimated odds of vaginal birth for babies born at a gestational age > 40 weeks in the sample?

D What is the estimated odds ratio of vaginal birth in a comparison of babies born at a gestational age ≤ 40 and babies born at a gestational age > 40?

E Interpret the odds ratio in words.

F Construct a 95% confidence interval for the true odds ratio, and interpret the confidence interval in words.

G Use the confidence interval for the odds ratio to test the null hypothesis. Be sure to clearly state the conclusion.

H How do the results based on the confidence interval of the odds ratio compare with the results based on the two-sample test of proportions and the chi-square test?

Part seven

Investigate whether there is a linear relationship between a mother's age and the amount of weight gained during pregnancy for the population of babies born in the United States in 2010. The two variables that we will be working with are *mothers_age* and *wt_gain*.

A Create a scatterplot of mother's age versus weight gain. Let weight gain be on the y-axis. Be sure to label each axis properly.

B Does there appear to be a linear relationship between the two variables?

C What is the Pearson coefficient of correlation?

D Use the sample Pearson correlation coefficient to test the null hypothesis that there is no linear relationship between the two variables. State the null and alternative hypotheses for the test.

E What is the p-value of the test statistic?

F Draw a conclusion for the test.

G What is the Spearman's rank correlation coefficient?

H Now, we will use the Spearman's correlation coefficient to test the same hypothesis. What is the p-value of the test statistic?

I Draw a conclusion for the test.

J Do the conclusions of the two tests agree? Briefly explain why you think that is so.

K Under what situations should we use Spearman's correlation coefficient in place of the Pearson?

Part eight

Suppose that we are interested in the relationship between mother's weight gain during pregnancy and gestational age. For all analyses, let weight gain be the dependent variable.

A Create a scatterplot of gestational age and weight gain during pregnancy. What can we say about the relationship between weight gain and gestational age?

B What would be the equation for the true population regression line predicting weight gain from gestational age?

C Obtain the least squares regression line.

D What is the least squares estimate of the true population intercept ($\hat{\alpha}$)? Interpret this value in words.

E What is the least squares estimate of the true population slope ($\hat{\beta}$)? Interpret this value in words.

F Test whether there is a significant linear relationship between the mother's weight gain and gestational age. State the null and alternative hypotheses, calculate the test statistic, state the distribution of the test statistic, state the *p*-value, and draw a conclusion.

G Calculate a 95% confidence interval for the slope of the true population regression line.

H How does it reflect the result of the hypothesis test?

I Now recreate the scatterplot, this time including the fitted values from the regression.
- First, we must create a predicted value for each observation.
- Then, create a scatterplot with the predicted values overlaid.
- Label each axis.

J What is the predicted mean weight gain ($\hat{y}$) for all mothers with babies born at 29 weeks gestational age?

K What is the coefficient of determination for the model, and how does it indicate the adequacy of this model in fitting the data?

L Produce a scatterplot of the residuals versus the fitted values. How does it indicate that assumptions of simple linear regression are met or violated?

Part nine

We now wish to determine whether the mother's weight gain also depends on the age of the mother.

A Write the form of the population regression model in terms of the predictor variables. Keep gestational age in the model, but add mother's age as an explanatory variable.

B Fit the model using SAS or Stata. Keep gestational age in the model, and add mother's age as an additional explanatory variable.

C What is the equation of the estimated line?

D At the $\alpha = 0.05$ level of significance, test the null hypothesis that the slope associated with each gestational age and mother's age is equal to 0 while holding the other factor constant. (Note: two separate tests.)

E What percentage of the variability do gestational age and mother's age together explain?

F Is this the most appropriate measure for models with more than one explanatory variable? If not, what is the most appropriate measure?

G Find the most appropriate measure in this case, and discuss how the change in its value indicates whether adding mother's age as an explanatory variable may or may not improve the ability to predict mother's weight gain for infants in the population.

H Would you leave mother's age in a final model to predict weight gain? Why or why not?

Part ten

Now add a variable indicating pregnancy-associated hypertension to the model that includes gestational age as the only other explanatory variable to see whether a mother's diagnosis of hypertension during pregnancy affects her weight gain after controlling for gestational age. Recode the *preg_htn* variable so that the values are $x_3 = 1$ for yes (pregnancy-associated hypertension), $x_3 = 0$ for no, and $x_3 =$ for unknown.

A Fit this model in SAS or Stata.
B Report the equation of the estimated regression line.

C At the $\alpha = 0.05$ significance level, test the null hypothesis that the coefficient associated with hypertension is equal to 0 using the output from your regression. What do you conclude?

D Interpret the estimated coefficients for gestational age and hypertension in words.

E Compare this to the model that contains only gestational age using the adjusted R^2. How has it changed by adding the indicator for hypertension?

F Plot the residuals of this model versus its fitted values, and comment on the appropriateness of the model.

G To determine whether an increase in gestational age has a different effect on weight gain for mothers who were diagnosed with hypertension versus mothers who were not, we could add an additional variable to the model. What is this additional variable?

H If this variable significantly added to the model, what does this mean in terms of how gestational age and hypertension each relate to the weight gain of mothers in this population?

I Create an interaction term for gestational age and hypertension. Examine the values of the interaction term. Add the interaction term into the previous model, and determine whether it improves our ability to predict the weight gain of a mother in the population using the following criteria:
  1 Test the null hypothesis that the variable's coefficient is 0.
  2 Examine the change in the value of the adjusted R^2 with previous models.

J Of the models examined, what model are you most comfortable using for prediction? Why did you choose it?

Reference

1. Vital Statistics Data Available Online. Hyattsville, MD: Centers for Disease Control and Prevention, National Center for Health Statistics. 2016. http://www.cdc.gov/nchs/data_access/vitalstatsonline .htm. Accessed November 22, 2016.

Appendix: Statistical tables

Table A.1 Binomial distribution probabilities

n	k	0.05	0.10	0.15	0.20	0.25	0.30	0.35	0.40	0.45	0.50
2	0	0.9020	0.8100	0.7225	0.6400	0.5625	0.4900	0.4225	0.3600	0.3025	0.2500
	1	0.0950	0.1800	0.2550	0.3200	0.3750	0.4200	0.4550	0.4800	0.4950	0.5000
	2	0.0025	0.0100	0.0225	0.0400	0.0625	0.0900	0.1225	0.1600	0.2025	0.2500
3	0	0.8574	0.7290	0.6141	0.5120	0.4219	0.3430	0.2746	0.2160	0.1664	0.1250
	1	0.1354	0.2430	0.3250	0.3840	0.4220	0.4410	0.4440	0.4320	0.4080	0.3750
	2	0.0071	0.0270	0.0574	0.0960	0.1406	0.1890	0.2389	0.2880	0.3341	0.3750
	3	0.0001	0.0010	0.0034	0.0080	0.0156	0.0270	0.0429	0.0640	0.0911	0.1250
4	0	0.8145	0.6561	0.5220	0.4096	0.3164	0.2401	0.1785	0.1296	0.0915	0.0625
	1	0.1715	0.2916	0.3685	0.4096	0.4219	0.4116	0.3845	0.3456	0.2995	0.2500
	2	0.0135	0.0486	0.0975	0.1536	0.2109	0.2646	0.3105	0.3456	0.3675	0.3750
	3	0.0005	0.0036	0.0115	0.0256	0.0469	0.0756	0.1115	0.1536	0.2005	0.2500
	4	0.0000	0.0001	0.0005	0.0016	0.0039	0.0081	0.0150	0.0256	0.0410	0.0625
5	0	0.7738	0.5905	0.4437	0.3277	0.2373	0.1681	0.1160	0.0778	0.0503	0.0313
	1	0.2036	0.3281	0.3915	0.4096	0.3955	0.3602	0.3124	0.2592	0.2059	0.1563
	2	0.0214	0.0729	0.1382	0.2048	0.2637	0.3087	0.3364	0.3456	0.3369	0.3125
	3	0.0011	0.0081	0.0244	0.0512	0.0879	0.1323	0.1811	0.2304	0.2757	0.3125
	4	0.0000	0.0005	0.0022	0.0064	0.0146	0.0284	0.0488	0.0768	0.1128	0.1563
	5	0.0000	0.0000	0.0001	0.0003	0.0010	0.0024	0.0053	0.0102	0.0185	0.0313
6	0	0.7351	0.5314	0.3771	0.2621	0.1780	0.1176	0.0754	0.0467	0.0277	0.0156
	1	0.2321	0.3543	0.3993	0.3932	0.3560	0.3025	0.2437	0.1866	0.1359	0.0938
	2	0.0305	0.0984	0.1762	0.2458	0.2966	0.3241	0.3280	0.3110	0.2780	0.2344
	3	0.0021	0.0146	0.0415	0.0819	0.1318	0.1852	0.2355	0.2765	0.3032	0.3125
	4	0.0001	0.0012	0.0055	0.0154	0.0330	0.0595	0.0951	0.1382	0.1861	0.2344

(Continued)

Table A.1 (Continued) Binomial distribution probabilities

n	*k*	*0.05*	*0.10*	*0.15*	*0.20*	*0.25*	*0.30*	*0.35*	*0.40*	*0.45*	*0.50*
	5	0.0000	0.0001	0.0004	0.0015	0.0044	0.0102	0.0205	0.0369	0.0609	0.0938
	6	0.0000	0.0000	0.0000	0.0001	0.0002	0.0007	0.0018	0.0041	0.0083	0.0156
7	0	0.6983	0.4783	0.3206	0.2097	0.1335	0.0824	0.0490	0.0280	0.0152	0.0078
	1	0.2573	0.3720	0.3960	0.3670	0.3115	0.2471	0.1848	0.1306	0.0872	0.0547
	2	0.0406	0.1240	0.2097	0.2753	0.3115	0.3177	0.2985	0.2613	0.2140	0.1641
	3	0.0036	0.0230	0.0617	0.1147	0.1730	0.2269	0.2679	0.2903	0.2918	0.2734
	4	0.0002	0.0026	0.0109	0.0287	0.0577	0.0972	0.1442	0.1935	0.2388	0.2734
	5	0.0000	0.0002	0.0012	0.0043	0.0115	0.0250	0.0466	0.0774	0.1172	0.1641
	6	0.0000	0.0000	0.0001	0.0004	0.0013	0.0036	0.0084	0.0172	0.0320	0.0547
	7	0.0000	0.0000	0.0000	0.0000	0.0001	0.0002	0.0006	0.0016	0.0037	0.0078
8	0	0.6634	0.4305	0.2725	0.1678	0.1001	0.0576	0.0319	0.0168	0.0084	0.0039
	1	0.2793	0.3826	0.3847	0.3355	0.2670	0.1977	0.1373	0.0896	0.0548	0.0313
	2	0.0515	0.1488	0.2376	0.2936	0.3115	0.2965	0.2587	0.2090	0.1569	0.1094
	3	0.0054	0.0331	0.0839	0.1468	0.2076	0.2541	0.2786	0.2787	0.2568	0.2188
	4	0.0004	0.0046	0.0185	0.0459	0.0865	0.1361	0.1875	0.2322	0.2627	0.2734
	5	0.0000	0.0004	0.0026	0.0092	0.0231	0.0467	0.0808	0.1239	0.1719	0.2188
	6	0.0000	0.0000	0.0002	0.0011	0.0038	0.0100	0.0217	0.0413	0.0703	0.1094
	7	0.0000	0.0000	0.0000	0.0001	0.0004	0.0012	0.0033	0.0079	0.0164	0.0313
	8	0.0000	0.0000	0.0000	0.0000	0.0000	0.0001	0.0002	0.0007	0.0017	0.0039
9	0	0.6302	0.3874	0.2316	0.1342	0.0751	0.0404	0.0207	0.0101	0.0046	0.0020
	1	0.2985	0.3874	0.3679	0.3020	0.2253	0.1556	0.1004	0.0605	0.0339	0.0176
	2	0.0629	0.1722	0.2597	0.3020	0.3003	0.2668	0.2162	0.1612	0.1110	0.0703
	3	0.0077	0.0446	0.1069	0.1762	0.2336	0.2668	0.2716	0.2508	0.2119	0.1641
	4	0.0006	0.0074	0.0283	0.0661	0.1168	0.1715	0.2194	0.2508	0.2600	0.2461

(Continued)

Table A.1 (Continued) Binomial distribution probabilities

n	k	0.05	0.10	0.15	0.20	0.25	0.30	0.35	0.40	0.45	0.50
	5	0.0000	0.0008	0.0050	0.0165	0.0389	0.0735	0.1181	0.1672	0.2128	0.2461
	6	0.0000	0.0001	0.0006	0.0028	0.0087	0.0210	0.0424	0.0743	0.1160	0.1641
	7	0.0000	0.0000	0.0000	0.0003	0.0012	0.0039	0.0098	0.0212	0.0407	0.0703
	8	0.0000	0.0000	0.0000	0.0000	0.0001	0.0004	0.0013	0.0035	0.0083	0.0176
	9	0.0000	0.0000	0.0000	0.0000	0.0000	0.0000	0.0001	0.0003	0.0008	0.0020
10	0	0.5987	0.3487	0.1969	0.1074	0.0563	0.0282	0.0135	0.0060	0.0025	0.0010
	1	0.3151	0.3874	0.3474	0.2684	0.1877	0.1211	0.0725	0.0403	0.0207	0.0098
	2	0.0746	0.1937	0.2759	0.3020	0.2816	0.2335	0.1757	0.1209	0.0763	0.0439
	3	0.0105	0.0574	0.1298	0.2013	0.2503	0.2668	0.2522	0.2150	0.1665	0.1172
	4	0.0010	0.0112	0.0401	0.0881	0.1460	0.2001	0.2377	0.2508	0.2384	0.2051
	5	0.0001	0.0015	0.0085	0.0264	0.0584	0.1029	0.1536	0.2007	0.2340	0.2461
	6	0.0000	0.0001	0.0012	0.0055	0.0162	0.0368	0.0689	0.1115	0.1596	0.2051
	7	0.0000	0.0000	0.0001	0.0008	0.0031	0.0090	0.0212	0.0425	0.0746	0.1172
	8	0.0000	0.0000	0.0000	0.0001	0.0004	0.0014	0.0043	0.0106	0.0229	0.0439
	9	0.0000	0.0000	0.0000	0.0000	0.0000	0.0001	0.0005	0.0016	0.0042	0.0098
	10	0.0000	0.0000	0.0000	0.0000	0.0000	0.0000	0.0000	0.0001	0.0003	0.0010
11	0	0.5688	0.3138	0.1673	0.0859	0.0422	0.0198	0.0088	0.0036	0.0014	0.0005
	1	0.3293	0.3835	0.3248	0.2362	0.1549	0.0932	0.0518	0.0266	0.0125	0.0054
	2	0.0867	0.2131	0.2866	0.2953	0.2581	0.1998	0.1395	0.0887	0.0513	0.0269
	3	0.0137	0.0710	0.1517	0.2215	0.2581	0.2568	0.2254	0.1774	0.1259	0.0806
	4	0.0014	0.0158	0.0536	0.1107	0.1721	0.2201	0.2428	0.2365	0.2060	0.1611
	5	0.0001	0.0025	0.0132	0.0388	0.0803	0.1321	0.1830	0.2207	0.2360	0.2256
	6	0.0000	0.0003	0.0023	0.0097	0.0268	0.0566	0.0985	0.1471	0.1931	0.2256
	7	0.0000	0.0000	0.0003	0.0017	0.0064	0.0173	0.0379	0.0701	0.1128	0.1611
	8	0.0000	0.0000	0.0000	0.0002	0.0011	0.0037	0.0102	0.0234	0.0462	0.0806

(Continued)

Table A.1 (Continued) Binomial distribution probabilities

n	*k*	*0.05*	*0.10*	*0.15*	*0.20*	*0.25*	*0.30*	*0.35*	*0.40*	*0.45*	*0.50*
	9	0.0000	0.0000	0.0000	0.0000	0.0001	0.0005	0.0018	0.0052	0.0126	0.0269
	10	0.0000	0.0000	0.0000	0.0000	0.0000	0.0000	0.0002	0.0007	0.0021	0.0054
	11	0.0000	0.0000	0.0000	0.0000	0.0000	0.0000	0.0000	0.0000	0.0002	0.0005
12	0	0.5404	0.2824	0.1422	0.0687	0.0317	0.0138	0.0057	0.0022	0.0008	0.0002
	1	0.3413	0.3766	0.3012	0.2062	0.1267	0.0712	0.0368	0.0174	0.0075	0.0029
	2	0.0988	0.2301	0.2924	0.2835	0.2323	0.1678	0.1088	0.0639	0.0339	0.0161
	3	0.0173	0.0852	0.1720	0.2362	0.2581	0.2397	0.1954	0.1419	0.0923	0.0537
	4	0.0021	0.0213	0.0683	0.1329	0.1936	0.2311	0.2367	0.2128	0.1700	0.1208
	5	0.0002	0.0038	0.0193	0.0532	0.1032	0.1585	0.2039	0.2270	0.2225	0.1934
	6	0.0000	0.0005	0.0040	0.0155	0.0401	0.0792	0.1281	0.1766	0.2124	0.2256
	7	0.0000	0.0000	0.0006	0.0033	0.0115	0.0291	0.0591	0.1009	0.1489	0.1934
	8	0.0000	0.0000	0.0001	0.0005	0.0024	0.0078	0.0199	0.0420	0.0762	0.1208
	9	0.0000	0.0000	0.0000	0.0001	0.0004	0.0015	0.0048	0.0125	0.0277	0.0537
	10	0.0000	0.0000	0.0000	0.0000	0.0000	0.0002	0.0008	0.0025	0.0068	0.0161
	11	0.0000	0.0000	0.0000	0.0000	0.0000	0.0000	0.0001	0.0003	0.0010	0.0029
	12	0.0000	0.0000	0.0000	0.0000	0.0000	0.0000	0.0000	0.0000	0.0001	0.0002
13	0	0.5133	0.2542	0.1209	0.0550	0.0238	0.0097	0.0037	0.0013	0.0004	0.0001
	1	0.3512	0.3672	0.2774	0.1787	0.1029	0.0540	0.0259	0.0113	0.0045	0.0016
	2	0.1109	0.2448	0.2937	0.2680	0.2059	0.1388	0.0836	0.0453	0.0220	0.0095
	3	0.0214	0.0997	0.1900	0.2457	0.2517	0.2181	0.1651	0.1107	0.0660	0.0349
	4	0.0028	0.0277	0.0838	0.1535	0.2097	0.2337	0.2222	0.1845	0.1350	0.0873
	5	0.0003	0.0055	0.0266	0.0691	0.1258	0.1803	0.2154	0.2214	0.1989	0.1571
	6	0.0000	0.0008	0.0063	0.0230	0.0559	0.1030	0.1546	0.1968	0.2169	0.2095
	7	0.0000	0.0001	0.0011	0.0058	0.0186	0.0442	0.0833	0.1312	0.1775	0.2095
	8	0.0000	0.0000	0.0001	0.0011	0.0047	0.0142	0.0336	0.0656	0.1089	0.1571

(*Continued*)

Table A.1 (Continued) Binomial distribution probabilities

n	*k*	*0.05*	*0.10*	*0.15*	*0.20*	*0.25*	*0.30*	*0.35*	*0.40*	*0.45*	*0.50*
	9	0.0000	0.0000	0.0000	0.0001	0.0009	0.0034	0.0101	0.0243	0.0495	0.0873
	10	0.0000	0.0000	0.0000	0.0000	0.0001	0.0006	0.0022	0.0065	0.0162	0.0349
	11	0.0000	0.0000	0.0000	0.0000	0.0000	0.0001	0.0003	0.0012	0.0036	0.0095
	12	0.0000	0.0000	0.0000	0.0000	0.0000	0.0000	0.0000	0.0001	0.0005	0.0016
	13	0.0000	0.0000	0.0000	0.0000	0.0000	0.0000	0.0000	0.0000	0.0000	0.0001
14	0	0.4877	0.2288	0.1028	0.0440	0.0178	0.0068	0.0024	0.0008	0.0002	0.0001
	1	0.3593	0.3559	0.2539	0.1539	0.0832	0.0407	0.0181	0.0073	0.0027	0.0009
	2	0.1229	0.2570	0.2912	0.2501	0.1802	0.1134	0.0634	0.0317	0.0141	0.0056
	3	0.0259	0.1142	0.2056	0.2501	0.2402	0.1943	0.1366	0.0845	0.0462	0.0222
	4	0.0037	0.0349	0.0998	0.1720	0.2202	0.2290	0.2022	0.1549	0.1040	0.0611
	5	0.0004	0.0078	0.0352	0.0860	0.1468	0.1963	0.2178	0.2066	0.1701	0.1222
	6	0.0000	0.0013	0.0093	0.0322	0.0734	0.1262	0.1759	0.2066	0.2088	0.1833
	7	0.0000	0.0002	0.0019	0.0092	0.0280	0.0618	0.1082	0.1574	0.1952	0.2095
	8	0.0000	0.0000	0.0003	0.0020	0.0082	0.0232	0.0510	0.0918	0.1398	0.1833
	9	0.0000	0.0000	0.0000	0.0003	0.0018	0.0066	0.0183	0.0408	0.0762	0.1222
	10	0.0000	0.0000	0.0000	0.0000	0.0003	0.0014	0.0049	0.0136	0.0312	0.0611
	11	0.0000	0.0000	0.0000	0.0000	0.0000	0.0002	0.0010	0.0033	0.0093	0.0222
	12	0.0000	0.0000	0.0000	0.0000	0.0000	0.0000	0.0001	0.0005	0.0019	0.0056
	13	0.0000	0.0000	0.0000	0.0000	0.0000	0.0000	0.0000	0.0001	0.0002	0.0009
	14	0.0000	0.0000	0.0000	0.0000	0.0000	0.0000	0.0000	0.0000	0.0000	0.0001
15	0	0.4633	0.2059	0.0874	0.0352	0.0134	0.0047	0.0016	0.0005	0.0001	0.0000
	1	0.3658	0.3432	0.2312	0.1319	0.0668	0.0305	0.0126	0.0047	0.0016	0.0005
	2	0.1348	0.2669	0.2856	0.2309	0.1559	0.0916	0.0476	0.0219	0.0090	0.0032
	3	0.0307	0.1285	0.2184	0.2501	0.2252	0.1700	0.1110	0.0634	0.0318	0.0139
	4	0.0049	0.0428	0.1156	0.1876	0.2252	0.2186	0.1792	0.1268	0.0780	0.0417

(Continued)

Table A.1 (Continued) Binomial distribution probabilities

n	*k*	*0.05*	*0.10*	*0.15*	*0.20*	*0.25*	*0.30*	*0.35*	*0.40*	*0.45*	*0.50*
	5	0.0006	0.0105	0.0449	0.1032	0.1651	0.2061	0.2123	0.1859	0.1404	0.0916
	6	0.0000	0.0019	0.0132	0.0430	0.0917	0.1472	0.1906	0.2066	0.1914	0.1527
	7	0.0000	0.0003	0.0030	0.0138	0.0393	0.0811	0.1319	0.1771	0.2013	0.1964
	8	0.0000	0.0000	0.0005	0.0035	0.0131	0.0348	0.0710	0.1181	0.1647	0.1964
	9	0.0000	0.0000	0.0001	0.0007	0.0034	0.0116	0.0298	0.0612	0.1048	0.1527
	10	0.0000	0.0000	0.0000	0.0001	0.0007	0.0030	0.0096	0.0245	0.0515	0.0916
	11	0.0000	0.0000	0.0000	0.0000	0.0001	0.0006	0.0024	0.0074	0.0191	0.0417
	12	0.0000	0.0000	0.0000	0.0000	0.0000	0.0001	0.0004	0.0016	0.0052	0.0139
	13	0.0000	0.0000	0.0000	0.0000	0.0000	0.0000	0.0001	0.0003	0.0010	0.0032
	14	0.0000	0.0000	0.0000	0.0000	0.0000	0.0000	0.0000	0.0000	0.0001	0.0005
	15	0.0000	0.0000	0.0000	0.0000	0.0000	0.0000	0.0000	0.0000	0.0000	0.0000
16	0	0.4401	0.1853	0.0743	0.0281	0.0100	0.0033	0.0010	0.0003	0.0001	0.0000
	1	0.3706	0.3294	0.2097	0.1126	0.0535	0.0228	0.0087	0.0030	0.0009	0.0002
	2	0.1463	0.2745	0.2775	0.2111	0.1336	0.0732	0.0353	0.0150	0.0056	0.0018
	3	0.0359	0.1423	0.2285	0.2463	0.2079	0.1465	0.0888	0.0468	0.0215	0.0085
	4	0.0061	0.0514	0.1311	0.2001	0.2252	0.2040	0.1553	0.1014	0.0572	0.0278
	5	0.0008	0.0137	0.0555	0.1201	0.1802	0.2099	0.2008	0.1623	0.1123	0.0667
	6	0.0001	0.0028	0.0180	0.0550	0.1101	0.1649	0.1982	0.1983	0.1684	0.1222
	7	0.0000	0.0004	0.0045	0.0197	0.0524	0.1010	0.1524	0.1889	0.1969	0.1746
	8	0.0000	0.0001	0.0009	0.0055	0.0197	0.0487	0.0923	0.1417	0.1812	0.1964
	9	0.0000	0.0000	0.0001	0.0012	0.0058	0.0185	0.0442	0.0840	0.1318	0.1746
	10	0.0000	0.0000	0.0000	0.0002	0.0014	0.0056	0.0167	0.0392	0.0755	0.1222
	11	0.0000	0.0000	0.0000	0.0000	0.0002	0.0013	0.0049	0.0142	0.0337	0.0667
	12	0.0000	0.0000	0.0000	0.0000	0.0000	0.0002	0.0011	0.0040	0.0115	0.0278
	13	0.0000	0.0000	0.0000	0.0000	0.0000	0.0000	0.0002	0.0008	0.0029	0.0085
	14	0.0000	0.0000	0.0000	0.0000	0.0000	0.0000	0.0000	0.0001	0.0005	0.0018

(Continued)

Table A.1 (Continued) Binomial distribution probabilities

n	*k*	*0.05*	*0.10*	*0.15*	*0.20*	*0.25*	*0.30*	*0.35*	*0.40*	*0.45*	*0.50*
	15	0.0000	0.0000	0.0000	0.0000	0.0000	0.0000	0.0000	0.0000	0.0001	0.0002
	16	0.0000	0.0000	0.0000	0.0000	0.0000	0.0000	0.0000	0.0000	0.0000	0.0000
17	0	0.4181	0.1668	0.0631	0.0225	0.0075	0.0023	0.0007	0.0002	0.0000	0.0000
	1	0.3741	0.3150	0.1893	0.0957	0.0426	0.0169	0.0060	0.0019	0.0005	0.0001
	2	0.1575	0.2800	0.2673	0.1914	0.1136	0.0581	0.0260	0.0102	0.0035	0.0010
	3	0.0415	0.1556	0.2359	0.2393	0.1893	0.1245	0.0701	0.0341	0.0144	0.0052
	4	0.0076	0.0605	0.1457	0.2093	0.2209	0.1868	0.1320	0.0796	0.0411	0.0182
	5	0.0010	0.0175	0.0668	0.1361	0.1914	0.2081	0.1849	0.1379	0.0875	0.0472
	6	0.0001	0.0039	0.0236	0.0680	0.1276	0.1784	0.1991	0.1839	0.1432	0.0944
	7	0.0000	0.0007	0.0065	0.0267	0.0668	0.1201	0.1685	0.1927	0.1841	0.1484
	8	0.0000	0.0001	0.0014	0.0084	0.0279	0.0644	0.1134	0.1606	0.1883	0.1855
	9	0.0000	0.0000	0.0003	0.0021	0.0093	0.0276	0.0611	0.1070	0.1540	0.1855
	10	0.0000	0.0000	0.0000	0.0004	0.0025	0.0095	0.0263	0.0571	0.1008	0.1484
	11	0.0000	0.0000	0.0000	0.0001	0.0005	0.0026	0.0090	0.0242	0.0525	0.0944
	12	0.0000	0.0000	0.0000	0.0000	0.0001	0.0006	0.0024	0.0081	0.0215	0.0472
	13	0.0000	0.0000	0.0000	0.0000	0.0000	0.0001	0.0005	0.0021	0.0068	0.0182
	14	0.0000	0.0000	0.0000	0.0000	0.0000	0.0000	0.0001	0.0004	0.0016	0.0052
	15	0.0000	0.0000	0.0000	0.0000	0.0000	0.0000	0.0000	0.0001	0.0003	0.0010
	16	0.0000	0.0000	0.0000	0.0000	0.0000	0.0000	0.0000	0.0000	0.0000	0.0001
	17	0.0000	0.0000	0.0000	0.0000	0.0000	0.0000	0.0000	0.0000	0.0000	0.0000
18	0	0.3972	0.1501	0.0536	0.0180	0.0056	0.0016	0.0004	0.0001	0.0000	0.0000
	1	0.3763	0.3002	0.1704	0.0811	0.0338	0.0126	0.0042	0.0012	0.0003	0.0001

(*Continued*)

Table A.1 (Continued) Binomial distribution probabilities

n	*k*	*0.05*	*0.10*	*0.15*	*0.20*	*0.25*	*0.30*	*0.35*	*0.40*	*0.45*	*0.50*
	2	0.1683	0.2835	0.2556	0.1723	0.0958	0.0458	0.0190	0.0069	0.0022	0.0006
	3	0.0473	0.1680	0.2406	0.2297	0.1704	0.1046	0.0547	0.0246	0.0095	0.0031
	4	0.0093	0.0700	0.1592	0.2153	0.2130	0.1681	0.1104	0.0614	0.0291	0.0117
	5	0.0014	0.0218	0.0787	0.1507	0.1988	0.2017	0.1664	0.1146	0.0666	0.0327
	6	0.0002	0.0052	0.0301	0.0816	0.1436	0.1873	0.1941	0.1655	0.1181	0.0708
	7	0.0000	0.0010	0.0091	0.0350	0.0820	0.1376	0.1792	0.1892	0.1657	0.1214
	8	0.0000	0.0002	0.0022	0.0120	0.0376	0.0811	0.1327	0.1734	0.1864	0.1669
	9	0.0000	0.0000	0.0004	0.0033	0.0139	0.0386	0.0794	0.1284	0.1694	0.1855
	10	0.0000	0.0000	0.0001	0.0008	0.0042	0.0149	0.0385	0.0771	0.1248	0.1669
	11	0.0000	0.0000	0.0000	0.0001	0.0010	0.0046	0.0151	0.0374	0.0742	0.1214
	12	0.0000	0.0000	0.0000	0.0000	0.0002	0.0012	0.0047	0.0145	0.0354	0.0708
	13	0.0000	0.0000	0.0000	0.0000	0.0000	0.0002	0.0012	0.0045	0.0134	0.0327
	14	0.0000	0.0000	0.0000	0.0000	0.0000	0.0000	0.0002	0.0011	0.0039	0.0117
	15	0.0000	0.0000	0.0000	0.0000	0.0000	0.0000	0.0000	0.0002	0.0009	0.0031
	16	0.0000	0.0000	0.0000	0.0000	0.0000	0.0000	0.0000	0.0000	0.0001	0.0006
	17	0.0000	0.0000	0.0000	0.0000	0.0000	0.0000	0.0000	0.0000	0.0000	0.0001
	18	0.0000	0.0000	0.0000	0.0000	0.0000	0.0000	0.0000	0.0000	0.0000	0.0000
19	0	0.3774	0.1351	0.0456	0.0144	0.0042	0.0011	0.0003	0.0001	0.0000	0.0000
	1	0.3774	0.2852	0.1529	0.0685	0.0268	0.0093	0.0029	0.0008	0.0002	0.0000
	2	0.1787	0.2852	0.2428	0.1540	0.0803	0.0358	0.0138	0.0046	0.0013	0.0003
	3	0.0533	0.1796	0.2428	0.2182	0.1517	0.0869	0.0422	0.0175	0.0062	0.0018
	4	0.0112	0.0798	0.1714	0.2182	0.2023	0.1491	0.0909	0.0467	0.0203	0.0074
	5	0.0018	0.0266	0.0907	0.1636	0.2023	0.1916	0.1468	0.0933	0.0497	0.0222
	6	0.0002	0.0069	0.0374	0.0955	0.1574	0.1916	0.1844	0.1451	0.0949	0.0518
	7	0.0000	0.0014	0.0122	0.0443	0.0974	0.1525	0.1844	0.1797	0.1443	0.0961
	8	0.0000	0.0002	0.0032	0.0166	0.0487	0.0981	0.1489	0.1797	0.1771	0.1442

(*Continued*)

Table A.1 (Continued) Binomial distribution probabilities

n	*k*	*0.05*	*0.10*	*0.15*	*0.20*	*0.25*	*0.30*	*0.35*	*0.40*	*0.45*	*0.50*
	9	0.0000	0.0000	0.0007	0.0051	0.0198	0.0514	0.0980	0.1464	0.1771	0.1762
	10	0.0000	0.0000	0.0001	0.0013	0.0066	0.0220	0.0528	0.0976	0.1449	0.1762
	11	0.0000	0.0000	0.0000	0.0003	0.0018	0.0077	0.0233	0.0532	0.0970	0.1442
	12	0.0000	0.0000	0.0000	0.0000	0.0004	0.0022	0.0083	0.0237	0.0529	0.0961
	13	0.0000	0.0000	0.0000	0.0000	0.0001	0.0005	0.0024	0.0085	0.0233	0.0518
	14	0.0000	0.0000	0.0000	0.0000	0.0000	0.0001	0.0006	0.0024	0.0082	0.0222
	15	0.0000	0.0000	0.0000	0.0000	0.0000	0.0000	0.0001	0.0005	0.0022	0.0074
	16	0.0000	0.0000	0.0000	0.0000	0.0000	0.0000	0.0000	0.0001	0.0005	0.0018
	17	0.0000	0.0000	0.0000	0.0000	0.0000	0.0000	0.0000	0.0000	0.0001	0.0003
	18	0.0000	0.0000	0.0000	0.0000	0.0000	0.0000	0.0000	0.0000	0.0000	0.0000
	19	0.0000	0.0000	0.0000	0.0000	0.0000	0.0000	0.0000	0.0000	0.0000	0.0000

Table A.2 Poisson distribution probabilities

	λ									
k	*0.5*	*1*	*1.5*	*2*	*2.5*	*3*	*3.5*	*4*	*4.5*	*5*
0	0.6065	0.3679	0.2231	0.1353	0.0821	0.0498	0.0302	0.0183	0.0111	0.0067
1	0.3033	0.3679	0.3347	0.2707	0.2052	0.1494	0.1057	0.0733	0.0500	0.0337
2	0.0758	0.1839	0.2510	0.2707	0.2565	0.2240	0.1850	0.1465	0.1125	0.0842
3	0.0126	0.0613	0.1255	0.1804	0.2138	0.2240	0.2158	0.1954	0.1687	0.1404
4	0.0016	0.0153	0.0471	0.0902	0.1336	0.1680	0.1888	0.1954	0.1898	0.1755
5	0.0002	0.0031	0.0141	0.0361	0.0668	0.1008	0.1322	0.1563	0.1708	0.1755
6	0.0000	0.0005	0.0035	0.0120	0.0278	0.0504	0.0771	0.1042	0.1281	0.1462
7	0.0000	0.0001	0.0008	0.0034	0.0099	0.0216	0.0385	0.0595	0.0824	0.1044
8	0.0000	0.0000	0.0001	0.0009	0.0031	0.0081	0.0169	0.0298	0.0463	0.0653
9	0.0000	0.0000	0.0000	0.0002	0.0009	0.0027	0.0066	0.0132	0.0232	0.0363
10	0.0000	0.0000	0.0000	0.0000	0.0002	0.0008	0.0023	0.0053	0.0104	0.0181
11	0.0000	0.0000	0.0000	0.0000	0.0000	0.0002	0.0007	0.0019	0.0043	0.0082
12	0.0000	0.0000	0.0000	0.0000	0.0000	0.0001	0.0002	0.0006	0.0016	0.0034
13	0.0000	0.0000	0.0000	0.0000	0.0000	0.0000	0.0001	0.0002	0.0006	0.0013
14	0.0000	0.0000	0.0000	0.0000	0.0000	0.0000	0.0000	0.0001	0.0002	0.0005
15	0.0000	0.0000	0.0000	0.0000	0.0000	0.0000	0.0000	0.0000	0.0001	0.0002
16	0.0000	0.0000	0.0000	0.0000	0.0000	0.0000	0.0000	0.0000	0.0000	0.0000
17	0.0000	0.0000	0.0000	0.0000	0.0000	0.0000	0.0000	0.0000	0.0000	0.0000
18	0.0000	0.0000	0.0000	0.0000	0.0000	0.0000	0.0000	0.0000	0.0000	0.0000
19	0.0000	0.0000	0.0000	0.0000	0.0000	0.0000	0.0000	0.0000	0.0000	0.0000
20	0.0000	0.0000	0.0000	0.0000	0.0000	0.0000	0.0000	0.0000	0.0000	0.0000
21	0.0000	0.0000	0.0000	0.0000	0.0000	0.0000	0.0000	0.0000	0.0000	0.0000
22	0.0000	0.0000	0.0000	0.0000	0.0000	0.0000	0.0000	0.0000	0.0000	0.0000
23	0.0000	0.0000	0.0000	0.0000	0.0000	0.0000	0.0000	0.0000	0.0000	0.0000
24	0.0000	0.0000	0.0000	0.0000	0.0000	0.0000	0.0000	0.0000	0.0000	0.0000

(*Continued*)

Table A.2 (Continued) Poisson distribution probabilities

	λ									
k	*0.5*	*1*	*1.5*	*2*	*2.5*	*3*	*3.5*	*4*	*4.5*	*5*
25	0.0000	0.0000	0.0000	0.0000	0.0000	0.0000	0.0000	0.0000	0.0000	0.0000
26	0.0000	0.0000	0.0000	0.0000	0.0000	0.0000	0.0000	0.0000	0.0000	0.0000
27	0.0000	0.0000	0.0000	0.0000	0.0000	0.0000	0.0000	0.0000	0.0000	0.0000
28	0.0000	0.0000	0.0000	0.0000	0.0000	0.0000	0.0000	0.0000	0.0000	0.0000
29	0.0000	0.0000	0.0000	0.0000	0.0000	0.0000	0.0000	0.0000	0.0000	0.0000
30	0.0000	0.0000	0.0000	0.0000	0.0000	0.0000	0.0000	0.0000	0.0000	0.0000
31	0.0000	0.0000	0.0000	0.0000	0.0000	0.0000	0.0000	0.0000	0.0000	0.0000
32	0.0000	0.0000	0.0000	0.0000	0.0000	0.0000	0.0000	0.0000	0.0000	0.0000
33	0.0000	0.0000	0.0000	0.0000	0.0000	0.0000	0.0000	0.0000	0.0000	0.0000

	λ									
k	*5.5*	*6*	*6.5*	*7*	*7.5*	*8*	*8.5*	*9*	*9.5*	*10*
0	0.0041	0.0025	0.0015	0.0009	0.0006	0.0003	0.0002	0.0001	0.0001	0.0000
1	0.0225	0.0149	0.0098	0.0064	0.0041	0.0027	0.0017	0.0011	0.0007	0.0005
2	0.0618	0.0446	0.0318	0.0223	0.0156	0.0107	0.0074	0.0050	0.0034	0.0023
3	0.1133	0.0892	0.0688	0.0521	0.0389	0.0286	0.0208	0.0150	0.0107	0.0076
4	0.1558	0.1339	0.1118	0.0912	0.0729	0.0573	0.0443	0.0337	0.0254	0.0189
5	0.1714	0.1606	0.1454	0.1277	0.1094	0.0916	0.0752	0.0607	0.0483	0.0378
6	0.1571	0.1606	0.1575	0.1490	0.1367	0.1221	0.1066	0.0911	0.0764	0.0631
7	0.1234	0.1377	0.1462	0.1490	0.1465	0.1396	0.1294	0.1171	0.1037	0.0901
8	0.0849	0.1033	0.1188	0.1304	0.1373	0.1396	0.1375	0.1318	0.1232	0.1126
9	0.0519	0.0688	0.0858	0.1014	0.1144	0.1241	0.1299	0.1318	0.1300	0.1251
10	0.0285	0.0413	0.0558	0.0710	0.0858	0.0993	0.1104	0.1186	0.1235	0.1251
11	0.0143	0.0225	0.0330	0.0452	0.0585	0.0722	0.0853	0.0970	0.1067	0.1137

(*Continued*)

Table A.2 (Continued) Poisson distribution probabilities

	λ									
k	*5.5*	*6*	*6.5*	*7*	*7.5*	*8*	*8.5*	*9*	*9.5*	*10*
12	0.0065	0.0113	0.0179	0.0263	0.0366	0.0481	0.0604	0.0728	0.0844	0.0948
13	0.0028	0.0052	0.0089	0.0142	0.0211	0.0296	0.0395	0.0504	0.0617	0.0729
14	0.0011	0.0022	0.0041	0.0071	0.0113	0.0169	0.0240	0.0324	0.0419	0.0521
15	0.0004	0.0009	0.0018	0.0033	0.0057	0.0090	0.0136	0.0194	0.0265	0.0347
16	0.0001	0.0003	0.0007	0.0014	0.0026	0.0045	0.0072	0.0109	0.0157	0.0217
17	0.0000	0.0001	0.0003	0.0006	0.0012	0.0021	0.0036	0.0058	0.0088	0.0128
18	0.0000	0.0000	0.0001	0.0002	0.0005	0.0009	0.0017	0.0029	0.0046	0.0071
19	0.0000	0.0000	0.0000	0.0001	0.0002	0.0004	0.0008	0.0014	0.0023	0.0037
20	0.0000	0.0000	0.0000	0.0000	0.0001	0.0002	0.0003	0.0006	0.0011	0.0019
21	0.0000	0.0000	0.0000	0.0000	0.0000	0.0001	0.0001	0.0003	0.0005	0.0009
22	0.0000	0.0000	0.0000	0.0000	0.0000	0.0000	0.0001	0.0001	0.0002	0.0004
23	0.0000	0.0000	0.0000	0.0000	0.0000	0.0000	0.0000	0.0000	0.0001	0.0002
24	0.0000	0.0000	0.0000	0.0000	0.0000	0.0000	0.0000	0.0000	0.0000	0.0001
25	0.0000	0.0000	0.0000	0.0000	0.0000	0.0000	0.0000	0.0000	0.0000	0.0000
26	0.0000	0.0000	0.0000	0.0000	0.0000	0.0000	0.0000	0.0000	0.0000	0.0000
27	0.0000	0.0000	0.0000	0.0000	0.0000	0.0000	0.0000	0.0000	0.0000	0.0000
28	0.0000	0.0000	0.0000	0.0000	0.0000	0.0000	0.0000	0.0000	0.0000	0.0000
29	0.0000	0.0000	0.0000	0.0000	0.0000	0.0000	0.0000	0.0000	0.0000	0.0000
30	0.0000	0.0000	0.0000	0.0000	0.0000	0.0000	0.0000	0.0000	0.0000	0.0000
31	0.0000	0.0000	0.0000	0.0000	0.0000	0.0000	0.0000	0.0000	0.0000	0.0000
32	0.0000	0.0000	0.0000	0.0000	0.0000	0.0000	0.0000	0.0000	0.0000	0.0000
33	0.0000	0.0000	0.0000	0.0000	0.0000	0.0000	0.0000	0.0000	0.0000	0.0000

(Continued)

Table A.2 (Continued) Poisson distribution probabilities

	λ									
k	*10.5*	*11*	*11.5*	*12*	*12.5*	*13*	*13.5*	*14*	*14.5*	*15*
0	0.0000	0.0000	0.0000	0.0000	0.0000	0.0000	0.0000	0.0000	0.0000	0.0000
1	0.0003	0.0002	0.0001	0.0001	0.0000	0.0000	0.0000	0.0000	0.0000	0.0000
2	0.0015	0.0010	0.0007	0.0004	0.0003	0.0002	0.0001	0.0001	0.0001	0.0000
3	0.0053	0.0037	0.0026	0.0018	0.0012	0.0008	0.0006	0.0004	0.0003	0.0002
4	0.0139	0.0102	0.0074	0.0053	0.0038	0.0027	0.0019	0.0013	0.0009	0.0006
5	0.0293	0.0224	0.0170	0.0127	0.0095	0.0070	0.0051	0.0037	0.0027	0.0019
6	0.0513	0.0411	0.0325	0.0255	0.0197	0.0152	0.0115	0.0087	0.0065	0.0048
7	0.0769	0.0646	0.0535	0.0437	0.0353	0.0281	0.0222	0.0174	0.0135	0.0104
8	0.1009	0.0888	0.0769	0.0655	0.0551	0.0457	0.0375	0.0304	0.0244	0.0194
9	0.1177	0.1085	0.0982	0.0874	0.0765	0.0661	0.0563	0.0473	0.0394	0.0324
10	0.1236	0.1194	0.1129	0.1048	0.0956	0.0859	0.0760	0.0663	0.0571	0.0486
11	0.1180	0.1194	0.1181	0.1144	0.1087	0.1015	0.0932	0.0844	0.0753	0.0663
12	0.1032	0.1094	0.1131	0.1144	0.1132	0.1099	0.1049	0.0984	0.0910	0.0829
13	0.0834	0.0926	0.1001	0.1056	0.1089	0.1099	0.1089	0.1060	0.1014	0.0956
14	0.0625	0.0728	0.0822	0.0905	0.0972	0.1021	0.1050	0.1060	0.1051	0.1024
15	0.0438	0.0534	0.0630	0.0724	0.0810	0.0885	0.0945	0.0989	0.1016	0.1024
16	0.0287	0.0367	0.0453	0.0543	0.0633	0.0719	0.0798	0.0866	0.0920	0.0960
17	0.0177	0.0237	0.0306	0.0383	0.0465	0.0550	0.0633	0.0713	0.0785	0.0847
18	0.0104	0.0145	0.0196	0.0255	0.0323	0.0397	0.0475	0.0554	0.0632	0.0706
19	0.0057	0.0084	0.0119	0.0161	0.0213	0.0272	0.0337	0.0409	0.0483	0.0557
20	0.0030	0.0046	0.0068	0.0097	0.0133	0.0177	0.0228	0.0286	0.0350	0.0418
21	0.0015	0.0024	0.0037	0.0055	0.0079	0.0109	0.0146	0.0191	0.0242	0.0299
22	0.0007	0.0012	0.0020	0.0030	0.0045	0.0065	0.0090	0.0121	0.0159	0.0204
23	0.0003	0.0006	0.0010	0.0016	0.0024	0.0037	0.0053	0.0074	0.0100	0.0133
24	0.0001	0.0003	0.0005	0.0008	0.0013	0.0020	0.0030	0.0043	0.0061	0.0083

(Continued)

Table A.2 (Continued) Poisson distribution probabilities

	λ									
k	10.5	11	11.5	12	12.5	13	13.5	14	14.5	15
25	0.0001	0.0001	0.0002	0.0004	0.0006	0.0010	0.0016	0.0024	0.0035	0.0050
26	0.0000	0.0000	0.0001	0.0002	0.0003	0.0005	0.0008	0.0013	0.0020	0.0029
27	0.0000	0.0000	0.0000	0.0001	0.0001	0.0002	0.0004	0.0007	0.0011	0.0016
28	0.0000	0.0000	0.0000	0.0000	0.0001	0.0001	0.0002	0.0003	0.0005	0.0009
29	0.0000	0.0000	0.0000	0.0000	0.0000	0.0001	0.0001	0.0002	0.0003	0.0004
30	0.0000	0.0000	0.0000	0.0000	0.0000	0.0000	0.0000	0.0001	0.0001	0.0002
31	0.0000	0.0000	0.0000	0.0000	0.0000	0.0000	0.0000	0.0000	0.0001	0.0001
32	0.0000	0.0000	0.0000	0.0000	0.0000	0.0000	0.0000	0.0000	0.0000	0.0001
33	0.0000	0.0000	0.0000	0.0000	0.0000	0.0000	0.0000	0.0000	0.0000	0.0000
34	0.0000	0.0000	0.0000	0.0000	0.0000	0.0000	0.0000	0.0000	0.0000	0.0000
35	0.0000	0.0000	0.0000	0.0000	0.0000	0.0000	0.0000	0.0000	0.0000	0.0000

	λ									
k	15.5	16	16.5	17	17.5	18	18.5	19	19.5	20
0	0.0000	0.0000	0.0000	0.0000	0.0000	0.0000	0.0000	0.0000	0.0000	0.0000
1	0.0000	0.0000	0.0000	0.0000	0.0000	0.0000	0.0000	0.0000	0.0000	0.0000
2	0.0000	0.0000	0.0000	0.0000	0.0000	0.0000	0.0000	0.0000	0.0000	0.0000
3	0.0001	0.0001	0.0001	0.0000	0.0000	0.0000	0.0000	0.0000	0.0000	0.0000
4	0.0004	0.0003	0.0002	0.0001	0.0001	0.0001	0.0000	0.0000	0.0000	0.0000
5	0.0014	0.0010	0.0007	0.0005	0.0003	0.0002	0.0002	0.0001	0.0001	0.0001
6	0.0036	0.0026	0.0019	0.0014	0.0010	0.0007	0.0005	0.0004	0.0003	0.0002
7	0.0079	0.0060	0.0045	0.0034	0.0025	0.0019	0.0014	0.0010	0.0007	0.0005
8	0.0153	0.0120	0.0093	0.0072	0.0055	0.0042	0.0031	0.0024	0.0018	0.0013
9	0.0264	0.0213	0.0171	0.0135	0.0107	0.0083	0.0065	0.0050	0.0038	0.0029
10	0.0409	0.0341	0.0281	0.0230	0.0186	0.0150	0.0120	0.0095	0.0074	0.0058

(Continued)

Table A.2 (Continued) Poisson distribution probabilities

	λ									
k	*15.5*	*16*	*16.5*	*17*	*17.5*	*18*	*18.5*	*19*	*19.5*	*20*
11	0.0577	0.0496	0.0422	0.0355	0.0297	0.0245	0.0201	0.0164	0.0132	0.0106
12	0.0745	0.0661	0.0580	0.0504	0.0432	0.0368	0.0310	0.0259	0.0214	0.0176
13	0.0888	0.0814	0.0736	0.0658	0.0582	0.0509	0.0441	0.0378	0.0322	0.0271
14	0.0983	0.0930	0.0868	0.0800	0.0728	0.0655	0.0583	0.0514	0.0448	0.0387
15	0.1016	0.0992	0.0955	0.0906	0.0849	0.0786	0.0719	0.0650	0.0582	0.0516
16	0.0984	0.0992	0.0985	0.0963	0.0929	0.0884	0.0831	0.0772	0.0710	0.0646
17	0.0897	0.0934	0.0956	0.0963	0.0956	0.0936	0.0904	0.0863	0.0814	0.0760
18	0.0773	0.0830	0.0876	0.0909	0.0929	0.0936	0.0930	0.0911	0.0882	0.0844
19	0.0630	0.0699	0.0761	0.0814	0.0856	0.0887	0.0905	0.0911	0.0905	0.0888
20	0.0489	0.0559	0.0628	0.0692	0.0749	0.0798	0.0837	0.0866	0.0883	0.0888
21	0.0361	0.0426	0.0493	0.0560	0.0624	0.0684	0.0738	0.0783	0.0820	0.0846
22	0.0254	0.0310	0.0370	0.0433	0.0496	0.0560	0.0620	0.0676	0.0727	0.0769
23	0.0171	0.0216	0.0265	0.0320	0.0378	0.0438	0.0499	0.0559	0.0616	0.0669
24	0.0111	0.0144	0.0182	0.0226	0.0275	0.0328	0.0385	0.0442	0.0500	0.0557
25	0.0069	0.0092	0.0120	0.0154	0.0193	0.0237	0.0285	0.0336	0.0390	0.0446
26	0.0041	0.0057	0.0076	0.0101	0.0130	0.0164	0.0202	0.0246	0.0293	0.0343
27	0.0023	0.0034	0.0047	0.0063	0.0084	0.0109	0.0139	0.0173	0.0211	0.0254
28	0.0013	0.0019	0.0028	0.0038	0.0053	0.0070	0.0092	0.0117	0.0147	0.0181
29	0.0007	0.0011	0.0016	0.0023	0.0032	0.0044	0.0058	0.0077	0.0099	0.0125
30	0.0004	0.0006	0.0009	0.0013	0.0019	0.0026	0.0036	0.0049	0.0064	0.0083
31	0.0002	0.0003	0.0005	0.0007	0.0010	0.0015	0.0022	0.0030	0.0040	0.0054
32	0.0001	0.0001	0.0002	0.0004	0.0006	0.0009	0.0012	0.0018	0.0025	0.0034
33	0.0000	0.0001	0.0001	0.0002	0.0003	0.0005	0.0007	0.0010	0.0015	0.0020
34	0.0000	0.0000	0.0001	0.0001	0.0002	0.0002	0.0004	0.0006	0.0008	0.0012
35	0.0000	0.0000	0.0000	0.0000	0.0001	0.0001	0.0002	0.0003	0.0005	0.0007
36	0.0000	0.0000	0.0000	0.0000	0.0000	0.0001	0.0001	0.0002	0.0003	0.0004
37	0.0000	0.0000	0.0000	0.0000	0.0000	0.0000	0.0001	0.0001	0.0001	0.0002
38	0.0000	0.0000	0.0000	0.0000	0.0000	0.0000	0.0000	0.0000	0.0001	0.0001

Table A.3 Standard normal probability distribution, area in the upper tail

z	*0.0*	*0.01*	*0.02*	*0.03*	*0.04*	*0.05*	*0.06*	*0.07*	*0.08*	*0.09*
0.0	0.500	0.496	0.492	0.488	0.484	0.480	0.476	0.472	0.468	0.464
0.1	0.460	0.456	0.452	0.448	0.444	0.440	0.436	0.433	0.429	0.425
0.2	0.421	0.417	0.413	0.409	0.405	0.401	0.397	0.394	0.390	0.386
0.3	0.382	0.378	0.374	0.371	0.367	0.363	0.359	0.356	0.352	0.348
0.4	0.345	0.341	0.337	0.334	0.330	0.326	0.323	0.319	0.316	0.312
0.5	0.309	0.305	0.302	0.298	0.295	0.291	0.288	0.284	0.281	0.278
0.6	0.274	0.271	0.268	0.264	0.261	0.258	0.255	0.251	0.248	0.245
0.7	0.242	0.239	0.236	0.233	0.230	0.227	0.224	0.221	0.218	0.215
0.8	0.212	0.209	0.206	0.203	0.200	0.198	0.195	0.192	0.189	0.187
0.9	0.184	0.181	0.179	0.176	0.174	0.171	0.169	0.166	0.164	0.161
1.0	0.159	0.156	0.154	0.152	0.149	0.147	0.145	0.142	0.140	0.138
1.1	0.136	0.133	0.131	0.129	0.127	0.125	0.123	0.121	0.119	0.117
1.2	0.115	0.113	0.111	0.109	0.107	0.106	0.104	0.102	0.100	0.099
1.3	0.097	0.095	0.093	0.092	0.090	0.089	0.087	0.085	0.084	0.082
1.4	0.081	0.079	0.078	0.076	0.075	0.074	0.072	0.071	0.069	0.068
1.5	0.067	0.066	0.064	0.063	0.062	0.061	0.059	0.058	0.057	0.056
1.6	0.055	0.054	0.053	0.052	0.051	0.049	0.048	0.047	0.046	0.046
1.7	0.045	0.044	0.043	0.042	0.041	0.040	0.039	0.038	0.038	0.037
1.8	0.036	0.035	0.034	0.034	0.033	0.032	0.031	0.031	0.030	0.029

(*Continued*)

Table A.3 (Continued) Standard normal probability distribution, area in the upper tail

z	*0.0*	*0.01*	*0.02*	*0.03*	*0.04*	*0.05*	*0.06*	*0.07*	*0.08*	*0.09*
1.9	0.029	0.028	0.027	0.027	0.026	0.026	0.025	0.024	0.024	0.023
2.0	0.023	0.022	0.022	0.021	0.021	0.020	0.020	0.019	0.019	0.018
2.1	0.018	0.017	0.017	0.017	0.016	0.016	0.015	0.015	0.015	0.014
2.2	0.014	0.014	0.013	0.013	0.013	0.012	0.012	0.012	0.011	0.011
2.3	0.011	0.010	0.010	0.010	0.010	0.009	0.009	0.009	0.009	0.008
2.4	0.008	0.008	0.008	0.008	0.007	0.007	0.007	0.007	0.007	0.006
2.5	0.006	0.006	0.006	0.006	0.006	0.005	0.005	0.005	0.005	0.005
2.6	0.005	0.005	0.004	0.004	0.004	0.004	0.004	0.004	0.004	0.004
2.7	0.003	0.003	0.003	0.003	0.003	0.003	0.003	0.003	0.003	0.003
2.8	0.003	0.002	0.002	0.002	0.002	0.002	0.002	0.002	0.002	0.002
2.9	0.002	0.002	0.002	0.002	0.002	0.002	0.002	0.001	0.001	0.001
3.0	0.001	0.001	0.001	0.001	0.001	0.001	0.001	0.001	0.001	0.001
3.1	0.001	0.001	0.001	0.001	0.001	0.001	0.001	0.001	0.001	0.001
3.2	0.001	0.001	0.001	0.001	0.001	0.001	0.001	0.001	0.001	0.001
3.3	0.000	0.000	0.000	0.000	0.000	0.000	0.000	0.000	0.000	0.000
3.4	0.000	0.000	0.000	0.000	0.000	0.000	0.000	0.000	0.000	0.000

Table A.4 t Distribution, area in the upper tail

df	*0.10*	*0.05*	*0.025*	*0.01*	*0.005*	*0.0005*
1	3.078	6.314	12.706	31.821	63.657	636.619
2	1.886	2.920	4.303	6.965	9.925	31.599
3	1.638	2.353	3.182	4.541	5.841	12.924
4	1.533	2.132	2.776	3.747	4.604	8.610
5	1.476	2.015	2.571	3.365	4.032	6.869
6	1.440	1.943	2.447	3.143	3.707	5.959
7	1.415	1.895	2.365	2.998	3.499	5.408
8	1.397	1.860	2.306	2.896	3.355	5.041
9	1.383	1.833	2.262	2.821	3.250	4.781
10	1.372	1.812	2.228	2.764	3.169	4.587
11	1.363	1.796	2.201	2.718	3.106	4.437
12	1.356	1.782	2.179	2.681	3.055	4.318
13	1.350	1.771	2.160	2.650	3.012	4.221
14	1.345	1.761	2.145	2.624	2.977	4.140
15	1.341	1.753	2.131	2.602	2.947	4.073
16	1.337	1.746	2.120	2.583	2.921	4.015
17	1.333	1.740	2.110	2.567	2.898	3.965
18	1.330	1.734	2.101	2.552	2.878	3.922
19	1.328	1.729	2.093	2.539	2.861	3.883
20	1.325	1.725	2.086	2.528	2.845	3.850
21	1.323	1.721	2.080	2.518	2.831	3.819
22	1.321	1.717	2.074	2.508	2.819	3.792
23	1.319	1.714	2.069	2.500	2.807	3.768
24	1.318	1.711	2.064	2.492	2.797	3.745
25	1.316	1.708	2.060	2.485	2.787	3.725
26	1.315	1.706	2.056	2.479	2.779	3.707
27	1.314	1.703	2.052	2.473	2.771	3.690
28	1.313	1.701	2.048	2.467	2.763	3.674
29	1.311	1.699	2.045	2.462	2.756	3.659
30	1.310	1.697	2.042	2.457	2.750	3.646
40	1.303	1.684	2.021	2.423	2.704	3.551
50	1.299	1.676	2.009	2.403	2.678	3.496
60	1.296	1.671	2.000	2.390	2.660	3.460
70	1.294	1.667	1.994	2.381	2.648	3.435
80	1.292	1.664	1.990	2.374	2.639	3.416
90	1.291	1.662	1.987	2.368	2.632	3.402
100	1.290	1.660	1.984	2.364	2.626	3.390
110	1.289	1.659	1.982	2.361	2.621	3.381
120	1.289	1.658	1.980	2.358	2.617	3.373
∞	1.282	1.645	1.960	2.327	2.576	3.291

Table A.5 Chi-squared distribution, area in the upper tail

df	*0.1*	*0.05*	*0.025*	*0.01*	*0.001*
1	2.71	3.84	5.02	6.63	10.83
2	4.61	5.99	7.38	9.21	13.82
3	6.25	7.81	9.35	11.34	16.27
4	7.78	9.49	11.14	13.28	18.47
5	9.24	11.07	12.83	15.09	20.52
6	10.64	12.59	14.45	16.81	22.46
7	12.02	14.07	16.01	18.48	24.32
8	13.36	15.51	17.53	20.09	26.12
9	14.68	16.92	19.02	21.67	27.88
10	15.99	18.31	20.48	23.21	29.59
11	17.28	19.68	21.92	24.72	31.26
12	18.55	21.03	23.34	26.22	32.91
13	19.81	22.36	24.74	27.69	34.53
14	21.06	23.68	26.12	29.14	36.12
15	22.31	25.00	27.49	30.58	37.70
16	23.54	26.30	28.85	32.00	39.25
17	24.77	27.59	30.19	33.41	40.79
18	25.99	28.87	31.53	34.81	42.31
19	27.20	30.14	32.85	36.19	43.82
20	28.41	31.41	34.17	37.57	45.31
21	29.62	32.67	35.48	38.93	46.80
22	30.81	33.92	36.78	40.29	48.27
23	32.01	35.17	38.08	41.64	49.73
24	33.20	36.42	39.36	42.98	51.18
25	34.38	37.65	40.65	44.31	52.62

Table A.6 F Distribution, area in upper tail

Den. df (df_2)	Area in upper tail	Num. df (df_1)										
		1	2	3	4	5	6	7	8	12	24	∞
2	0.100	8.53	9.00	9.16	9.24	9.29	9.33	9.35	9.37	9.41	9.45	9.49
	0.050	18.51	19.00	19.16	19.25	19.30	19.33	19.35	19.37	19.41	19.45	19.50
	0.025	38.51	39.00	39.17	39.25	39.30	39.33	39.36	39.37	39.41	39.46	39.50
	0.010	98.50	99.00	99.17	99.25	99.30	99.33	99.36	99.37	99.42	99.46	99.50
	0.005	198.50	199.00	199.17	199.25	199.30	199.33	199.36	199.37	199.42	199.46	199.50
	0.001	998.50	999.00	999.17	999.25	999.30	999.33	999.36	999.37	999.42	999.46	999.50
3	0.100	5.54	5.46	5.39	5.34	5.31	5.28	5.27	5.25	5.22	5.18	5.13
	0.050	10.13	9.55	9.28	9.12	9.01	8.94	8.89	8.85	8.74	8.64	8.53
	0.025	17.44	16.04	15.44	15.10	14.88	14.73	14.62	14.54	14.34	14.12	13.90
	0.010	34.12	30.82	29.46	28.71	28.24	27.91	27.67	27.49	27.05	26.60	26.13
	0.005	55.55	49.80	47.47	46.19	45.39	44.84	44.43	44.13	43.39	42.62	41.83
	0.001	167.03	148.50	141.11	137.10	134.58	132.85	131.58	130.62	128.32	125.94	123.50
4	0.100	4.54	4.32	4.19	4.11	4.05	4.01	3.98	3.95	3.90	3.83	3.76
	0.050	7.71	6.94	6.59	6.39	6.26	6.16	6.09	6.04	5.91	5.77	5.63
	0.025	12.22	10.65	9.98	9.60	9.36	9.20	9.07	8.98	8.75	8.51	8.26
	0.010	21.20	18.00	16.69	15.98	15.52	15.21	14.98	14.80	14.37	13.93	13.46
	0.005	31.33	26.28	24.26	23.15	22.46	21.97	21.62	21.35	20.70	20.03	19.32
	0.001	74.14	61.25	56.18	53.44	51.71	50.53	49.66	49.00	47.41	45.77	44.05
5	0.100	4.06	3.78	3.62	3.52	3.45	3.40	3.37	3.34	3.27	3.19	3.10
	0.050	6.61	5.79	5.41	5.19	5.05	4.95	4.88	4.82	4.68	4.53	4.36
	0.025	10.01	8.43	7.76	7.39	7.15	6.98	6.85	6.76	6.52	6.28	6.02
	0.010	16.26	13.27	12.06	11.39	10.97	10.67	10.46	10.29	9.89	9.47	9.02
	0.005	22.78	18.31	16.53	15.56	14.94	14.51	14.20	13.96	13.38	12.78	12.14
	0.001	47.18	37.12	33.20	31.09	29.75	28.83	28.16	27.65	26.42	25.13	23.79
6	0.100	3.78	3.46	3.29	3.18	3.11	3.05	3.01	2.98	2.90	2.82	2.72

(*Continued*)

Table A.6 (Continued) F Distribution, area in upper tail

Den. df (df_2)	Area in upper tail	Num. df (df_1)										
		1	2	3	4	5	6	7	8	12	24	∞
	0.050	5.99	5.14	4.76	4.53	4.39	4.28	4.21	4.15	4.00	3.84	3.67
	0.025	8.81	7.26	6.60	6.23	5.99	5.82	5.70	5.60	5.37	5.12	4.85
	0.010	13.75	10.92	9.78	9.15	8.75	8.47	8.26	8.10	7.72	7.31	6.88
	0.005	18.63	14.54	12.92	12.03	11.46	11.07	10.79	10.57	10.03	9.47	8.88
	0.001	35.51	27.00	23.70	21.92	20.80	20.03	19.46	19.03	17.99	16.90	15.75
7	0.100	3.59	3.26	3.07	2.96	2.88	2.83	2.78	2.75	2.67	2.58	2.47
	0.050	5.59	4.74	4.35	4.12	3.97	3.87	3.79	3.73	3.57	3.41	3.23
	0.025	8.07	6.54	5.89	5.52	5.29	5.12	4.99	4.90	4.67	4.41	4.14
	0.010	12.25	9.55	8.45	7.85	7.46	7.19	6.99	6.84	6.47	6.07	5.65
	0.005	16.24	12.40	10.88	10.05	9.52	9.16	8.89	8.68	8.18	7.64	7.08
	0.001	29.25	21.69	18.77	17.20	16.21	15.52	15.02	14.63	13.71	12.73	11.70
8	0.100	3.46	3.11	2.92	2.81	2.73	2.67	2.62	2.59	2.50	2.40	2.29
	0.050	5.32	4.46	4.07	3.84	3.69	3.58	3.50	3.44	3.28	3.12	2.93
	0.025	7.57	6.06	5.42	5.05	4.82	4.65	4.53	4.43	4.20	3.95	3.67
	0.010	11.26	8.65	7.59	7.01	6.63	6.37	6.18	6.03	5.67	5.28	4.86
	0.005	14.69	11.04	9.60	8.81	8.30	7.95	7.69	7.50	7.01	6.50	5.95
	0.001	25.41	18.49	15.83	14.39	13.48	12.86	12.40	12.05	11.19	10.30	9.33
9	0.100	3.36	3.01	2.81	2.69	2.61	2.55	2.51	2.47	2.38	2.28	2.16
	0.050	5.12	4.26	3.86	3.63	3.48	3.37	3.29	3.23	3.07	2.90	2.71
	0.025	7.21	5.71	5.08	4.72	4.48	4.32	4.20	4.10	3.87	3.61	3.33
	0.010	10.56	8.02	6.99	6.42	6.06	5.80	5.61	5.47	5.11	4.73	4.31
	0.005	13.61	10.11	8.72	7.96	7.47	7.13	6.88	6.69	6.23	5.73	5.19
	0.001	22.86	16.39	13.90	12.56	11.71	11.13	10.70	10.37	9.57	8.72	7.81
10	0.100	3.29	2.92	2.73	2.61	2.52	2.46	2.41	2.38	2.28	2.18	2.06
	0.050	4.96	4.10	3.71	3.48	3.33	3.22	3.14	3.07	2.91	2.74	2.54

(Continued)

Table A.6 (Continued) *F* Distribution, area in upper tail

Den. df (df_2)	Area in upper tail	Num. df (df_1)										
		1	2	3	4	5	6	7	8	12	24	∞
	0.025	6.94	5.46	4.83	4.47	4.24	4.07	3.95	3.85	3.62	3.37	3.08
	0.010	10.04	7.56	6.55	5.99	5.64	5.39	5.20	5.06	4.71	4.33	3.91
	0.005	12.83	9.43	8.08	7.34	6.87	6.54	6.30	6.12	5.66	5.17	4.64
	0.001	21.04	14.91	12.55	11.28	10.48	9.93	9.52	9.20	8.45	7.64	6.76
12	0.100	3.18	2.81	2.61	2.48	2.39	2.33	2.28	2.24	2.15	2.04	1.90
	0.050	4.75	3.89	3.49	3.26	3.11	3.00	2.91	2.85	2.69	2.51	2.30
	0.025	6.55	5.10	4.47	4.12	3.89	3.73	3.61	3.51	3.28	3.02	2.72
	0.010	9.33	6.93	5.95	5.41	5.06	4.82	4.64	4.50	4.16	3.78	3.36
	0.005	11.75	8.51	7.23	6.52	6.07	5.76	5.52	5.35	4.91	4.43	3.90
	0.001	18.64	12.97	10.80	9.63	8.89	8.38	8.00	7.71	7.00	6.25	5.42
14	0.100	3.10	2.73	2.52	2.39	2.31	2.24	2.19	2.15	2.05	1.94	1.80
	0.050	4.60	3.74	3.34	3.11	2.96	2.85	2.76	2.70	2.53	2.35	2.13
	0.025	6.30	4.86	4.24	3.89	3.66	3.50	3.38	3.29	3.05	2.79	2.49
	0.010	8.86	6.51	5.56	5.04	4.69	4.46	4.28	4.14	3.80	3.43	3.00
	0.005	11.06	7.92	6.68	6.00	5.56	5.26	5.03	4.86	4.43	3.96	3.44
	0.001	17.14	11.78	9.73	8.62	7.92	7.44	7.08	6.80	6.13	5.41	4.60
16	0.100	3.05	2.67	2.46	2.33	2.24	2.18	2.13	2.09	1.99	1.87	1.72
	0.050	4.49	3.63	3.24	3.01	2.85	2.74	2.66	2.59	2.42	2.24	2.01
	0.025	6.12	4.69	4.08	3.73	3.50	3.34	3.11	3.12	2.89	2.63	2.32
	0.010	8.53	6.23	5.29	4.77	4.44	4.20	4.03	3.89	3.55	3.18	2.75
	0.005	10.58	7.51	6.30	5.64	5.21	4.91	4.69	4.52	4.10	3.64	3.11
	0.001	16.12	10.97	9.01	7.94	7.27	6.80	6.46	6.19	5.55	4.85	4.06
18	0.100	3.01	2.62	2.42	2.29	2.20	2.13	2.08	2.04	1.93	1.81	1.66
	0.050	4.41	3.55	3.16	2.93	2.77	2.66	2.58	2.51	2.34	2.15	1.92
	0.025	5.98	4.56	3.95	3.61	3.38	3.22	3.10	3.01	2.77	2.50	2.19

(*Continued*)

Table A.6 (Continued) F Distribution, area in upper tail

Den. df (df_2)	Area in upper tail	Num. df (df_1)										
		1	2	3	4	5	6	7	8	12	24	∞
	0.010	8.29	6.01	5.09	4.58	4.25	4.01	3.84	3.71	3.37	3.00	2.57
	0.005	10.22	7.21	6.03	5.37	4.96	4.66	4.44	4.28	3.86	3.40	2.87
	0.001	15.38	10.39	8.49	7.46	6.81	6.35	6.02	5.76	5.13	4.45	3.67
20	0.100	2.97	2.59	2.38	2.25	2.16	2.09	2.04	2.00	1.89	1.77	1.61
	0.050	4.35	3.49	3.10	2.87	2.71	2.60	2.51	2.45	2.28	2.08	1.84
	0.025	5.87	4.46	3.86	3.51	3.29	3.13	3.01	2.91	2.68	2.41	2.09
	0.010	8.10	5.85	4.94	4.43	4.10	3.87	3.70	3.56	3.23	2.86	2.42
	0.005	9.94	6.99	5.82	5.17	4.76	4.47	4.26	4.09	3.68	3.22	2.69
	0.001	14.82	9.95	8.10	7.10	6.46	6.02	5.69	5.44	4.82	4.15	3.38
30	0.100	2.88	2.49	2.28	2.14	2.05	1.98	1.93	1.88	1.77	1.64	1.46
	0.050	4.17	3.32	2.92	2.69	2.53	2.42	2.33	2.27	2.09	1.89	1.62
	0.025	5.57	4.18	3.59	3.25	3.03	2.87	2.75	2.65	2.41	2.14	1.79
	0.010	7.56	5.39	4.51	4.02	3.70	3.47	3.30	3.17	2.84	2.47	2.01
	0.005	9.18	6.35	5.24	4.62	4.23	3.95	3.74	3.58	3.18	2.73	2.18
	0.001	13.29	8.77	7.05	6.12	5.53	5.12	4.82	4.58	4.00	3.36	2.59
40	0.100	2.84	2.44	2.23	2.09	2.00	1.93	1.87	1.83	1.71	1.57	1.38
	0.050	4.08	3.23	2.84	2.61	2.45	2.34	2.25	2.18	2.00	1.79	1.51
	0.025	5.42	4.05	3.46	3.13	2.90	2.74	2.62	2.53	2.29	2.01	1.64
	0.010	7.31	5.18	4.31	3.83	3.51	3.29	3.12	2.99	2.66	2.29	1.80
	0.005	8.83	6.07	4.98	4.37	3.99	3.71	3.51	3.35	2.95	2.50	1.93
	0.001	12.61	8.25	6.59	5.70	5.13	4.73	4.44	4.21	3.64	3.01	2.23
60	0.100	2.79	2.39	2.18	2.04	1.95	1.87	1.82	1.77	1.66	1.51	1.29
	0.050	4.00	3.15	2.76	2.53	2.37	2.25	2.17	2.10	1.92	1.70	1.39
	0.025	5.29	3.93	3.34	3.01	2.79	2.63	2.51	2.41	2.17	1.88	1.48
	0.010	7.08	4.98	4.13	3.65	3.34	3.12	2.95	2.82	2.50	2.12	1.60

(Continued)

Table A.6 (Continued) F Distribution, area in upper tail

Den. df (df_2)	*Area in upper tail*	*Num. df* (df_1)										
		1	*2*	*3*	*4*	*5*	*6*	*7*	*8*	*12*	*24*	∞
	0.005	8.49	5.79	4.73	4.14	3.76	3.49	3.29	3.13	2.74	2.29	1.69
	0.001	11.97	7.77	6.17	5.31	4.76	4.37	4.09	3.86	3.32	2.69	1.89
80	0.100	2.77	2.37	2.15	2.02	1.92	1.85	1.79	1.75	1.63	1.48	1.24
	0.050	3.96	3.11	2.72	2.49	2.33	2.21	2.13	2.06	1.88	1.65	1.32
	0.025	5.22	3.86	3.28	2.95	2.73	2.57	2.45	2.35	2.11	1.82	1.40
	0.010	6.96	4.88	4.04	3.56	3.26	3.04	2.87	2.74	2.42	2.03	1.49
	0.005	8.33	5.67	4.61	4.03	3.65	3.39	3.19	3.03	2.64	2.19	1.56
	0.001	11.67	7.54	5.97	5.12	4.58	4.20	3.92	3.70	3.16	2.54	1.72
100	0.100	2.76	2.36	2.14	2.00	1.91	1.83	1.78	1.73	1.61	1.46	1.21
	0.050	3.94	3.09	2.70	2.46	2.31	2.19	2.10	2.03	1.85	1.63	1.28
	0.025	5.18	3.83	3.25	2.92	2.70	2.54	2.42	2.32	2.08	1.78	1.35
	0.010	6.90	4.82	3.98	3.51	3.21	2.99	2.82	2.69	2.37	1.98	1.43
	0.005	8.24	5.59	4.54	3.96	3.59	3.33	3.13	2.97	2.58	2.13	1.49
	0.001	11.50	7.41	5.86	5.02	4.48	4.11	3.83	3.61	3.07	2.46	1.62
120	0.100	2.75	2.35	2.13	1.99	1.90	1.82	1.77	1.72	1.60	1.45	1.19
	0.050	3.92	3.07	2.68	2.45	2.29	2.18	2.09	2.02	1.83	1.61	1.25
	0.025	5.15	3.80	3.23	2.89	2.67	2.52	2.39	2.30	2.05	1.76	1.31
	0.010	6.85	4.79	3.95	3.48	3.17	2.96	2.79	2.66	2.34	1.95	1.38
	0.005	8.18	5.54	4.50	3.92	3.55	3.28	3.09	2.93	2.54	2.09	1.43
	0.001	11.38	7.32	5.78	4.95	4.42	4.04	3.77	3.55	3.02	2.40	1.54
∞	0.100	2.71	2.30	2.08	1.94	1.85	1.77	1.72	1.67	1.55	1.38	1.00
	0.050	3.84	3.00	2.60	2.37	2.21	2.10	2.01	1.94	1.75	1.52	1.00
	0.025	5.02	3.69	3.12	2.79	2.57	2.41	2.29	2.19	1.94	1.64	1.00
	0.010	6.63	4.61	3.78	3.32	3.02	2.80	2.64	2.51	2.18	1.79	1.00
	0.005	7.88	5.30	4.28	3.72	3.35	3.09	2.90	2.74	2.36	1.90	1.00
	0.001	10.83	6.91	5.42	4.62	4.10	3.74	3.47	3.27	2.74	2.13	1.00

Table A.7 T, the Wilcoxon signed-rank, distribution

	Sample size										
T_0	*2*	*3*	*4*	*5*	*6*	*7*	*8*	*9*	*10*	*11*	*12*
1	0.5000	0.2500	0.1250	0.0625	0.0313	0.0157	0.0079	0.0040	0.0020	0.0010	0.0005
2		0.3750	0.1875	0.0938	0.0469	0.0235	0.0118	0.0059	0.0030	0.0015	0.0008
3		0.6250	0.3125	0.1563	0.0782	0.0391	0.0196	0.0098	0.0049	0.0025	0.0013
4			0.4375	0.2188	0.1094	0.0547	0.0274	0.0137	0.0069	0.0035	0.0018
5			0.5625	0.3125	0.1563	0.0782	0.0391	0.0196	0.0098	0.0049	0.0025
6				0.4063	0.2188	0.1094	0.0547	0.0274	0.0137	0.0069	0.0035
7				0.5000	0.2813	0.1485	0.0743	0.0372	0.0186	0.0093	0.0047
8					0.3438	0.1875	0.0977	0.0489	0.0245	0.0123	0.0062
9					0.4219	0.2344	0.1250	0.0645	0.0323	0.0162	0.0081
10					0.5000	0.2891	0.1563	0.0821	0.0420	0.0210	0.0105
11						0.3438	0.1915	0.1016	0.0528	0.0269	0.0135
12						0.4063	0.2305	0.1250	0.0655	0.0337	0.0171
13						0.4688	0.2735	0.1504	0.0801	0.0416	0.0213
14						0.5313	0.3204	0.1797	0.0967	0.0508	0.0262
15							0.3711	0.2129	0.1163	0.0616	0.0320
16							0.4219	0.2481	0.1377	0.0738	0.0386
17							0.4727	0.2852	0.1612	0.0875	0.0462
18							0.5274	0.3262	0.1875	0.1031	0.0550
19								0.3672	0.2159	0.1202	0.0647
20								0.4102	0.2461	0.1392	0.0757
21								0.4551	0.2784	0.1602	0.0882
22								0.5000	0.3125	0.1827	0.1019
23									0.3477	0.2066	0.1167
24									0.3848	0.2325	0.1331
25									0.4229	0.2598	0.1507

(*Continued*)

Table A.7 (Continued) T, the Wilcoxon signed-rank, distribution

T_0	Sample size										
	2	*3*	*4*	*5*	*6*	*7*	*8*	*9*	*10*	*11*	*12*
26									0.4610	0.2886	0.1697
27									0.5000	0.3189	0.1902
28										0.3501	0.2120
29										0.3824	0.2349
30										0.4156	0.2593
31										0.4493	0.2847
32										0.4830	0.3111
33										0.5171	0.3387
34											0.3667
35											0.3956
36											0.4251
37											0.4549
38											0.4849
39											0.5152

Table A.8 W, the Wilcoxon rank-sum, distribution

W_0	$n_2 = 3$		
	$n_1 = 1$	$n_1 = 2$	$n_1 = 3$
1	0.25		
2	0.50		
3		0.10	
4		0.20	
5		0.40	
6		0.60	0.05
7			0.10
8			0.20
9			0.35
10			0.50

W_0	$n_2 = 4$			
	$n_1 = 1$	$n_1 = 2$	$n_1 = 3$	$n_1 = 4$
1	0.20			
2	0.40			
3	0.60	0.0667		
4		0.1333		
5		0.2667		
6		0.4000	0.0286	
7		0.6000	0.0571	
8			0.1143	
9			0.2000	
10			0.3143	0.0143
11			0.4286	0.0286

(Continued)

Table A.8 (Continued) W, the Wilcoxon rank-sum, distribution

W_0	$n_2 = 4$			
	$n_1 = 1$	$n_1 = 2$	$n_1 = 3$	$n_1 = 4$
12			0.5714	0.0571
13				0.1000
14				0.1714
15				0.2429
16				0.3429
17				0.4429
18				0.5571

W_0	$n_2 = 5$				
	$n_1 = 1$	$n_1 = 2$	$n_1 = 3$	$n_1 = 4$	$n_1 = 5$
1	0.1667				
2	0.3333				
3	0.5000	0.0476			
4		0.0952			
5		0.1905			
6		0.2857	0.0179		
7		0.4286	0.0357		
8		0.5714	0.0714		
9			0.1250		
10			0.1964	0.0079	
11			0.2857	0.0159	
12			0.3929	0.0317	
13			0.5000	0.0556	
14				0.0952	

(Continued)

Table A.8 (Continued) W, the Wilcoxon rank-sum, distribution

W_0	$n_2 = 5$				
	$n_1 = 1$	$n_1 = 2$	$n_1 = 3$	$n_1 = 4$	$n_1 = 5$
15				0.1429	0.0040
16				0.2063	0.0079
17				0.2778	0.0159
18				0.3651	0.0278
19				0.4524	0.0476
20				0.5476	0.0754
21					0.1111
22					0.1548
23					0.2103
24					0.2738
25					0.3452
26					0.4206
27					0.5000

W_0	$n_2 = 6$					
	$n_1 = 1$	$n_1 = 2$	$n_1 = 3$	$n_1 = 4$	$n_1 = 5$	$n_1 = 6$
1	0.1429					
2	0.2857					
3	0.4286	0.0357				
4	0.5714	0.0714				
5		0.1429				
6		0.2143	0.0119			
7		0.3214	0.0238			
8		0.4286	0.0476			

(Continued)

Table A.8 (Continued) W, the Wilcoxon rank-sum, distribution

	$n_2 = 6$					
W_0	$n_1 = 1$	$n_1 = 2$	$n_1 = 3$	$n_1 = 4$	$n_1 = 5$	$n_1 = 6$
9		0.5714	0.0833			
10			0.1310	0.0048		
11			0.1905	0.0095		
12			0.2738	0.0190		
13			0.3571	0.0333		
14			0.4524	0.0571		
15			0.5476	0.0857	0.0022	
16				0.1286	0.0043	
17				0.1762	0.0087	
18				0.2381	0.0152	
19				0.3048	0.0260	
20				0.3810	0.0411	
21				0.4571	0.0628	0.0011
22				0.5429	0.0887	0.0022
23					0.1234	0.0043
24					0.1645	0.0076
25					0.2143	0.0130
26					0.2684	0.0206
27					0.3312	0.0325
28					0.3961	0.0465
29					0.4654	0.0660
30					0.5346	0.0898
31						0.1201
32						0.1548
33						0.1970

(Continued)

Table A.8 (Continued) W, the Wilcoxon rank-sum, distribution

W_0	$n_2 = 6$					
	$n_1 = 1$	$n_1 = 2$	$n_1 = 3$	$n_1 = 4$	$n_1 = 5$	$n_1 = 6$
34						0.2424
35						0.2944
36						0.3496
37						0.4091
38						0.4686
39						0.5314

W_0	$n_2 = 7$						
	$n_1 = 1$	$n_1 = 2$	$n_1 = 3$	$n_1 = 4$	$n_1 = 5$	$n_1 = 6$	$n_1 = 7$
1	0.125						
2	0.250						
3	0.375	0.0278					
4	0.500	0.0556					
5		0.1111					
6		0.1667	0.0083				
7		0.2500	0.0167				
8		0.3333	0.0333				
9		0.4444	0.0583				
10		0.5556	0.0917	0.0030			
11			0.1333	0.0061			
12			0.1917	0.0121			
13			0.2583	0.0212			
14			0.3333	0.0364			
15			0.4167	0.0545	0.0013		

(*Continued*)

Table A.8 (Continued) W, the Wilcoxon rank-sum, distribution

	$n_2 = 7$						
W_0	$n_1 = 1$	$n_1 = 2$	$n_1 = 3$	$n_1 = 4$	$n_1 = 5$	$n_1 = 6$	$n_1 = 7$
16			0.5000	0.0818	0.0025		
17				0.1152	0.0051		
18				0.1576	0.0088		
19				0.2061	0.0152		
20				0.2636	0.0240		
21				0.3242	0.0366	0.0006	
22				0.3939	0.0530	0.0012	
23				0.4636	0.0745	0.0023	
24				0.5364	0.1010	0.0041	
25					0.1338	0.0070	
26					0.1717	0.0111	
27					0.2159	0.0175	
28					0.2652	0.0256	0.0003
29					0.3194	0.0367	0.0006
30					0.3775	0.0507	0.0012
31					0.4381	0.0688	0.0020
32					0.5000	0.0903	0.0035
33						0.1171	0.0055
34						0.1474	0.0087
35						0.1830	0.0131
36						0.2226	0.0189
37						0.2669	0.0265
38						0.3141	0.0364
39						0.3654	0.0487
40						0.4178	0.0641

(Continued)

Table A.8 (Continued) W, the Wilcoxon rank-sum, distribution

	$n_2 = 7$						
W_0	$n_1 = 1$	$n_1 = 2$	$n_1 = 3$	$n_1 = 4$	$n_1 = 5$	$n_1 = 6$	$n_1 = 7$
41						0.4726	0.0825
42						0.5274	0.1043
43							0.1297
44							0.1588
45							0.1914
46							0.2279
47							0.2675
48							0.3100
49							0.3552
50							0.4024
51							0.4508
52							0.5000

	$n_2 = 8$							
W_0	$n_1 = 1$	$n_1 = 2$	$n_1 = 3$	$n_1 = 4$	$n_1 = 5$	$n_1 = 6$	$n_1 = 7$	$n_1 = 8$
1	0.1111							
2	0.2222							
3	0.3333	0.0222						
4	0.4444	0.0444						
5	0.5556	0.0889						
6		0.1333	0.0061					
7		0.2000	0.0121					
8		0.2667	0.0242					
9		0.3556	0.0424					

(Continued)

Table A.8 (Continued) W, the Wilcoxon rank-sum, distribution

	$n_2 = 8$							
W_0	$n_1 = 1$	$n_1 = 2$	$n_1 = 3$	$n_1 = 4$	$n_1 = 5$	$n_1 = 6$	$n_1 = 7$	$n_1 = 8$
10		0.4444	0.0667	0.0020				
11		0.5556	0.0970	0.0040				
12			0.1394	0.0081				
13			0.1879	0.0141				
14			0.2485	0.0242				
15			0.3152	0.0364	0.0008			
16			0.3879	0.0545	0.0016			
17			0.4606	0.0768	0.0031			
18			0.5394	0.1071	0.0054			
19				0.1414	0.0093			
20				0.1838	0.0148			
21				0.2303	0.0225	0.0003		
22				0.2848	0.0326	0.0007		
23				0.3414	0.0466	0.0013		
24				0.4040	0.0637	0.0023		
25				0.4667	0.0855	0.0040		
26				0.5333	0.1111	0.0063		
27					0.1422	0.0100		
28					0.1772	0.0147	0.0002	
29					0.2176	0.0213	0.0003	
30					0.2618	0.0296	0.0006	
31					0.3108	0.0406	0.0011	
32					0.3621	0.0539	0.0019	
33					0.4165	0.0709	0.0030	
34					0.4716	0.0906	0.0047	

(Continued)

Table A.8 (Continued) W, the Wilcoxon rank-sum, distribution

W_0	$n_2 = 8$							
	$n_1 = 1$	$n_1 = 2$	$n_1 = 3$	$n_1 = 4$	$n_1 = 5$	$n_1 = 6$	$n_1 = 7$	$n_1 = 8$
35					0.5284	0.1142	0.0070	
36						0.1412	0.0103	0.0001
37						0.1725	0.0145	0.0002
38						0.2068	0.0200	0.0003
39						0.2454	0.0270	0.0005
40						0.2864	0.0361	0.0009
41						0.3310	0.0469	0.0015
42						0.3773	0.0603	0.0023
43						0.4259	0.0760	0.0035
44						0.4749	0.0946	0.0052
45						0.5251	0.1159	0.0074
46							0.1405	0.0103
47							0.1678	0.0141
48							0.1984	0.0190
49							0.2317	0.0249
50							0.2679	0.0325
51							0.3063	0.0415
52							0.3472	0.0524
53							0.3894	0.0652
54							0.4333	0.0803
55							0.4775	0.0974
56							0.5225	0.1172
57								0.1393
58								0.1641
59								0.1911

(Continued)

Table A.8 (Continued) W, the Wilcoxon rank-sum, distribution

W_0	$n_2 = 8$							
	$n_1 = 1$	$n_1 = 2$	$n_1 = 3$	$n_1 = 4$	$n_1 = 5$	$n_1 = 6$	$n_1 = 7$	$n_1 = 8$
60								0.2209
61								0.2527
62								0.2869
63								0.3227
64								0.3605
65								0.3992
66								0.4392
67								0.4796
68								0.5204

W_0	$n_2 = 9$								
	$n_1 = 1$	$n_1 = 2$	$n_1 = 3$	$n_1 = 4$	$n_1 = 5$	$n_1 = 6$	$n_1 = 7$	$n_1 = 8$	$n_1 = 9$
1	0.1000								
2	0.2000								
3	0.3000	0.0182							
4	0.4000	0.0364							
5	0.5000	0.0727							
6		0.1091	0.0045						
7		0.1636	0.0091						
8		0.2182	0.0182						
9		0.2909	0.0318						
10		0.3636	0.0500	0.0014					
11		0.4545	0.0727	0.0028					
12		0.5455	0.1045	0.0056					

(*Continued*)

Table A.8 (Continued) W, the Wilcoxon rank-sum, distribution

	$n_2 = 9$								
W_0	$n_1 = 1$	$n_1 = 2$	$n_1 = 3$	$n_1 = 4$	$n_1 = 5$	$n_1 = 6$	$n_1 = 7$	$n_1 = 8$	$n_1 = 9$
13			0.1409	0.0098					
14			0.1864	0.0168					
15			0.2409	0.0252	0.0005				
16			0.3000	0.0378	0.0010				
17			0.3636	0.0531	0.0020				
18			0.4318	0.0741	0.0035				
19			0.5000	0.0993	0.0060				
20				0.1301	0.0095				
21				0.1650	0.0145	0.0002			
22				0.2070	0.0210	0.0004			
23				0.2517	0.0300	0.0008			
24				0.3021	0.0415	0.0014			
25				0.3552	0.0559	0.0024			
26				0.4126	0.0734	0.0038			
27				0.4699	0.0949	0.0060			
28				0.5301	0.1199	0.0088	0.0001		
29					0.1489	0.0128	0.0002		
30					0.1818	0.0180	0.0003		
31					0.2188	0.0248	0.0006		
32					0.2592	0.0332	0.0010		
33					0.3032	0.0440	0.0017		
34					0.3497	0.0567	0.0026		
35					0.3986	0.0723	0.0039		
36					0.4491	0.0905	0.0058	0.0000	
37					0.5000	0.1119	0.0082	0.0001	

(Continued)

Table A.8 (Continued) W, the Wilcoxon rank-sum, distribution

	$n_2 = 9$								
W_0	$n_1 = 1$	$n_1 = 2$	$n_1 = 3$	$n_1 = 4$	$n_1 = 5$	$n_1 = 6$	$n_1 = 7$	$n_1 = 8$	$n_1 = 9$
38						0.1361	0.0115	0.0002	
39						0.1638	0.0156	0.0003	
40						0.1942	0.0209	0.0005	
41						0.2280	0.0274	0.0008	
42						0.2643	0.0356	0.0012	
43						0.3035	0.0454	0.0019	
44						0.3445	0.0571	0.0028	
45						0.3878	0.0708	0.0039	0.0000
46						0.4320	0.0869	0.0056	0.0000
47						0.4773	0.1052	0.0076	0.0001
48						0.5227	0.1261	0.0103	0.0001
49							0.1496	0.0137	0.0002
50							0.1755	0.0180	0.0004
51							0.2039	0.0232	0.0006
52							0.2349	0.0296	0.0009
53							0.2680	0.0372	0.0014
54							0.3032	0.0464	0.0020
55							0.3403	0.0570	0.0028
56							0.3788	0.0694	0.0039
57							0.4185	0.0836	0.0053
58							0.4591	0.0998	0.0071
59							0.5000	0.1179	0.0094
60								0.1383	0.0122
61								0.1606	0.0157
62								0.1852	0.0200

(Continued)

Table A.8 (Continued) W, the Wilcoxon rank-sum, distribution

	$n_2 = 9$								
W_0	$n_1 = 1$	$n_1 = 2$	$n_1 = 3$	$n_1 = 4$	$n_1 = 5$	$n_1 = 6$	$n_1 = 7$	$n_1 = 8$	$n_1 = 9$
63								0.2117	0.0252
64								0.2404	0.0313
65								0.2707	0.0385
66								0.3029	0.0470
67								0.3365	0.0567
68								0.3715	0.0680
69								0.4074	0.0807
70								0.4442	0.0951
71								0.4813	0.1112
72								0.5187	0.1290
73									0.1487
74									0.1701
75									0.1933
76									0.2181
77									0.2447
78									0.2729
79									0.3024
80									0.3332
81									0.3652
82									0.3981
83									0.4317
84									0.4657
85									0.5000

(Continued)

Table A.8 (Continued) W, the Wilcoxon rank-sum, distribution

W_0	$n_2 = 10$									
	$n_1 = 1$	$n_1 = 2$	$n_1 = 3$	$n_1 = 4$	$n_1 = 5$	$n_1 = 6$	$n_1 = 7$	$n_1 = 8$	$n_1 = 9$	$n_1 = 10$
1	0.0909									
2	0.1818									
3	0.2727	0.0152								
4	0.3636	0.0303								
5	0.4545	0.0606								
6	0.5455	0.0909	0.0035							
7		0.1364	0.0070							
8		0.1818	0.0140							
9		0.2424	0.0245							
10		0.3030	0.0385	0.0010						
11		0.3788	0.0559	0.0020						
12		0.4545	0.0804	0.0040						
13		0.5455	0.1084	0.0070						
14			0.1434	0.0120						
15			0.1853	0.0180	0.0003					
16			0.2343	0.0270	0.0007					
17			0.2867	0.0380	0.0013					
18			0.3462	0.0529	0.0023					
19			0.4056	0.0709	0.0040					
20			0.4685	0.0939	0.0063					
21			0.5315	0.1199	0.0097	0.0001				
22				0.1518	0.0140	0.0002				
23				0.1868	0.0200	0.0005				
24				0.2268	0.0276	0.0009				
25				0.2697	0.0376	0.0015				

(*Continued*)

Table A.8 (Continued) W, the Wilcoxon rank-sum, distribution

	$n_2 = 10$									
$\mathbf{W}_0$	$n_1 = 1$	$n_1 = 2$	$n_1 = 3$	$n_1 = 4$	$n_1 = 5$	$n_1 = 6$	$n_1 = 7$	$n_1 = 8$	$n_1 = 9$	$n_1 = 10$
26				0.3177	0.0496	0.0024				
27				0.3666	0.0646	0.0037				
28				0.4196	0.0823	0.0055	0.0001			
29				0.4725	0.1023	0.0080	0.0001			
30				0.5275	0.1272	0.0112	0.0002			
31					0.1548	0.0156	0.0004			
32					0.1855	0.0210	0.0006			
33					0.2198	0.0280	0.0010			
34					0.2567	0.0363	0.0015			
35					0.2970	0.0467	0.0023			
36					0.3393	0.0589	0.0034	0.0000		
37					0.3839	0.0736	0.0048	0.0000		
38					0.4296	0.0903	0.0068	0.0001		
39					0.4765	0.1099	0.0093	0.0002		
40					0.5235	0.1317	0.0125	0.0003		
41						0.1566	0.0165	0.0004		
42						0.1838	0.0215	0.0007		
43						0.2139	0.0277	0.0010		
44						0.2461	0.0351	0.0015		
45						0.2811	0.0439	0.0022	0.0000	
46						0.3177	0.0544	0.0031	0.0000	
47						0.3564	0.0665	0.0043	0.0000	
48						0.3962	0.0806	0.0058	0.0001	
49						0.4374	0.0966	0.0078	0.0001	
50						0.4789	0.1148	0.0103	0.0002	

(Continued)

Table A.8 (Continued) W, the Wilcoxon rank-sum, distribution

	$n_2 = 10$									
$\mathbf{W}_0$	$n_1 = 1$	$n_1 = 2$	$n_1 = 3$	$n_1 = 4$	$n_1 = 5$	$n_1 = 6$	$n_1 = 7$	$n_1 = 8$	$n_1 = 9$	$n_1 = 10$
51						0.5211	0.1349	0.0133	0.0003	
52							0.1574	0.0171	0.0005	
53							0.1819	0.0217	0.0007	
54							0.2087	0.0273	0.0011	
55							0.2374	0.0338	0.0015	0.0000
56							0.2681	0.0416	0.0021	0.0000
57							0.3004	0.0506	0.0028	0.0000
58							0.3345	0.0610	0.0038	0.0000
59							0.3698	0.0729	0.0051	0.0001
60							0.4063	0.0864	0.0066	0.0001
61							0.4434	0.1015	0.0086	0.0002
62							0.4811	0.1185	0.0110	0.0002
63							0.5189	0.1371	0.0140	0.0004
64								0.1577	0.0175	0.0005
65								0.1800	0.0217	0.0008
66								0.2041	0.0267	0.0010
67								0.2299	0.0326	0.0014
68								0.2574	0.0394	0.0019
69								0.2863	0.0474	0.0026
70								0.3167	0.0564	0.0034

(Continued)

Table A.8 (Continued) W, the Wilcoxon rank-sum, distribution

	$n_2 = 10$									
W_0	$n_1 = 1$	$n_1 = 2$	$n_1 = 3$	$n_1 = 4$	$n_1 = 5$	$n_1 = 6$	$n_1 = 7$	$n_1 = 8$	$n_1 = 9$	$n_1 = 10$
71								0.3482	0.0667	0.0045
72								0.3809	0.0782	0.0057
73								0.4143	0.0912	0.0073
74								0.4484	0.1055	0.0093
75								0.4827	0.1214	0.0116
76								0.5173	0.1388	0.0144
77									0.1577	0.0177
78									0.1781	0.0216
79									0.2001	0.0262
80									0.2235	0.0315
81									0.2483	0.0376
82									0.2745	0.0446
83									0.3019	0.0526
84									0.3304	0.0615
85									0.3598	0.0716
86									0.3901	0.0827
87									0.4211	0.0952
88									0.4524	0.1088
89									0.4841	0.1237
90									0.5159	0.1399

(*Continued*)

Table A.8 (Continued) W, the Wilcoxon rank-sum, distribution

	$n_2 = 10$									
W_0	$n_1 = 1$	$n_1 = 2$	$n_1 = 3$	$n_1 = 4$	$n_1 = 5$	$n_1 = 6$	$n_1 = 7$	$n_1 = 8$	$n_1 = 9$	$n_1 = 10$
91										0.1575
92										0.1763
93										0.1965
94										0.2179
95										0.2406
96										0.2644
97										0.2894
98										0.3153
99										0.3421
100										0.3697
101										0.3980
102										0.4267
103										0.4559
104										0.4853
105										0.5147

Index

Page numbers followed by f and t indicate figures and tables, respectively.

D

E

H

I

K

L

M

P

Q

R